W9-CFO-997

THE TEENAGE BODY BOOK

Other Books by Kathy McCoy, Ph.D.

Life Happens: A Teenager's Guide to Friends, Failure, Sexuality, Love, Rejection, Addiction, Peer Pressure, Families, Loss, Depression, Change and Other Challenges of Living (with Charles Wibbelsman, M.D.)

Understanding Your Teenager's Depression: Issues, Insights and Practical Guidance for Parents

Changes and Choices: A Junior High Survival Guide

Solo Parenting: Your Essential Guide

Coping with Teenage Depression

The Teenage Survival Guide

The Teenage Body Book Guide to Sexuality

The Teenage Body Book Guide to Dating

Growing and Changing: A Guide for Preteens (with Charles Wibbelsman, M.D.)

Crisis-Proof Your Teenager (with Charles Wibbelsman, M.D.)

Most Perigee Books are available at special quantity discounts for bulk purchases for sales promotions, premiums, fund-raising, or educational use. Special books or book excerpts can also be created to fit specific needs.

For details, write to Special Markets, The Berkley Publishing Group, 375 Hudson Street, New York, New York 10014.

THE TEENAGE BODY BOOK

REVISED AND UPDATED

■

Kathy McCoy, Ph.D., and Charles Wibbelsman, M.D.

Illustrations by
Bob Stover, Kelly Grady, and Jennifer Rourke

PERIGEE

A Perigee Book
Published by The Berkley Publishing Group
A division of Penguin Putnam Inc.
375 Hudson Street
New York, New York 10014

Copyright © 1992 by Kathy McCoy, Ph.D., and Charles Wibbelsman, M.D.
Book design by Pauline Neuwirth, Neuwirth & Associates, Inc.
Cover design by Miguel Santana
Cover photo copyright © by Lisette Le Bon/Superstock

All rights reserved. This book, or parts thereof,
may not be reproduced in any form without permission.

First edition: March 1992
Revised and updated edition: September 1999

Published simultaneously in Canada.

The Penguin Putnam Inc. World Wide Web site address is
http://www.penguinputnam.com

Library of Congress Cataloging-in-Publication Data

McCoy, Kathy.
   The teenage body book / Kathy McCoy & Charles
 Wibbelsman ; illustrations by Bob Stover, Kelly Grady, and Jennifer Rourke—[Rev. ed.]
       p.   cm.
   "A Perigee Book"
   Includes bibliographical references and index.
   Summary: A handbook for teenagers discussing such
topics as the male and female bodies, health, grooming,
emotions, various aspects of sex, eating disorders,
depression, drugs, and sexually transmitted diseases.
   ISBN 0-399-52535-1 (trade paperback)
   1. Teenagers—Health and hygiene.
2. Adolescence. [1. Health. 2. Sex instruction for
youth. 3. Adolescence.] I. Wibbelsman, Charles.
II. Stover, Bob; Grady, Kelly; Rourke, Jennifer, ill. III. Title.
RA777.M33 1992   91-35962 CIP AC
613'.0433—dc20

Printed in the United States of America

10 9 8 7 6 5 4 3 2

Acknowledgments

Our special thanks to . . .

- Bob Stover, the artist for the original edition of this book in 1979 and all subsequent editions. His creative talents, hard work, and generosity over the years have been much appreciated and have contributed significantly to the book's success. This time, he contributed even more—as the main artist, as art coordinator working with our two young co-illustrators, and as a full participant in the production of the manuscript, volunteering to type a number of the original chapters into the computer so that our revision process could proceed more quickly and smoothly. For his practical help, advice, and many long, tedious hours at the computer (broken by dashes to his drawing board to produce another illustration), we extend our love and deep gratitude. We couldn't have done this without you, Bob!
- Our two young artists, Kelly Grady and Jennifer Rourke, for their wonderful work done under considerable deadline pressures—and we wish them much future success!
- Roxanne Camron, executive editor of 'TEEN magazine, for her friendship over the years. The Teenage Body Book had its beginnings when we were on the staff of 'TEEN, and most of the letters in our original edition came from 'TEEN readers. It means a great deal to us that, for this 20th anniversary edition, Roxanne offered a great selection of reader letters to supplement those we had received personally. We are also grateful to Robert MacLeod, recently retired publisher of 'TEEN, for his courage, insight, and wonderful support as he made possible our first collaboration efforts so many years ago.
- Our agent, Susan Ann Protter, for believing in us and our book before anyone else did!
- Our publisher, John Duff, for his commitment and support in keeping The Teenage Body Book in print and responsive to changing times.
- Our copy editor Amy Schneider for her excellent and painstaking work on the manuscript.
- Some special professionals who gave us their time and expertise as we planned this new edition: Dean Blumberg, Karen Blanpied (and her students at University High in San Francisco who offered comments on how this book could be more helpful to teens), and psychotherapists Mary Breiner, M.A.; Joan Powers, M.A.; Virginia Andrews, M.A.; and Kathleen Lake, Ph.D. We're also grateful to Rev. Lynn Jay and her associates Lili Bush and Peg Bradley at St. Stephen's Episcopal Church in Valencia, California, for their valu-

able feedback and advice on teen and family issues.

■ Michael Scavio, Ph.D., chancellor at the California School of Professional Psychology in Los Angeles, for his warm encouragement and support. Thanks, too, to our CSPP colleagues Linda Beckman, Ph.D.; Carlton Parks, Ph.D.; Michael Jospe, Ph.D.; Ellin Bloch, Ph.D.; Shelly Harrell, Ph.D.; Carmen Ortiz; Leticia Keenan; Kelly Hogancamp; and Rosemary Abend, Ph.D.

■ Some special young people in our lives who have given us insights into the turn-of-the-century teen generation: Ryan Grady; Angie and Amanda Arellano (and their mom, Marci!); Aryana Mareld; and Michelle, Nicholas, and Caroline Wibbelsman.

■ Supportive family members and friends who have helped in a myriad of ways as we dealt with deadline pressure: Elizabeth McCoy, Angie Fisher, Tai Mareld, Cecilia Wibbelsman, David Hyman, Joe Rourke, Dan and Lydie Colonello, and Michael McCog, M.D.

■ Elizabeth Canfield, who introduced us so many years ago . . . loving thanks, Liz!

■ All the teens whose letters appear on these pages. Thanks for sharing your questions, your thoughts, and your feelings with us!

Contents

INTRODUCTION 1

Welcome . . . to a New Century and a Special Generation 1

CHAPTER ONE: Am I Normal? 3

Is My Growth Normal? 3

Is My Body Normal? 3

Are My Feelings Normal? 4

It's Normal to Be Changing in All Ways! 4

Quick Scan 5

CHAPTER TWO: A Woman's Body 7

Female Anatomy 7

Physical Development 9

Breasts 12

Menstruation 15

Menstrual Problems 16

Sanitary Products 20

Vaginal Health and Infections 22

Vaginal Infections 23

Growing from Girl to Woman 24

Quick Scan 25

CHAPTER THREE: A Man's Body 27

Male Anatomy 27

Physical Development 29

Special Problems 31

Short Stature 31

Adolescent Nodule/Adolescent Gynecomastia 32

Prostatitis 32

Pink Pearly Papules 33

Undescended Testicle(s) 33

Testicular Cancer 33

Benign Scrotal Masses 34

Foreskin Problems 34

Pain in the Groin 35

Ejaculation Problems 35

Growing from Boy to Man 37

Quick Scan 37

CHAPTER FOUR: Feelings 39

Feelings About Yourself 40

Feelings About Your Parents 42

Feelings About Your Changing Family 43

Love 44

Anger 46

Shyness 47

Boredom 48

Feelings and Cyberspace 49

Stress 49

Defiance and Self-Defeating Behavior 51

Feelings About the "Isms" 52

Physical, Emotional, and Sexual Abuse 54

Date Rape 55

If You Are Raped 56

Depression 56

Major Depressive Disorder, Single Episode or Recurrent 56

Dysthymic Disorder 57

Bipolar Disorder 57

If You're Grieving a Loss 57

If You're in a Depressed Mood 58

If Your Depressed Mood Persists 58

Suicidal Feelings 59

If You Are Feeling Suicidal 60

Feelings and Your Health 60

Quick Facts for Parents 62

CHAPTER FIVE: Eating for Good Health 63

Are You What You Eat? 63

Improving Your Eating Habits (Painlessly!) 66

Reaching and Maintaining Your Best Weight 67

If You Feel You're Underweight 67

If You Feel You're Overweight 68

Quick Scan 74

CHAPTER SIX: Exercising for Good Health 75

Your Best Exercise Plan 75

For a Successful Start to Your Active New Life 76

Exercising for—and in—Good Health 81

Quick Scan 81

Chapter Seven: Good Health and Good Looks 83

Healthy Skin 83

Acne 83

Eczema 86

Psoriasis 86

Warts 87

Moles 88

A Sun-Lover's Guide to Protecting Your Skin 88

Healthy Feet, Nails, and Hair 90

Feet 90

Nails 91

Hair 91

Healthy Eyes 92

Contacts 92

Eye Surgery 93

Caring for Your Eyes 93

Healthy Teeth and Gums 93

Periodontal (Gum) Disease and Its Prevention 94

Bleaching, Bonding, Invisible Braces, and Other Dental Innovations 96

Special Help for Good Looks 98

Plastic Surgery 98

Cosmetics 101

Special Problems 103

Ear and Body Piercing 103

Excess Hair 104

Perspiration 105

Questionable Beauty Aids 106

Creating a Beautiful, Healthy Future 107

Quick Scan 109

CHAPTER EIGHT: Drugs, Drinking, and Smoking 111

Why Saying No Is Vital to Your Health 111

What Does All This Mean for You? 113

The Real Dangers of These Problem Substances 114

These Substances Are Hazardous to Your Health—And Your Life! 114

Smoking 114

Smokeless Tobacco 115

Alcohol 115

    Marijuana   117
    Inhalants   118
    Stimulants   118
    LSD   119
    Heroin   119
    Anabolic-Androgenic Steroids   119
  Making a Decision About Drugs, Drinking, and Smoking   120
    Saying No from the Beginning   120
    Saying "No Thanks" Without Transforming into a Dork   121
    Stopping a Harmful Habit   121
    Quick Scan   124

CHAPTER NINE: Mind over Body   125
  The Stress Connection   126
  Headaches   126
    Tension Headaches   127
    Depression Headaches   127
    Migraine Headaches   127
  Stress and Your Stomach   128
    Irritable Bowel Syndrome   128
  Stress and Eating Disorders   129
    Fear-of-Obesity Syndrome   130
    Anorexia Nervosa   130
    Bulimia   131
    Compulsive Overeating   132
  Hypertension (High Blood Pressure)   132
  Alternative Medicine: New/Old Ways of Healing   133
  Making Sense of the Mind-Body Connection   136
    Quick Scan   136

CHAPTER TEN: Your Special Medical Needs   137
  Allergies   138
  Anemia   139
    Iron-Deficiency Anemia   140
    Sickle Cell Anemia   140
  Asthma   141
  Bed Wetting (Nocturnal Enuresis)   142
  Diabetes   143
  Epilepsy   146
  Infectious Mononucleosis   147
  Osgood-Schlatter Disease   148
  Scoliosis   149
  Urinary Tract Infections   150
  Living with Special Medical Needs   151

Quick Scan 151

CHAPTER ELEVEN: You and Your Sexuality 153
Sexuality As Part of Your Life 153
Your Sexual Orientation 154
Sex Education and Your Sexual Choices 158
Making Sexual Choices 159
Masturbation 160
Relating to Others 161
    A Few Words About Dating Violence and Date Rape 162
    How to Know When You're Ready for Sex 163
    Sex vs. Intimacy 165
    Quick Scan 166

CHAPTER TWELVE: The Truth About Sexually Transmitted Diseases 167
AIDS 168
Bacterial Vaginosis 171
Chlamydia 171
Genital Herpes 173
Genital Warts 174
Gonorrhea 175
Molluscum Contagiosum 176
Pubic Lice 177
Scabies 177
Syphilis 177
Tinea Cruris (Jock Itch) 178
Trichomoniasis 179
The ABCs of Hepatitis 179
    If You Have Been Exposed to Hepatitis A 180
    If You Have Been Exposed to Hepatitis B 180
    Avoiding Hepatitis C 180
What Is "Safe Sex"? 180
Ten Safe-Sex Guidelines 181
    Quick Scan 184

CHAPTER THIRTEEN: Birth Control: An Ounce of Prevention 185
Five Lame Excuses for Not Using Birth Control 185
You *Can* Get Pregnant If . . . 186
Teens *Can* Get Birth Control Products 187
    Legal Aspects of Your Access to Birth Control 187
Which Methods Work? 188
    The Pill (Oral Contraceptives) 189
    Depo-Provera 191
    The Norplant System 192

The Diaphragm 193

The Cervical Cap 194

The Condom (Male) 195

The Condom (Female) 197

Spermicidal Jelly, Cream, and Foam 198

Natural Family Planning 199

Sterilization 200

In an Emergency . . . 201

Birth Control of the Future 202

Quick Scan 203

CHAPTER FOURTEEN: Pregnancy and Parenthood 205

Considering Parenthood 205

If You Think You Might Be Pregnant 207

Making Decisions About Your Pregnancy 208

Having the Baby and Marrying the Father 208

Having the Baby and Raising It As a Single Parent 209

Having the Baby and Giving It Up for Adoption 209

Having an Abortion 210

Why Follow-Up Medical Care Is Vital—Whatever Your Choice 211

If You Are Continuing Your Pregnancy 211

If You Are Terminating Your Pregnancy 211

Living with Your Choice 211

Quick Scan 212

CHAPTER FIFTEEN: Help! When You Need It (And How to Ask for It) 213

In an Emergency 213

If You're Sexually Active 214

As Part of Your Regular Health Maintenance 214

If You Have Questions About Your Body 215

Legal Aspects of Your Medical Care 215

Communicating with Your Doctor 217

The Physical Examination 219

The General Examination 219

Male Genital Examination 220

Female Pelvic Examination 220

Rectal Examination 221

Continuing the General Examination 222

Lab Tests 222

Getting Help from Medical Web Sites 222

Getting Help for Your Mental Health 222

Why Do People See Therapists Anyway? 223

Who Are These Mental Health Professionals? 223

How Do You Find a Therapist? 224

What to Expect/How to Make the Most of Therapy   225
Growing Toward a Healthy Future   226
Quick Scan   227

APPENDIX: Help! Where to Find It   229
Crisis Counseling   229
General Adolescent Health   229
General Health   229
Special-Needs Resources   230
Abortion   230
Adoption   230
AIDS   230
Alcohol/Alcoholism   230
Alternative Medicine   230
Anemia (Sickle Cell)   231
Anorexia Nervosa, Bulimia, and General Eating Disorders   231
Asthma   231
Birth Control   231
Diet, Nutrition, and Fitness   231
Drug Abuse   232
Epilepsy   232
Gay and Lesbian Teens   232
Grief   232
Headaches   233
Melanoma   233
Mental Health   233
Parenting (New)   233
Plastic Surgery   233
PMS   233
Sex Education   233
Sexually Transmitted Diseases   234
Smoking   234
Stress   234

Index   235

Introduction

WELCOME . . . TO A NEW CENTURY AND A SPECIAL GENERATION

You're special—part of the first generation of teenagers to greet the 21st century. While some aspects of adolescent life and health are timeless, your lifestyle, your choices, and your challenges aren't quite like those of any generation of teens before you.

So *The Teenage Body Book* is changing with the times—to meet the needs of *your* time as you come of age at the dawn of a new century.

Some aspects of adolescence have stayed much the same since the first edition of this book was published 20 years ago: the timing and facts of physical development, the pain of feeling different or losing a love, the risks of substance abuse, the difficulties of having a chronic medical condition, the challenge of making decisions about sex that are right for *you*. But so much has changed and so much is unique about you:

- *You're part of the most diverse, multicultural teen population ever*—and this new edition of *The Teenage Body Book* will reflect more of the realities, needs, and challenges of your life today as part of this new generation.
- *You're busier than your older brothers and sisters were.* More teens are working while going to school or struggling to balance school, special interests, community service, and time to hang out with friends. When you're looking for information, you need it fast. This new edition recognizes that fact; we've put all you need to know about your body and your health at your fingertips with our "Quick Scan" feature. You now have a choice: You can read an entire chapter word for word *or* you can get the basic facts fast in the "Quick Scan" box at the end of that chapter.
- *You're the most cyberwise generation yet!* You've grown up with computers, and the Internet is likely to be part of your everyday life. So our "Help! Where to Find It" appendix has lots of e-mail addresses and Web sites that can help you get all kinds of great information whenever you need it.
- *New discoveries can change your life.* Medical advances are being made all the time—and you can benefit! We'll tell you the most recent findings about treatment for diseases such as asthma, epilepsy, and diabetes so you can live a happier, healthier life. We'll help you keep up to date on the latest diet and fitness news, the truth about beauty aids, how to handle difficult feelings and situations, and how to get the best possible medical care when you need it.
- *You have the power to change history.* The health

history of teens in the last few decades of the 20th century was not the greatest: Your older brothers and sisters have been hooked on junk food, cigarettes, and risky behavior. The suicide rate has continued to climb and teens continue to die in accidents at a tragic rate. By making smart choices, you can begin to change this reality and become part of the healthiest generation of teens ever. By eating and exercising for good health (it *is* possible to do that and still have a good time with your friends); by making wise choices about your friends, activities, sexuality, and behaviors; and by knowing, understanding, and respecting your body's needs, you can help change history in a positive way.

We're here to help—as you face the exciting new possibilities of coming of age in a new century. We know that it isn't easy to be a teen. These years can be painful, exciting, boring, fun, and challenging. They will probably not be the best years of your life (no matter what anyone says!), but they can be very important to your whole life. Think about it:

- Now is when you make a choice—either actively or passively—about how much education you will get and which general career direction your life will take. Choices you make now can affect your life for years to come.

- Now is when you set a health pattern for your life. Your eating patterns and exercise habits are often set in these years. Similarly, those who will be habitual smokers or problem drinkers in adulthood often start these behaviors in the teen years, establishing patterns that are harder to break than those started in adulthood. Those who are active and maintain a normal weight in adolescence are less likely to get certain cancers and to experience obesity in later life. So what you do now is important—not only for today, but also for years to come.

- Now is when you become your own person—or not. Developing a strong sense of who you are and what you want can be a vital step both to independence *and* to the capacity to have truly intimate relationships (because when you have good feelings about and a strong sense of who you are, you don't have to worry about losing yourself in a relationship).

We're here to help . . . with your health and fitness concerns, your feelings, your relationship issues, your questions about sexuality, your plans and dreams for the future. We're with you in all the changes and challenges you're facing—today and in the years to come!

CHAPTER ONE

Am I Normal?

What's normal? Good question. In fact, that's the one question teens have asked us over and over, in many different ways, during the past 20 years. This may be *your* most pressing question as you:

- Find yourself making quiet comparisons between you and your friends, calculating how you compare in your growth and development, and wondering who's normal and who's not.
- Feel uncomfortable about the way you look.
- Wonder if your feelings—such as loving and hating your parents at the same time or feeling up and feeling down more than you used to—are normal or a sign that something is secretly (or, worse yet, very obviously) wrong with you.

If you've ever wondered "Am I normal?" you have a lot of company. Most teens ask this question in the following ways:

Is My Growth Normal?

You may wonder this for a lot of reasons. Boys may watch girls tower above them at junior high dances and wonder if things will always be this way. Girls may notice that one classmate begins to look like a teenager in third or fourth grade while another may

still look like a kid when starting high school—with everyone else in between. And everyone is normal!

The fact is, normal rates of development vary widely and are based, in part, on your genetic heritage. Ask your parents about their adolescent changes and you may get some important clues to what's normal for you. Look at friends who share your ethnicity, and you may discover some important similarities. For example, it's quite normal for many African Americans to start showing very normal signs of puberty at age 8 or 9. And, as a teen of the 21st century, your normal rate of development is quite different from that of teens a century ago. Then, it was normal for young people to start puberty in the mid- to late teens! Now, due to better general health and nutrition, both boys and girls are larger and become physically mature at earlier ages.

Is My Body Normal?

Besides the changes of adolescence, young people worry a lot about how they look: whether they're too fat, too thin, too tall, or too short and whether they're attractive. Teasing by classmates or looking in the mirror and knowing, without a doubt, that you'll never look like the media ideal of beauty or hunkiness can cause a lot of pain. If you worry about your body, you're far from alone. Very few people look like models or movie stars. There are a number of different and quite normal body types. You can be healthy and attractive whatever body type you have!

Are My Feelings Normal?

New feelings come as your body and your social world change. You may have very different feelings about the opposite sex these days, with boys (or girls) looking a lot more interesting to you than they used to. And you find yourself having conflicting feelings about the parents you once admired without question: They have turned embarrassing and clueless at times, wise and comforting at other times. You admire them one minute and can't stand them the next. What's going on?

It's all part of the normal passage of adolescence. Due to hormonal changes, you may have fairly dramatic mood swings—feeling on top of the world one minute and really upset and depressed the next. And, in your changing world, relationships aren't as simple as they used to be. You both love and hate, have a desire for independence from and a longing to stay attached to your parents. Your friends are more important than ever—but friendships, too, can have significant ups and downs. And because you're beginning to *look* like an adult, people expect more of you. You're growing up faster and facing more challenges at an earlier age than your teen counterparts of a century ago.

It's Normal to Be Changing in All Ways!

Change is the natural order of things in adolescence and young adulthood. In fact, the Latin root of the word *adolescence* is *esco*, which means "becoming." This period of becoming is a long transition time between childhood and adulthood. This is a time of life when there can be dramatic differences between you and your friends. It's a huge temptation to look at someone who is your age and say to yourself: "That person seems to be normal. But I'm different. So I'm not normal."

The fact is, you can be both different and normal. Normal covers an incredibly wide spectrum. The physical changes of adolescence are quite distinct and universal, but the *timing* of these changes is entirely your own. And how other changes happen is unique to you, too. For example, some people mature socially and emotionally before they have any signs of physical maturity—and you see a young adult in a child's body. The opposite is true, too: Some people grow physically into young adults before their social and emotional development has a chance to catch up—and so you see an adult-sized child. And there are a lot of people in between.

At this time of life, feelings of confusion and self-consciousness and fears about being normal or not are common. It can help a lot to share these fears. Talk with your parents about their own growing-up experiences. These are important because they may hold clues for your own physical growth timetable—and help you feel more normal. Your doctor or school nurse can help by answering your questions and concerns about your body; a counselor—at school or outside of school—can help you sort out your feelings if they trouble you a lot. Your friends can help, too, by sharing their own experiences with you and listening to yours. In sharing your fears and feelings, you will learn that you're not so different after all, that what used to seem abnormal is looking more normal all the time.

If talking with others seems too risky right now, try this: Sit back in the privacy of your room or wherever you are, and read this book. You'll discover what other teens are thinking and asking. The questions in this book come from hundreds of teens we have met in schools, in clinics, in interviews, and through letters they have sent to us or to 'TEEN magazine begging for information, advice, and reassurance. As you read, you'll realize that you're both normal *and* unique.

When you see that you're as normal as the next person, then you can begin to appreciate the ways you are special. You may begin to give yourself permission *not* to be perfect. You may begin to appreciate who you are and who you may grow to become. You may become newly aware of what's happening with your changing body and life and see some of your anxieties in a new light. As you read this book, you may find that many people share your feelings. You may realize that, although you're special and unique, you're also, in many ways, just like anyone else. And most important, you're not alone!

AM I NORMAL?

✔ Teens worry about whether their physical changes, body size and shape, and feelings are normal. There is a very wide range of what is normal—especially in adolescence.

✔ The timing of your physical changes is linked to genetics: You may mature at the same rate your mom or dad did or, if you are African American, you may quite normally begin puberty before your white classmates. Good health and nutrition can also be factors in earlier puberty. (Those in poor countries or who keep body fat unusually low due to physical pursuits such as ballet, figure skating, or gymnastics may experience rates of physical changes more like that of teens a century ago—looking like kids until their late teens!)

✔ Having ups and downs in feelings and relationships is a normal part of adolescence. Part of it may be hormonal. And part of it may be social changes: You still love and need your parents, but you want to be your own independent person; your friends are even more important to you—and what they think or say can hurt or help you a lot.

✔ Talking with your parents, your physician, a counselor, and/or your friends can help reassure you that you're normal and not alone. So can reading the letters in this book! The fact is: You're both normal *and* unique!

A Woman's Body

I used to feel good about being me, but now I'm not so sure. My body has changed a lot the last year (I'm almost 13) and I got my period two months ago. I feel so different and embarrassed about how I look, and having my period isn't as cool as I thought it would be. How can I start feeling better about myself?

Ashley

Change *can* be unsettling, even change you've anticipated. It's not at all unusual for girls to have mixed feelings about their changing bodies. You may, for example, feel pleasure and pride in your growing strength and adult appearance while feeling self-conscious about changes people notice (such as breast development), especially if they tease or make embarrassing comments. You may be happy to be a young woman, but dislike the inconvenience of menstrual periods. You may realize that puberty brings a new shape to your body, but feel fat with those curves. And with all the physical changes going on, your body may be something of a mystery. This chapter will help clear up this mystery and help you understand more about your body and the way it works. Knowing and understanding your anatomy, the process of physical change, and the common concerns and problems women have about their bodies can help you to feel more comfortable and normal.

FEMALE ANATOMY

Maybe these illustrations—and the terms for parts of the female anatomy—are very familiar to you. If not, you might want to read this section closely (and maybe even examine yourself with a mirror in the process).

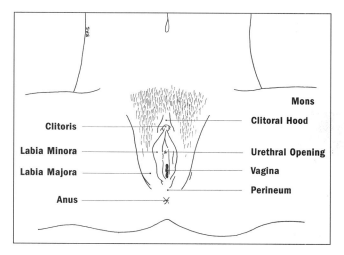

Clitoris

Labia Minora

Labia Majora

Anus

Mons

Clitoral Hood

Urethral Opening

Vagina

Perineum

External Female Genitalia

The external female genital area, called the *vulva*, includes the *labia majora*, which are covered with hair if you have reached a certain stage of development, and which protect the genital area within. Inside these are the *labia minora*. Sometimes these lips protrude from the outer lips and may be wrinkled or smooth. They may vary in color from pink to brown. The *clitoris* is located at the juncture where the labia minora connect. The clitoris is tiny but very sensitive and plays a vital role in a woman's sexual arousal and pleasure.

Below the clitoris is the *urethra* or urinary opening; beneath that is the *vaginal opening*. This may be ringed or partially covered by the *hymen*. The hymen may be very evident or hardly visible. It may have one opening or several.

The presence or absence of a hymen is not definitive proof of virginity. A doctor can't tell whether or not you are a virgin. A virgin is a person who has not had sexual intercourse. Some women who are virgins may have been born without a noticeable hymen or may have stretched the hymen during vigorous sports activities or masturbation or other sexual activities. Other women who are having sexual intercourse may have intact, though stretched, hymens. Only in very rare instances is there no opening in the hymen. This condition, which is usually discovered early in life and which requires surgery, is called *imperforate hymen* and is very rare.

The vaginal opening is the point connecting your external and internal genitals. What is beyond this opening? First, of course, is the *vagina*, a canal that stretches from the vaginal

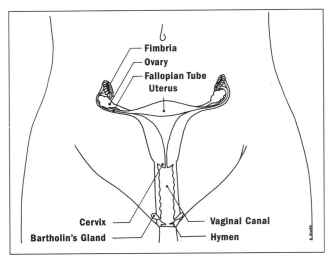

Front View of Female Reproductive System

opening to the *cervix* or neck of the uterus. In the center of the cervix is the *os*, or opening, which feels like a small dimple. This tiny opening can open (or dilate) wide enough to allow a baby to pass through, but, under ordinary circumstances, it is so small that it makes the upper end of the vagina seem closed. This fact may give some comfort to those who fear that tampons or other objects can get lost inside them. They can't. They have nowhere to go unless you remove or expel them from your vaginal opening.

The *uterus* is small, muscular, and pear-shaped. It's amazingly elastic—with the cavity in the non-pregnant state slimmer than the width of your little finger. After expanding to many times its original size during pregnancy, the uterus becomes quite small again after the baby is born.

At the upper portion of the uterus are the *Fallopian tubes*, passageways from the uterus to the *ovaries*, which hold the egg cells. Each month, an egg cell is released from one of the two ovaries in a process called *ovulation* and then begins its journey to the uterus. If the egg is met by male sperm and fertilized (a process called *conception*), this is the beginning of a baby. This tiny collection of cells will travel on through the tubes to the uterus where it will attach itself to the rich *endometrial walls* (lining of the uterus) to grow and develop.

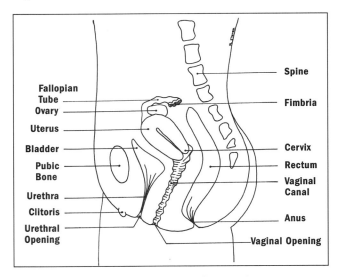

Side View of Female Reproductive System

The unfertilized egg, on the other hand, disintegrates, as does the endometrial tissue that has been building up in anticipation of receiving a fertilized egg to nourish. This material makes up the menstrual flow (*period*).

We have been describing, of course, the anatomy and monthly cycle of a mature or maturing female. Much of adolescence is spent in transit to maturity and it is the process of this journey that is a source of concern for many teens.

PHYSICAL DEVELOPMENT

What is the normal age for body changes like getting breasts and your period? I have two friends who got their periods and were wearing bras in fifth grade, others who began to look like teenagers last year in seventh grade and then there's me—almost 13 and nothing. Well, actually, I *do* have very small breasts. And I've grown a lot in the past year but I don't have my period yet! My friend Madison (who is 13 and doesn't have her period yet either) and I are worried that something is the matter with us. Among the friends I've told you about, who's normal?

Kelsey J.

All of the people Kelsey describes fall within the range of normal when it comes to physical development. Each person has his or her own special biological time clock that dictates when the various stages of puberty will occur. There is a very wide range of normal. One person might begin puberty as young as 8 and another might be in junior high or even high school before she notices any physical changes. In both cases, the timing of these changes is entirely normal.

Why do normal people vary so in the timing of their physical changes? Sometimes this variation is due to ethnic differences. For example, studies show that nearly *half* of African American girls begin the changes of puberty by the age of 8 (compared with 15 percent of white girls). At age 8, 48.3 percent of African American girls and 14.7 percent of white girls had begun developing breasts, pubic hair, or both. (This study was referenced in the April 1997 issue of *Pediatrics*, published by the American Academy of Pediatrics.) We don't know why such differences occur. There are some theories that exposure to chemicals that mimic the female hormone estrogen or actual estrogens (which are used in some hair products made primarily for African Americans) may play a role. Other studies, notably those by Anne Petersen at the University of Minnesota, show that high stress can bring on puberty early in a girl. (And an argument can be made for the fact that being African American in a still-racist society is inherently stressful.)

How does the process of puberty work? While a baby girl is born with thousands of immature eggs (ova) in her ovaries, it isn't until about age 8 (on the average) that the *pituitary gland*—the master gland of the body, which is located in the brain—sends a special hormone called *follicle-stimulating hormone (FSH)* to the ovaries. The long-dormant ovaries begin to make the hormone *estrogen*, which is released into the bloodstream, triggering the long process of puberty. These physical changes, hardly noticeable at first, occur in predictable stages, no matter what an individual girl's development timetable. These stages were identified by a British doctor named J. M. Tanner, who noted that within each stage there are many small changes and steps in breast, genital, and pubic hair growth as well as changes in height and weight. By recognizing the changes characteristic for each of the five stages of puberty, you and your doctor can tell where you are physically in your adolescence and what is likely to happen next. The following charts will give you a map to the different stages of puberty (Chart 1) and the normal age range for each stage (Chart 2).

■ ■ ■

STAGES OF PUBERTY IN GIRLS

Stage	Ages	Internal	Breasts	Growth	Pubic Hair	Menstruation
One	8–11	Ovaries are enlarging and making the hormone estrogen	None	Nothing Unusual	None	None
Two	8–14	Estrogen is quite evident in bloodstream	Breast buds: nipples elevated and tender	Rapid growth; hips broaden; fat deposits give softer, rounder shape	First signs: fine, straight, and sparse	None
Three	9–15	Vagina is enlarging; chemistry of vaginal secretions is changing	Breasts continue to grow; areola (around nipple) enlarges	Height and weight increase	Hair becomes darker and coarser but is still sparse	First menstrual period may occur at the end of this stage
Four	10–16	Ovaries enlarge; ovulation may begin	Nipple and areola form separate mound	Still growing	Pubic hair looks like an adult's, but covers smaller area; underarm hair appears	First menstrual period now if not at end of stage three; most periods at this stage don't involve ovulation
Five	12–19	Fully mature ovaries; regular ovulation	Full breast development	Full (or near) adult height	Full adult pattern	Regular menstruation with ovulation

1. Breast buds begin.

2. Breast and areola grow.

3. Nipple and areola form separate mound, protruding from breast.

4. Areola rejoins breast contour and development is complete.

Female Breast Development

AGE RANGE OF CHANGES OF PUBERTY IN GIRLS

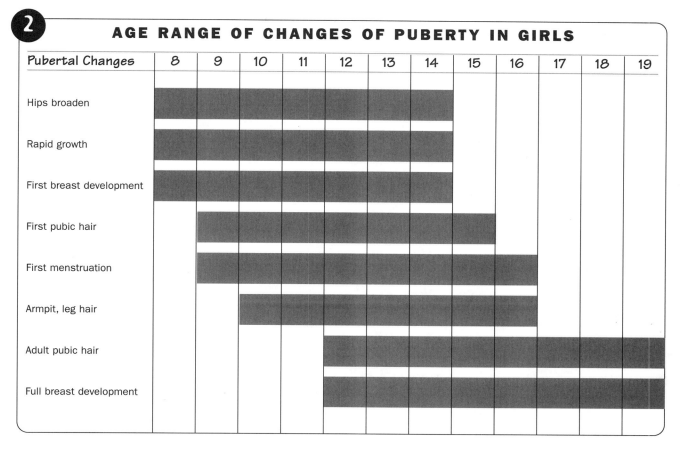

Pubertal Changes	8	9	10	11	12	13	14	15	16	17	18	19
Hips broaden												
Rapid growth												
First breast development												
First pubic hair												
First menstruation												
Armpit, leg hair												
Adult pubic hair												
Full breast development												

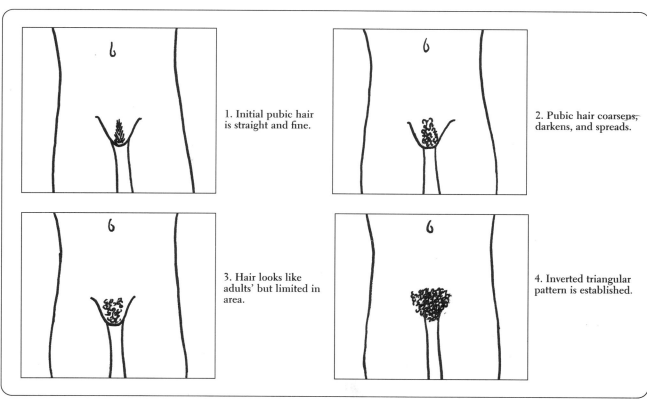

1. Initial pubic hair is straight and fine.

2. Pubic hair coarsens, darkens, and spreads.

3. Hair looks like adults' but limited in area.

4. Inverted triangular pattern is established.

Female Pubic Hair Development

When should you worry about lack of development?
Most physicians feel that if you're 16 or older and have no signs of puberty, such as pubic hair and breast development, or if you haven't yet started your period by this age, a medical checkup is in order.

What can cause delayed puberty? There are many possibilities, all of which will be considered during your physical exam. Some girls who are very physically active and have low body fat, especially gymnasts, ballet dancers, and figure skaters, may have delayed puberty. Typically, in the process of puberty, a girl will increase her body fat from 8 percent to 21–22 percent. Those who don't experience this increase in body fat due to restricted diets and/or heavy exercise may find puberty delayed. Still, it's a good idea to get a thorough checkup from your physician. In fact, the American Academy of Pediatrics is now recommending that young people age 11 and older see their physicians for an annual physical. This is a chance to ask questions and get information from your doctor about your body and your health.

BREASTS

What is normal breast size? I'm skinny and my breasts are small and everyone teases me. What can I do? Do those bust developers that are advertised in magazines really work? Help!

Embarrassed

"Normal breast size" is a relative term. Heredity plays a major role in determining what your normal size will be. Time can also be a factor. The average white American teen doesn't reach the final stage of breast growth until age 17 or older, while African American and Asian American teens may reach this stage a year or so earlier.

Weight can also be a factor in the size of your breasts—and gaining weight at any time in life may increase breast size. But it is heredity more than

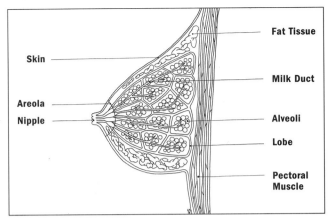

The Female Breast

weight that is the major determining factor in breast size. Heredity and skin tone can also affect the color of the *areola*, the area around the nipple. Teens with light skin tend to have very light pink areolas, while those with darker skin have brown-toned areolas. Those of any ethnicity who have been pregnant may notice a darkening of the skin of the areola. This is a normal change of pregnancy and is often permanent.

The breast is made up of fat and milk glands/ducts as well as nerves, arteries, veins, and lymph channels. Connective fibers help to give the breast its rounded shape, a shape it may not assume until late adolescence. There are no muscles in the breast itself, but there are pectoral muscles just beneath the breast on the chest wall. Any exercises you do—with or without "bust developer" devices—will not increase actual breast size. The most exercise can do is develop the pectoral muscles underneath the breast.

Some women notice a slight breast swelling while taking birth control pills, but this increase is very small and doesn't happen to everyone. In most cases, small breasts are the result of heredity, not hormone deficiency, so hormone therapy has little to offer.

Padded and uplift bras can make breasts appear larger, but the best method of long-term contentment is accepting and learning to love the uniqueness of your own body, whether you're small or large or somewhere in between.

My breasts are a different size. My left breast is quite a bit smaller than my right one. I feel lopsided and really embarrassed. Will they ever be the same size?

Lopsided

It's quite common, while breasts are growing and developing, to have one breast develop at a faster rate than the other. Generally, the slower breast will catch up. But breasts are rarely a perfect match, however. In most women, one breast may always be slightly larger than the other.

In rare instances, due to a congenital condition, one breast will remain undeveloped. In these cases, after the girl has reached full maturity, she may choose to have cosmetic surgery to increase the size of the undeveloped breast. However, such surgery should not be done during adolescence while one or both breasts are still developing.

I have gross nipples. Well, they're hardly nipples at all because they're inverted and look like little slits. Why does this happen and what can I do about it?

Dana Y.

Inverted nipples—nipples that turn inward instead of outward—are not uncommon and can appear in male or female breasts. This condition is usually caused by foreshortening of the milk ducts, with fibrous tissue strands binding the nipple down. This condition is usually present at birth, but becomes most noticeable later in life.

Sometimes the enlargement of breast tissue during puberty will cause one or both of the nipples to turn out after having been inverted since birth. This can also happen, too, during pregnancy. Even if it doesn't and a woman wants to breast-feed her baby, there are special shields made for women with inverted nipples to make it possible to breast-feed.

Can inverted nipples ever be a problem? Hygiene may be a special challenge, since secretions may dry and cake in the nipple crevices, and infections are also common. Some physicians recommend massage to help correct inverted nipples, but this usually isn't effective nor is surgery always successful. In surgery, the nipple is put in its normal position, but in the process, vital nerve fibers may have to be severed, causing the loss of some physical sensations in the breast.

If your nipples have always been turned out and then suddenly become inverted, this can be a sign of an underlying tumor and it's important to seek medical help immediately.

I have some dark hairs around my nipple. My mom said that pulling them out will cause cancer. How can I get rid of this hair?

Sue

Hair around the nipples is quite common and may be influenced both by ethnic origin and hormonal balance. It isn't necessarily a sign of underlying problems. The only cause for some concern would be if the hair appeared suddenly along with a number of masculine traits. Otherwise, if you have some hairs around your nipple that you find annoying or embarrassing, it's perfectly fine to remove them with no danger of cancer.

Can you get cancer if you get hit in the breasts with a soccer ball? I want to know because I got hit there last week and got a really bad bruise. My best friend says that getting bruised there can make you get breast cancer later on. Is that true? What can I do about it?

Leslie

Generally, breasts are pretty resilient, whether they are bruised by sports activities, accidents, or squeezing during sexual activity. However a more severe injury—caused by very hard squeezing or pinching—can cause some hemorrhage into the tissues. If such injuries happen over and over, with chronic irritation of the breast tissue, it's possible that, over a period of years, cancerous changes could take place.

Many women, including teens, worry about breast cancer. Even though breast cancer is not especially common in teenagers, it *is* a good idea to get into the habit of regular breast self-examinations (see the illustration in this section). Most breast lumps are benign, but it's vital to know how your breasts feel and to be able to notice changes immediately so that you can seek advice from your physician.

You should also seek medical advice if you notice a discharge from your nipple. While a small amount of discharge from the nipple is normal, it's usually not noticeable. What can an unusual discharge mean? If it contains pus, it can be a sign of an underlying infection. If it is bloody or pinkish and you're not pregnant, it could be a sign of an underlying breast disease. If the discharge is brownish, it could signal a sebaceous cyst with some infection.

One very common breast condition of puberty is an *adolescent nodule*. This is an enlargement and swelling, usually under the nipple, making the nipple very tender. It can happen in both males and females. No one knows for sure what causes it, but it may be due to an increased production of hormones. It will usually disappear in a short time. It should *never* be surgically removed; to do so could interfere with future breast development in a young girl.

Another breast condition that many women experience is called *fibrocystic disease*. It isn't really a disease, but a combination of breast changes, influenced by hormones, that results in fluid-filled cysts that enlarge, sometimes painfully, around the time of your menstrual period. Many women, in consultation with their physicians, find some relief in diet management. Abstaining from caffeine (found in colas, coffee, tea, and all forms of chocolate as well as some cold remedies) and cigarettes may relieve symptoms. Your physician may also prescribe drug or vitamin therapies.

Moles also commonly occur on the breasts. These should be watched; if they begin to change in color, increase in size, or bleed, they should be surgically removed.

1. Raise your arms, look in the mirror for changes in contour, skin texture, or color.

2. Examine your breasts, using a circular, clockwise motion to check for lumps.

Breast Self-Examination

It's important to begin the habit of breast self-examination right now, so that you know how your breasts normally change during your monthly cycle. That way, if anything unusual occurs later on, you'll notice right away. As well as feeling for lumps (see illustration for instruction), look for unusual changes such as:

- A dimple or pucker in the breast
- A previously normal nipple that has become inverted

- A change in skin texture or color
- Scaly skin around the nipple
- A change in breast shape
- A noticeable discharge from the nipple
- Swelling or redness in the breast
- A feeling of heat in the breast

When and how often should you do a breast self-exam? About once a month—perhaps a week or so after your menstrual period. If you do notice anything unusual, check with your physician. It's likely to be a minor problem, but only your doctor can confirm this. Although you're less likely to have serious problems with your breasts in the teen years than all other times of life, self-examination is a good habit to get into—one that could someday save your life.

MENSTRUATION

Menstruation isn't a curse or an illness. It's a positive sign of health, one of the best barometers you have to show that your body is healthy and functioning normally.

For centuries, there have been superstitions and myths about menstruation: that it is dirty, that one shouldn't bathe or swim during menstruation, that exercise is forbidden during the menstrual period. None of this is true. It's important to keep your routines as normal as possible during your period, whether this means bathing regularly, pursuing your usual exercise regimen, or doing any other activities. You *don't* have to put life on hold during menstruation. In fact, some Olympic athletes have given top performances during their menstrual

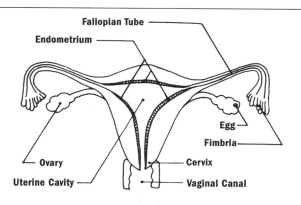

1. Hormonal levels rise and the uterine lining is prepared to receive a fertilized egg.

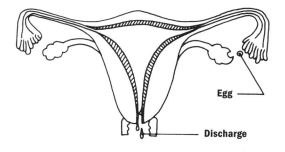

2. Around mid-cycle the ripened egg leaves the ovary and travels through the Fallopian tube.

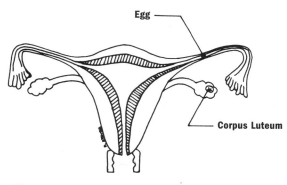

3. The egg approaches the uterine lining.

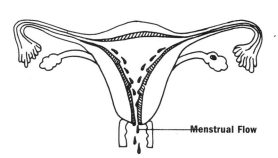

4. If conception has not taken place, the egg disintegrates and the lining is shed as menstruation.

The Menstrual Cycle

periods. So you can be your best, too, *any* day of the month!

What's the difference between the menstrual period and the menstrual cycle? Or are these both the same? What is the normal time between periods? Is it ever normal to skip a period—without being pregnant? There's so much I need to know!

Sheri A.

While most women equate menstruation with the actual menstrual period, the menstrual *cycle* is a continuous process involving ovulation, changes in the tissue lining of the uterus, and finally shedding that lining via the menstrual flow.

Menstruation involves the entire body, not just the uterus. The entire monthly cycle is controlled by a part of the brain known as the *hypothalamus* and by the *pituitary gland*. These control the ebb and flow of hormones—*estrogen* and *progesterone*—that cause women to develop and to have regular menstrual cycles. A regular cycle may vary widely from individual to individual. While a 28-day cycle might be considered *average*, a 21-, 30-, or even 60-day cycle may be normal for you.

How do you calculate your cycle length? Day 1 is the first day of your menstrual period. Start counting there. You may have your period an average of three to seven days. At this time, your estrogen level is low and you may feel a little short on energy.

When your period ends, keep counting. Now your estrogen level is rising once more, preparing the lining of your uterus to receive and nourish a fertilized egg. With this surge in your hormonal level, you may feel a sharp rise in energy and a sense of well-being.

Around mid-cycle—perhaps day 14 or 15—your cycle will begin to reach its peak. A second hormone, progesterone, joins estrogen in preparing the lush uterine lining for a fertilized egg. The egg itself has ripened and now receives the hormonal signal to leave the ovaries and begin its journey

through the Fallopian tubes to the uterus. It is during the egg's four-to-six-day journey to the uterus that it is most likely to be fertilized. If you have sexual intercourse during this time, you are much more likely to get pregnant than at other times. Relying on calculation of your "safe" times is risky, however. While the release of the egg (ovulation) is most likely to happen at mid-cycle, the exact timing is very difficult to calculate. It's wiser to assume that, if you're sexually active and not using a reliable method of birth control, pregnancy can occur at any time of the month. Please see Chapter 13 for birth control information.

At this mid-cycle time, with two hormones at top levels, you may feel unusually good. These hormones will reach a high level about day 20 and then start to drop if your egg has not been fertilized. The egg itself will begin to disintegrate and the lining of the uterus will start to break down. About day 28, this will begin to pass from your uterus, through your cervix, and out of your vagina as the menstrual flow.

Menstrual Problems

What does it mean if you skip a period or two and you're not having sex, so you couldn't be pregnant? I had two periods last year when I was 12 and then nothing for four months and then a period and then nothing again for the past two months. What's going on?

Jen

Just a quick question: Is PMS real or all in the head or what? My best friend and I have this bet. I say it's real because I know and she thinks it's just a bad attitude I've got. Who's right?

Annie P.

Annie and Jen describe two of the several conditions that may cause some concern to young teens. Among these are irregular periods, *secondary amenorrhea* (ceasing to have periods), endometriosis, PMS, and *dysmenorrhea* (menstrual cramps).

Irregular Periods

Symptoms: You have a period and then skip one or two. Or you may find yourself spotting between periods.

Causes: The most common cause for irregular periods is puberty itself. Your estrogen levels may be fluctuating more than usual and you may not yet be ovulating in the year or so after you have your first menstrual period. It may take several years to get a regular cycle established. Other causes of missed periods include emotional stress, jet lag, or an undisclosed physical problem. Spotting between periods may also be caused by emotional stress. Spotting is also a common side effect of birth control pills. It can also signal a physical problem such as an ovarian cyst or polyp.

What to Do: Keep track of your periods, as irregular as they might be, and any other symptoms you might have, to discuss with your physician.

Secondary Amenorrhea (Ceasing to Have Periods)

Symptoms: After having had menstrual periods, you suddenly stop.

Causes: Pregnancy, of course, is the first possibility to consider. But there are other common causes of secondary amenorrhea, including the following:

- *An unusual amount of stress in your life.* This may be the death of a loved one, a parental divorce, or a stressful change such as going away to college. Fear of pregnancy can fall into this category, too.
- *Heavy exercise.* Especially if you're involved in long-distance running, ballet, gymnastics, figure skating, or another sport where it's vital to have low body fat, your body fat may be too low

to allow you to have periods. In the long term, despite the benefits of exercise, this may take a toll on your body, with low estrogen levels, loss of calcium, and bone weakness (which can make you vulnerable to stress fractures).

- *A major weight change.* Up or down, a weight change of 10 to 15 percent of your total body weight can affect your menstrual cycle. Those with eating disorders such as anorexia or bulimia can stop menstruating due to malnutrition and iron deficiency. And because estrogen and progesterone can dissolve in excess fatty tissue, obese women can also have a disturbed hormone balance that translates into sporadic periods, heavy periods, or no menstruation at all for a time.
- *Use of drugs.* This would not only include possible drug abuse of tranquilizers (which can have a "down" effect on your menstrual cycle), but also normal use of prescription drugs. Birth control pills, for example, can cause lighter-than-normal periods, and some women may skip an occasional menstrual period.

What to Do: See your physician. If your amenorrhea is not due to any of the causes listed here, he or she will want to explore other possibilities such as tumors or polyps—growths in the uterus or ovaries—that may or may not require surgery. In most cases, however, amenorrhea is linked to stress, body weight, or possible drug influences. When the crisis has passed—for example, when your body fat has increased even slightly or your weight has otherwise stabilized—your periods may resume. If your doctor has found that your condition is not linked with birth control pills, pregnancy, or conditions such as ovarian cysts, he or she may give you the drug Provera to bring on your period. Provera or the hormones estrogen and progesterone, used in oral contraceptives, may be used to regulate the cycle for perhaps three months until the cycle is established again.

Endometriosis

Symptoms: Pelvic pain, prolonged menstrual periods, and, at times, pain during sexual intercourse.

Causes: There are a number of theories about this condition, which is not uncommon in teenagers. Endometriosis is an overgrowth of uterine lining outside the uterine cavity. Some think that it is caused by irregular ovarian function. Others believe that it may be hereditary. Some feel that endometriosis develops when menstrual blood containing endometrial tissue backs up and escapes from the uterus around the Fallopian tubes.

What to Do: See your physician. Endometriosis can be treated with painkillers, hormone therapy, or, in severe cases, surgery. (Laser surgery has been used increasingly to remove the overgrown endometrial tissues without harming the uterus or ovaries.) Birth control pills can also help alleviate symptoms.

Premenstrual Syndrome/Symptoms (PMS)

Symptoms: *Premenstrual changes* may include headaches, fatigue, increased appetite, mood changes with increased irritability, sadness or anger, and an increased sensitivity to pain. These may not be severe enough to be noticed by anyone but you. *Premenstrual syndrome* means that a number of these symptoms happen together premenstrually. These symptoms may be noticed by people close to you but may not be that obvious to anyone else. *Premenstrual disorder* means that the premenstrual symptoms are so severe that they seriously impair your ability to function at school or at work. *Premenstrual exacerbation* means that ongoing chronic conditions become worse just before menstruation. These conditions can include migraine headaches, allergies, or chronic depression.

Causes: Experts aren't yet entirely sure what causes PMS and other premenstrual problems. There may, in fact, be many causes. However, progress has been made in terms of alleviating or even eliminating some symptoms.

What to Do: First, keep track of your symptoms and your menstrual periods on a calendar for several months to see whether the symptoms are occurring in the week or so before your period. Understand that PMS is not in your head. It has definite physical links—and solutions. The following steps may help:

- *Eliminate potential problem foods and drinks from your diet.* These include caffeine-containing substances such as coffee, regular tea, chocolate, and cola drinks. These contain a substance that can increase your *prostaglandin* activity, which, in turn, can trigger cramps, breast tenderness, and nausea before and during your period. Also avoid salty foods such as chips, hot dogs, lunch meats, ham, canned foods (including canned soups), and frozen dinners, especially in the two weeks before your period. Read labels! Cutting down on salt can help to prevent premenstrual bloating and weight gain. Eat smaller, more frequent meals with lots of fresh fruits and vegetables, beans, fish, chicken, and whole-grain bread.
- *Learn to manage stress.* Do things that are calming, such as listening to music, meditating, or writing in your journal. Imagine yourself in a beautiful, peaceful place and let the fantasy of being in this place help to calm you.
- *Exercise regularly.* This is a good idea any time of the month, but aerobic exercise—whether it is dancing, cycling, swimming, running, or simply walking briskly for 30 minutes at least three times a week—can help alleviate a number of symptoms, including depression and anxiety.
- *See your doctor if symptoms persist.* While most women find relief with lifestyle changes such as improved diet, stress reduction, and increased exercise, see your doctor if doing all

of this doesn't help. Medication is considered a last resort. Sometimes hormone therapy, birth control pills, or special vitamin regimens (taken under a physician's supervision) may help. We can't emphasize too strongly that any medication *must* be taken only after seeing your doctor. Only your physician can rule out other possible causes of your symptoms and, given the current knowledge of the problem, determine which treatment is most appropriate for you.

Dysmenorrhea (Menstrual Cramps)

Symptoms: Abdominal pain as well as pain in the legs and back. Symptoms may also include chills, feeling shaky and sweaty, and feeling faint or nauseated.

Causes: Cramps caused by some sort of anatomical disorder or infection, ovarian tumor, or endometriosis is called *secondary dysmenorrhea*. However, it is much more common for women to have *primary dysmenorrhea*, or cramps not caused by an identifiable disorder.

In recent years, researchers have discovered that primary dysmenorrhea is often caused by an overproduction of prostaglandins. These hormonelike substances are manufactured throughout the body, including the lining of the uterus. Since these substances regulate the action of the body's involuntary muscles, they cause the muscular uterus to contract. Some contraction is necessary to expel the menstrual flow. But when too many prostaglandins are produced, the uterus contracts much more, causing painful cramps. Quite often, these contractions squeeze small blood vessels, causing the supply of blood and oxygen to the pelvic area to be reduced, resulting in lower back pain. If these excess prostaglandins get into the bloodstream, they can cause other involuntary muscles in the body—such as the stomach and intestines—to speed up contractions, causing nausea and diarrhea.

What to Do: Try taking an over-the-counter, low-dosage anti-prostaglandin medication such as Motrin, Advil, or Nuprin. You might also try Naprosyn or Ponstel. Some feel that Ponstel is most effective in relieving menstrual distress, since it inhibits the production of prostaglandins and the resulting cramps and is also effective in alleviating premenstrual and menstrual bloating and other uncomfortable symptoms.

How well these drugs work for you may depend on when and how often you take them. Your best plan of action is to take two of these nonprescription pills a day or two before your period even begins or, at the latest, at the very first sign of your period and then one every four to six hours as needed. If you wait until your cramps are severe, these drugs won't work nearly as well for you. And, if one brand doesn't seem effective, try another before you give up on nonprescription drugs.

If you get no relief from nonprescription medications, ask your doctor to prescribe the stronger, prescription variety of anti-prostaglandins. If those don't work for you, and especially if your cramps occur at other times besides your menstrual period, see your doctor for a thorough examination. You may have endometriosis or pelvic inflammatory disease. Both of these conditions can cause pain and can threaten your future fertility, so early diagnosis and treatment are a must. Other causes of secondary dysmenorrhea, such as ovarian cysts, also need prompt attention.

For persistent cramps that are not due to secondary dysmenorrhea, some doctors may prescribe estrogen/progesterone combination pills, which can regulate the cycle and decrease the number of days of flow and the cramps. Prescription painkillers are a last resort, usually prescribed only if a woman is allergic to aspirin or other anti-prostaglandins and also cannot take hormone pills.

Besides medication, many women find that exercise helps a lot. Yes, exercise! (Probably the last thing you were thinking of doing to alleviate cramps!) Actually, vigorous exercise such as brisk walking, swimming, or cycling can cause your body to release substances called *endorphins*, which tend to diminish pain. This approach doesn't work for everyone, but if you enjoy being active and can talk yourself into trying exercise during the most painful days of your period, you may be pleasantly surprised!

Meditation and relaxation exercises may also help you to ease muscle tension that can add to your discomfort. Trying these self-help measures can give you a feeling of control over your body and your life, no matter what day of the month it is.

Please Note: We've just devoted a lot of space to discussing menstrual problems and want to emphasize that, by definition, menstruation is a healthy process and is *not* a problem. We do tend to get more letters, calls, and complaints from girls having problems—and these problems are reflected in this section—but the fact is that most girls and women experience menstruation as just another part of their lives. Generally, there is no need to change your activities or your life in any way during the days you have your period. The only difference will be that you will be using a menstrual protection product—such as a sanitary napkin or tampon—and once you get used to that, it's no big deal. Remember that regular periods are a sign of health and physical maturity—both very positive aspects of your life today!

Sanitary Products

I recently started my period and want to use tampons but my mom won't let me because she says tampons give you a fatal disease and make you not a virgin anymore. Is any of this true or is it just crazy mom talk?

Jana K.

Choice of sanitary protection product is very much up to you. Your best choice is what *you're* most comfortable wearing. When your mother was a teen, there was a real difference between the comfort and convenience of pads and tam-

pons. Today, however, that difference is small or nonexistent.

Most of my friends use tampons and make fun of me for using pads, but I find them more comfortable. Are tampons better? Should I try them?

Tracy W.

In years past, pads were very bulky, had to be held on by uncomfortable belts and pins, and were not what you'd call discreetly portable. Today, all that has changed. Pads are made of thinner, more absorbent materials and attach to the underpants with a special adhesive. Some have special wrap-around panty protectors that keep the menstrual flow from spilling over the sides of the pad and staining clothing; some come individually wrapped in disposal packets or with a special carrying case to make pads just about as convenient to carry as tampons.

Various Types of Tampons and Pads

Many girls do prefer tampons, however, and these can be used from the first period on. Using a tampon does not make you a nonvirgin. Only having sexual

1. To insert a tampon, grasp tube with one hand and spread labia with the other.

2. Insert tampon, aiming at the small of the back.

3. Gently press inner tube into outer tube.

4. Withdraw both tubes, leaving the cord outside the body.

Inserting a Tampon

intercourse can do that. The hymen is elastic and stretches easily, in most cases, allowing the use of a tampon. Also, tampons are available in a number of sizes, including junior and slim regular sizes. These can make tampon use even easier.

Some fear that a tampon will "get lost" inside them, but that can't happen. The vaginal opening is the only genital opening large enough to admit a tampon. The cervical os, the opening leading to the uterus, is much too tiny to permit passage of a tampon.

Many new users of tampons find that those with applicators are easier to use, at least initially, than the ones inserted with a finger.

The menstrual cup—called Instead—is a new product that catches the menstrual flow in a soft flexible cup that is set into place over the cervix. This may be, at least initially, more difficult to insert than a tampon. Its advantage is that it gives you more protection time—for example, if you have to change a tampon every two hours, you can go about four hours without a change if you use Instead.

However, it's important to change whatever form of sanitary protection you use before the maximum time. This is particularly important with tampons and, quite possibly, any other internally worn product. The reason? You want to avoid the risk of a disease called *toxic shock syndrome (TSS)*. This was big in the news in 1980, when tampons were more absorbent and left in longer. TSS, a rare and sometimes fatal disease, is caused by a bacterium that can grow in surgical wounds, cuts, or skin abscesses or on tampons. You *can* use tampons safely, but keep the following safety tips in mind:

- If you're having your period and notice flu-like symptoms (a sudden fever of 102°F or higher, vomiting and diarrhea, headache, dizziness, sore throat, muscle aches, and a sunburnlike rash most commonly seen on the hands and feet), remove your tampon and seek medical help at once.
- Change tampons frequently—at least every three or four hours, even when the flow is light.
- Use tampons with the lowest possible absorbency. Even on heavy flow days, you might consider using a regular tampon with a mini-pad.
- Consider using tampons during the day and pads at night (when you will be sleeping and have a longer interval between changes).
- Avoid using tampons with plastic insertion tubes, especially those with the petal-shaped ends. Some of these have sharp edges that could scratch your vagina.
- Always wash your hands before inserting a tampon to make sure that you do not introduce bacteria into your vagina.
- Don't use tampons to absorb nonmenstrual vaginal secretions.

What kind of menstrual protection product to use comes down to personal choice—and you have a lot of choices today! Finding what works best for you may mean experimenting with a number of different products until you find the one—or several—you like best.

VAGINAL HEALTH AND INFECTIONS

What should I be doing as far as feminine hygiene goes? I'm not even sure what it means. But I heard my mother and her friend talking about douching and I don't know what it is and if I should be doing it, too. How can I prevent odors? I haven't noticed any myself, but I keep hearing about them in commercials. Help!

Andrea Y.

Simple soap and water—a daily bath or shower—is the best possible safeguard against unpleasant odors. Body odors are often caused by bacteria acting on perspiration and other normal secretions. Avoid clothes that increase perspiration, such as nylon underwear or pantyhose—unless they have cotton, ventilated crotches.

That's about all you need to do to avoid body odor: Bathe regularly and wear clean, absorbent, well-ventilated underwear. Forget the feminine sprays—they can irritate the delicate tissues of the vulva and vagina. And forget about douching, which is cleansing of the vagina with a solution of water and vinegar or a commercial douche preparation, using a douche bag or special squeeze bottle. The healthy vagina is essentially self-cleansing, making douching unnecessary. In fact, studies have found that excessive douching may actually make a woman more vulnerable to infection by altering the normal acidic balance of the vagina. For example, researchers at Mount Sinai School of Medicine in New York looked at 30 years of published research on the topic and found that women who douched had a 73 percent greater risk of pelvic inflammatory disease than women who did not. The only time a douche may be necessary is if it is a medicinal one prescribed by a physician for some varieties of vaginal infections.

Vaginal Infections

Help! I think I have an infection because I have this discharge. How do I know whether I have an infection or not without going to a doctor?

Cammie K.

It's normal to have a clear, whitish, nonirritating vaginal discharge. This mixture of mucus, bacteria, and discarded vaginal cells may turn from clear or white to pale yellow as it is exposed to the air. This discharge can become more noticeable under several circumstances, including during sexual excitement and during ovulation when the estrogen level is increased. This can also happen with women who are taking birth control pills.

How do you know whether you might have an infection? A vaginal discharge is *not* normal if it is irritating, causes itching, is mixed with nonmenstrual blood, has a foul odor, or is a different color from your normal discharge. These are usually symptoms of a vaginal infection and a sign that you should visit your doctor right away. Don't try to self-treat a vaginal infection if you're not sure what it is. Seek advice from your physician first.

The following chart will show you the most common types of vaginal infections and their symptoms and treatment.

If you have a persistent vaginal discharge that has not been diagnosed as an infection, you may have a more copious than usual vaginal discharge. What can help? Try alternating baths with showers, wearing cotton underwear, and avoiding tight jeans. Also, don't sleep in confining clothes (such as sweatsuits or underpants).

If you have painful urination, this could be a symptom of a bladder or urinary tract infection. Consult your physician.

If you have pain when you urinate, but don't feel the frequent urgency to urinate that characterizes urinary/bladder infections, you may have a small cut on your labia, or vaginal entrance, that burns when the acidic urine touches it. If you have a small cut, put a little petroleum jelly on it to protect it and thus promote healing.

Although the various types of vaginal infections may be identified by a specific discharge, tests by a physician are required to make absolutely sure that you have that specific infection. Since treatments vary widely from one type of vaginal infection to another, an accurate diagnosis is extremely

3 MOST COMMON VAGINAL INFECTIONS

Infection	Cause	Symptoms	Treatment
Bacterial vaginosis	Vulnerable during times of stress or while taking antibiotics. May also be sexually transmitted.	Heavy, creamy, gray-white discharge that has a foul, fishy odor.	See a physician. Treatment is usually prescription drug Flagyl (metronidazole) in pill form.
Candidiasis (yeast infection)	Imbalance of natural vaginal bacteria due to diabetes, tight clothing, prolonged use of antibiotics such as tetracycline, or birth control pills. Rarely sexually transmitted.	Thick, odorless, white discharge with the consistency of cottage cheese. Itching of the vulva and vagina and white patches of fungus over reddish, raw areas. Painful urination.	See a physician for correct diagnosis rather than trying to self-diagnose. Treatment of choice is either Monistat or Lotrimin in cream or suppository form. These are now available over the counter, but a correct diagnosis from your physician is crucial.
Trichomoniasis	Caused by a protozoan organism spread via shared washcloths, towels, wet bathing suits, toilet seats. Often sexually transmitted.	A frothy greenish-yellow, foul-smelling discharge, vaginal itching, inflammation of the vulva. There may also be frequent, painful urination and, in some cases, severe lower abdominal pain.	See a physician. The treatment is usually Flagyl in pill form. There are also Flagyl suppositories. Both forms are available only by prescription. If you're sexually active, your partner also needs to be treated.

important! Also, if you're having sex, even very infrequently, you are at risk for sexually transmitted diseases and must be examined by a physician to rule out that possibility. A number of sexually transmitted diseases, such as chlamydia and gonorrhea, must be promptly and correctly treated in order to preserve health and fertility. So if you have an unusual discharge or other troublesome symptoms, *don't* try to diagnose and treat yourself!

GROWING FROM GIRL TO WOMAN

I feel ugly and klutzy, not cute like my friends. I don't have a boyfriend like everyone else does even though I like one special boy a lot (but he doesn't notice me at all). I feel like a total loser and like there's something the matter with my body.

Hannah N.

Cultural expectations—to be popular, pretty, noticed by boys, sensitive to others, and "feminine" in the sense of not being too much of anything (too assertive or too strong or too smart)—hit teen girls especially hard. Many begin to lose their sense of self in a frenzy to meet others' expectations. Others rebel and remain very much themselves—sometimes at the price of acceptance by peers.

Women of all ages have insecurities about their bodies. Much of this is based on our society's unrealistic standards of beauty for women. Even young women who appear, to everyone else, to be slim and pretty all too often feel that they fall short of society's ideal. And those who look like themselves rather than a budding supermodel can suffer even more.

But who in normal, everyday life looks like a supermodel? Your beauty as a woman and your value as a person are expressed in many ways—more through who you are than how you look in terms of society's standards. Girls seem to suffer more than guys over society's "lookism." Some develop a poor body image as the result of comments and teasing from family and peers. Some, all

on their own, pick out a self-perceived flaw and feel that it overshadows whatever is good about their looks and themselves.

Having a negative body image can affect your life in many ways. Your confidence and self-esteem may suffer. You may feel insecure around guys—and not pretty unless some guy tells you that you are. Your self-consciousness may keep you from doing things you enjoy. You may even begin to believe that you're less deserving of love and happiness than other people are.

If this all sounds painfully familiar, what can you do?

- *Change your mind about your body before you try to change your looks.* It's important that you feel lovable and valuable as a person just as you are today. Otherwise, no amount of change will make any difference in how you feel about yourself. There are countless overweight people who lose weight and still feel fat. There are others who felt awkward and ugly in their preteens or teens and who have never outgrown these feelings, even as they have blossomed to lovely, healthy young adulthood. Accept and feel positive about the way you look right now. See exercising and eating healthy foods not as punishment, but as rewards—because you deserve tender loving care.

- *Realize that people who tease have their own insecurities.* Their comments have more to do with themselves than with you. Even though it's hard to turn a deaf ear to taunts, don't join the chorus. Don't give yourself a hard time for what can't be changed or what isn't perfect about your body, and start enjoying all of your great qualities. (And if you can't think of any, ask your parents or a trusted friend.)

- *Realize that in the real world, attractive people come in all sizes and shapes.* And what makes them most attractive goes far beyond the shape of their nose or body or the color of their hair.

Being active, friendly, kind, having a sense of humor, moving with confidence and grace, feeling at ease with yourself as you are—all of this can go a long way toward developing a positive body image. This positive image of yourself can do more for your appearance than all the cosmetic treatments put together.

Part of your growth as a woman is to find peace and acceptance of who you are physically and emotionally. In the chapters to come, we'll be sharing some useful ideas to maximize your changing body's health, fitness, and vitality. But it's up to you to discover your own unique beauty. That has nothing to do with being a certain weight or bra size and everything to do with good health, loving self-care of your body and your emotional needs, and your growth as a loving person. When you're able to love, accept, and appreciate yourself, others will too!

A WOMAN'S BODY

✔ There are many variations of normal when it comes to development. Your own timetable is based on your genetic and ethnic heritage (if you're African American, it is normal to develop a little earlier than friends of other ethnicities).

✔ If you're very physically active—in ballet, gymnastics, or figure skating, where body fat tends to be low—your physical development may be slowed by several years. But if you haven't started menstruating by age 16 or so, it's essential to see your physician to make sure all is well.

✔ Breast self-examination is an excellent health habit you should start today. (See the illustration on page 14 if you're not sure how to do it.)

✔ Learning how to manage stress, eating lots of fruits and vegetables, and getting regular exercise can help ease PMS and menstrual cramps.

✔ Don't try to self-diagnose vaginal infections; always see a doctor for a correct diagnosis.

✔ To decrease chances of vaginal infections, don't wear tight clothing or nylon underwear, don't share towels or damp bathing suits, and make personal hygiene (regular baths or showers) a priority.

CHAPTER
THREE

A Man's Body

My school sex ed class is, in a word, lame. My parents are too embarrassed to talk to me about anything personal and there are some things I'm too embarrassed to ask. But I have lots of questions. Like is it normal to have a hard-on a lot of times, off and on, throughout the day? What about the fact that I'm 14 and look pretty much like a man while my friend Eric, who is my age exactly, still looks like a little kid? Is there something wrong with him? I wonder about all the stuff that's going on with my body. Can you help me figure this all out?

Michael S.

Michael has lots of company. The changes of adolescence are dramatic and not always easy to understand. There is a much greater variation in male physical development from start to finish. One 14-year-old boy may be, indeed, still a boy, while his taller, more physically mature classmate may look very much like a man. Becoming a man is a complicated process. The better you understand the changes that your body is experiencing and what is normal, the more readily and completely you will begin to understand and accept yourself.

■ ■ ■

MALE ANATOMY

There are three parts to the male reproductive system. First, there are the organs of production—the *testicles*. At the beginning of puberty, on a chain-reaction signal from the *hypothalamus, pituitary*, and *pineal* glands, the testicles begin to produce the male hormone *testosterone*. This hormone triggers the common changes of adolescence such as enlargement of genital organs, growth of pubic hair, and deepening of the voice. As puberty progresses, the testicles also begin to mature and to produce sperm cells that, if united with a female's *ovum*, or egg, will produce a baby.

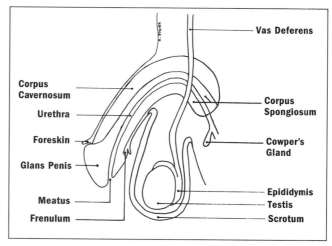

Side View of Male Genitalia

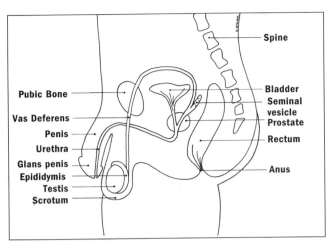

Side View of Male Reproductive System

The two testicles are encased in the *scrotum,* which hangs under the penis. It is quite common for one testicle to hang somewhat lower than the other. (There is a biological reason for this: If the testicles hung side by side, they would get constant friction from the legs. So, in a large percentage of men, one testicle—in 70 percent of such men, the left one—hangs a little lower than the other.)

The sperm cells are produced in a series of tiny chambers within the testicles, and as these sperm cells mature, they begin a long journey through the second part of the male reproductive system: the ducts for storage and transportation of sperm. First, there is the *epididymis,* a long, tightly coiled canal (uncoiled, it would stretch about 20 feet!) that lies over each testicle. Next, the sperm travel to the *vas deferens,* a shorter continuation of the epididymis. This brings the sperm from the scrotum to the abdominal cavity, passing to the back of the bladder and joining the *seminal vesicles,* forming the *ejaculatory duct* where sperm is stored.

The *prostate gland,* which lies against the bottom of the bladder, secretes much of the *seminal fluid,* which, combined with fluids from the seminal vesicles, carries the sperm from the body. The prostate gland enlarges dramatically during the changes of puberty. Other secretions come from the *bulbourethral glands,* two tiny structures on either side of the urethra, the passageway through which both urine and seminal fluid pass out of the penis. Dur-

ing sexual excitement, the bulbourethral glands produce a clear, sticky fluid that is thought to coat the urethra for the safe passage of the sperm. This is not seminal fluid, but it may contain a few stray sperm.

The third part of the male reproductive system is the *penis.*

When a mature or maturing man is sexually excited, he may ejaculate his seminal fluid out of the penis in a series of throbbing spurts. The total volume of this sticky white *ejaculate* is, on the average, about one teaspoon and is made up mostly of secretions from the prostate gland and the seminal vesicles. Although sperm make up only a small part of the total ejaculate, they are impressive in number. There may be about *400 million* sperm in one ejaculation! Obviously, the sperm cells are tiny. They are so small, in fact, that 400 million of them could fit on the head of a pin!

Another bit of sperm trivia: Your testicles may produce 200 million or more sperm cells a day! Obviously, only a few sperm cells, in any average man's lifetime, end up fertilizing an egg and producing a baby.

Penis Cross Section

A lot of people think that the penis is a skin-covered cylinder. That isn't so. The penis is made up of spongy tissues interlaced with large blood vessels (see cross-section illustration). There is a constant flow of blood in and out of the penis, which, despite a wide normal variation in size among men, *averages* three to four inches long and one and one-quarter inches in diameter—in the *flaccid,* or soft, state—in the mature male.

When a man becomes sexually excited, however, this even blood flow stops. The blood vessels expand, bringing more blood into the penis. Valves in the veins retain this blood under pressure, causing the spongy walls of the penis to expand and become hard. This is called an erection or hard-on.

Penis During Erection

The skin of the penis is loose to allow for expansion during erection. In some males, there is the *prepuce* or *foreskin*, which covers the head, or *glans*, of the penis. Although all males are born with this foreskin, many have it surgically removed, usually soon after birth, in a procedure called *circumcision*. All Jewish males are circumcised for religious reasons, but it has been common practice in this country until quite recently for the majority of hospital-born male infants to be circumcised. The practice today is becoming somewhat controversial, with some doctors questioning the automatic nature of this procedure and calling circumcision an option rather than a necessity. (In response to this changing feeling about circumcision, some insurance companies no longer cover the costs for this procedure, and the percentage of circumcised boys in this country is dropping. For example, while nearly all newborn boys in the United States were circumcised in the 1970s, by the mid-1980s that number was down to 59 percent—and it's still dropping.)

The circumcised and uncircumcised penis may look a bit different from each other in the flaccid state. Otherwise, each functions normally and there is no concrete evidence that circumcision—or lack of it—sharpens sexual response. The uncircumcised male, however, must take special care to keep his penis clean, since a foul-smelling substance called *smegma* may collect under the foreskin if the penis is not washed daily. Circumcised males don't experience this accumulation of smegma, and, according to some medical studies, may have a lower incidence of urinary tract infections.

Circumcised Penis   Uncircumcised Penis

As we mentioned earlier, circumcision is usually performed in the first few days of life. However, some teen boys and adult men elect to have this done, often due to a particularly tight foreskin—a problem we'll be discussing later on in this chapter.

We have just been describing the reproductive system of the mature male. It is important to know how your body is working—or will work—and it's also vital to know how you reach this point of maturity. For some, it is this journey, not the destination, that is of most concern right now.

PHYSICAL DEVELOPMENT

When is the normal time to start maturing? I'm almost 14 and I still look like a kid and get teased a lot. Should I see a doctor? Is something wrong with me?

Kevin T.

Males, as well as females, are subject to the highly individual rhythms of their own biological

STAGES OF PUBERTY IN BOYS

Stage	Ages	Internal	Genitals	Growth	Hair	Other
One	9–12	Male hormones are becoming active	No obvious change; testicles are maturing	Some start rapid growth late in this stage	No pubic or other body hair	None
Two	9–15	Hormonal changes cause new muscle tissue and fat to be added to body, changing the shape of the body	Testicles and scrotum are enlarging, but penis is not increasing much in size at this stage	Rapid growth, in height and in changing physique	Pubic hair appears at the base of the penis; will be straight and fine	The areola, the circle of darker skin around each nipple on the chest increases in size and darkens a little.
Three	11–16		Penis grows mostly in length; testicles and scrotum still growing	Adding more muscle tissue; still growing; shoulders broaden	Pubic hair is getting darker and coarse, spreading along the base of the penis; first traces of hair on upper lip	Voice starts deepening due to growth of larynx
Four	11–17	Sperm production begins; first ejaculation	Penis grows in width; testicles still growing		Underarm and facial hair increases; pubic hair looks more adult	Voice gets deeper and skin becomes more oily
Five	14–18	Full development	Adult in appearance	Near full adult height	Adult pubic hair; full beard	May get chest, body hair later

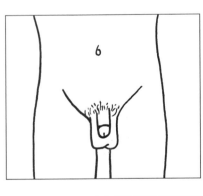

1. Straight hair appears at penis base. Testes increase in size and skin of scrotum reddens.

2. Pubic hair becomes curly and coarse. Penis grows in length.

3. Pubic hair is full, but limited in area. Penis grows in width.

4. Development of pubic hair and genitals is complete.

Male Pubic Hair and Genital Development

5 AGE RANGE OF CHANGES OF PUBERTY IN BOYS

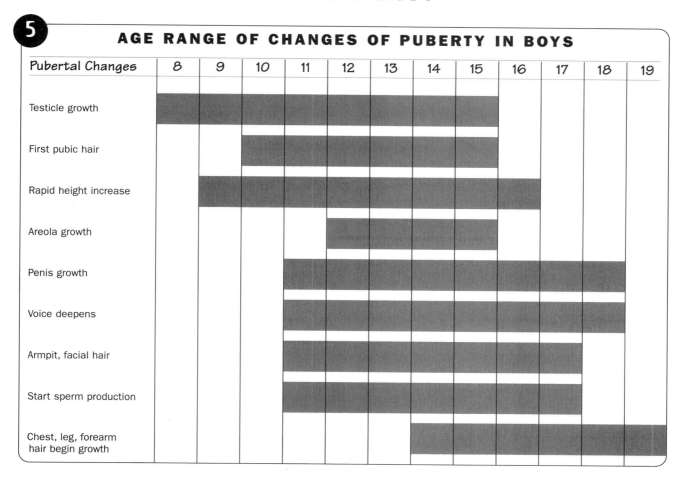

Pubertal Changes	8	9	10	11	12	13	14	15	16	17	18	19
Testicle growth	■	■	■	■	■	■	■	■				
First pubic hair			■	■	■	■	■	■				
Rapid height increase		■	■						■	■		
Areola growth					■	■	■	■				
Penis growth				■	■	■	■	■	■	■	■	
Voice deepens				■	■	■	■	■	■	■	■	
Armpit, facial hair				■	■	■	■	■	■	■		
Start sperm production				■	■	■	■	■				
Chest, leg, forearm hair begin growth							■	■	■	■	■	■

time clocks. The changes of puberty in the male may begin as early as age 8 or as late as age 15. Puberty may finish between ages 14 and 18. Therefore, some very normal 13- or 14-year-olds appear to be grown men, while some of their equally normal classmates still look like boys.

Slow development—often an inherited genetic characteristic—may be even more worrisome for a boy than for a girl. Girls tend to start puberty about a year or two earlier, on the average, than their male classmates. So the late-blooming male may feel really left behind. In most cases, however, the so-called late bloomer is entirely within the range of normal.

What are some of the age ranges for a boy's development into a man and what sequence do these changes follow? The stages of puberty were identified by a British doctor named J. M. Tanner, who noted that within each stage there are many small changes and steps in growth, genital devel-opment, and pubic hair development. There are many variations, of course, but the major changes follow a basic pattern shown in the following charts.

SPECIAL PROBLEMS

Short Stature

Please help me. I'm short and I get teased all the time. Is there anything I can do, like a treatment, that can make me taller?

Sean A.

There is a wide range of height among teen boys, but those on the lower end of the range may wonder whether they will always be shorter than average.

Heredity is a factor. If you're well along in your development and have shorter-than-average parents, chances are it's normal for you to be relatively short, too. If, on the other hand, you haven't begun much development and have a tall parent or parents, you may be due for a lot of growing.

You may wish to see your doctor for a complete physical, including thyroid testing, blood and urine analysis, and X rays to determine bone age. While hormone therapy can speed up a delayed puberty, physicians are reluctant to use this unnecessarily due to side effects. One of the side effects, ironically, in speeding up the process of puberty is that accelerating growth may cause a boy to be shorter as an adult than he would have been had he been allowed to mature on his own timetable. For this reason and others, many physicians prefer to let natural development take place in its own time whenever possible.

Society tends to put a premium on size in males. However, like a number of other societal expectations, this "tall, dark, and handsome" measure of desirable manhood is a myth. There are many very loving—and loved—men who are none of the above. Real men come in all sizes and physical types. You can be attractive even if you're far from tall or handsome. A lot has to do with how you develop your personality, your social skills, and your own good feelings about yourself.

Adolescent Nodule/ Adolescent Gynecomastia

What does it mean when you have swelling on your chest under the nipple area? It almost looks like I'm getting breasts. I'm too embarrassed to tell my parents or my doctor. Is something seriously wrong with me?

Travis T.

Several conditions can cause breast swelling in the adolescent male. First, there is the *adolescent nodule*. This small but firm swelling under the nipple may occur in one or both breasts and has been linked to increased secretion of the male sex hormone just before puberty begins. Although this

nodule may be tender and cause some concern, it doesn't require treatment. Most of these nodules go away within a year.

Second, and perhaps most common (occurring in 50 to 85 percent of all adolescent males) is a condition called *adolescent gynecomastia*. This breast enlargement, which looks much like female breast development, seems to be caused by an increase and, perhaps, a slight imbalance in the amount of hormones during early puberty. Less common types of this condition are found in boys with undescended testicles (who have, as a result, too few hormones in the bloodstream), and in boys with certain birth defects. It has also been linked with prolonged and heavy use of amphetamines (uppers). In its most common form, gynecomastia tends to subside as the teen boy progresses in his physical development, usually running its course within sixteen months. Several studies have found that several drugs—including Danazol—can be somewhat effective in reducing the size of a boy's breasts when symptoms of gynecomastia persist beyond sixteen months. However, more research needs to be done about the effectiveness and possible side effects of such drug therapy.

Prostatitis

I've been having a problem with pain when I piss. And I seem to be going to the bathroom a lot more than usual. I know it isn't any sexual disease because I'm not having sex. I'm more into weight lifting and sports in general. What should I do?

Brad C.

Brad's complaint sounds very much like prostatitis, and the cause may be his weight lifting. The symptoms? Frequent urination, often with pain. Since several sexually transmitted diseases have similar symptoms, it's always a good idea to see a physician for a correct diagnosis. Besides, prostatitis doesn't just go away. It requires treatment with antibiotics for several weeks—and swearing off weight lifting during the period of recovery.

Pink Pearly Papules

Can you have a disease without having sex? I'm 16 and haven't ever had sex but I just noticed these bumps in a circle around the head of my dick and I'm nervous that something serious may be wrong. This isn't something I can ask my mom about. What's going on?

Jared P.

What Jared is describing is called *pink pearly papules*. These benign lesions of the penile *corona* (the raised area of skin that separates the tip of the penis from the shaft of the penis) are not at all related to sexual activity and are not a disease of any kind. They usually grow in one to five rows along the corona of the penis and are pearly white in color. Uncircumcised males are somewhat more likely to have pearly papules; the highest incidence seems to be during major pubertal changes. About 15 percent of all adolescent males have these papules. They're completely harmless and no treatment is indicated.

However, especially if you are sexually active, it's important to see a doctor to confirm the fact that these are, indeed, pearly papules, since some sexually transmitted diseases show up as growths or lesions on the penis. Although all of these look quite different from the harmless papules, it may take a physician's practiced eye to tell the difference for sure.

Undescended Testicle(s)

Is it true if you have an undescended testicle, you can get cancer? That's all I want to know: Is it true?

Brandon H.

It's true that an undescended testicle is 10 to 40 percent more likely to become cancerous than a properly placed one. And testicular cancer does happen in young men.

What is an undescended testicle and how do you know if you have one? When a baby boy is developing in the womb, both of his testicles are in the abdomen. These usually descend into the scrotum before birth. However, in some cases, a boy may be born with one or both testicles undescended.

In many cases, this condition is detected right away and, if the testicle doesn't descend on its own between birth and puberty, medical intervention will be used to make sure it does get into the scrotum where it belongs. Only 1 boy in 500 will have a testicle still undescended by the time he starts puberty.

You can't always tell, simply by looking, whether your testicle is undescended. Some boys have testicles that move up into the groin area and then back to the scrotum from time to time. This is called a *floating testicle*. If you have this condition—or if you think or know that you have an undescended testicle—please see your doctor.

Some require surgery to correct this condition. Even if surgery means removing one testicle, that isn't going to interfere with your normal functioning as a male. You'll still be able to have sex and have children as easily as anyone else. You can manage just fine with one testicle. You don't even have to look different. Your doctor can put something called a *sialastic implant*, a special material made the size of a testicle, into your scrotum to make it look as if you have two testicles.

Testicular Cancer

I first heard about testicular cancer when the Olympic ice skating champion Scott Hamilton got it. I was sorry because I think he's pretty cool. But I didn't worry about it that much because he's as old as my dad. I heard from a friend recently that people my age (16) can get it, too, and that scared me. Is that true? How can I keep from getting it?

Scared in Spokane

According to the American Cancer Society, testicular cancer is one of the most common cancers in men between ages 15 and 35. It occurs in about 6,300 men each year, with 350 deaths. With early detection, however, the survival rate for the most common form of the disease is almost 100 percent; for all types of testicular cancer, there is a 78 to 85 percent five-year survival rate. Those with the best chance for survival are those whose cancer is discovered very early.

It's important, once you're well into puberty—generally between ages 13 and 15—to make a habit of examining your testicles about once a month. This is an important safeguard for your health and will take only about three minutes once you get used to doing it. It's best to do this self-exam after a warm bath or shower, when the scrotum is relaxed.

Testicular Self-Examination

How do you do the testicular self-exam? First, hold your scrotum in the palm of your hand, feeling one testicle at a time. Gently roll the testicle between the thumbs and fingers of both hands for several minutes. Then check the epididymis. This cord is behind your testicles. It will be a bit tender to the touch. That's normal. Next, check the vas deferens, which is above the epididymis and feels like a smooth, firm tube. Examine these cords on both sides.

It's important to get to know the feel and shape of your testicles. If you notice any nodules, lumps, swelling, or a severe, knifelike pain in the groin or testicles, see your doctor immediately! And, when you have regular physical exams, ask your doctor to examine your testicles as well. (This may be embarrassing the first time, but it's an important part of your exam, so be sure to speak up if your doctor doesn't include it in the exam process.)

Benign Scrotal Masses

I felt my balls when I was showering last night and felt something different like a bag of worms or something on the left side. Does this mean I have cancer or something horrible? Please answer me fast!

Todd L.

There are several benign conditions that can feel scary when you first notice them. One is *varicocele*, which is what Todd is describing. It is due to the dilation of veins in the scrotum and usually occurs on the left side. Surgery is done only in extreme cases where there is a major enlargement of the scrotum accompanied by pain. About 10 to 15 percent of adolescents experience this condition. Other conditions such as *spermatocele* (a benign cyst at the head of the epididymis with no treatment indicated), *hydrocele* (a fluid collection in the spermatic cord, with surgery indicated if hydrocele persists in adolescence), and *hernia* (a protrusion of intestine into the scrotum, resolved with surgery) are quite rare, each with less than 1 percent incidence in adolescents. If you notice any of these conditions, it's important to see your doctor for a correct diagnosis.

Foreskin Problems

I'm not circumcised and that's never been a problem for me until recently, when it has become harder to pull my foreskin back all the way when I wash. What can I do?

Clive K.

Clive—and anyone else who is suddenly having trouble pulling his foreskin back—should check with his doctor. It's possible that a physician could correct this by loosening the foreskin. This condition often develops because of poor hygiene. The foreskin needs to be pulled back daily to wash the head of the penis. This is an important preventive measure.

If you find that your penis is swollen and painful *and* you're unable to pull back your foreskin, seek medical help immediately. This condition, known as *paraphimosis*, and another condition called *phimosis*, where the foreskin adheres to the head of the penis and can't be pulled back at all, are best corrected by circumcision. Although circumcision in the adolescent or adult male may be more involved than it is for an infant, it is still a safe and minor surgical procedure.

Pain in the Groin

What does it mean when you have pain in your groin? I guess what I mean is, how serious is it?

Cameron J.

If you have pain in your groin, see your doctor immediately. The problem could be minor—or it could be major—and only your doctor can tell for sure. The reason we suggest *immediate* action is that severe, knifelike pain in the groin can be a symptom of *testicular torsion*. If this condition is not diagnosed and treated within a few hours of the onset of symptoms, the affected testicle will die, eventually shriveling to the size of a marble and becoming useless. In rare, but tragic cases, this has happened to some boys and men, at different times, in both testicles and was not treated in time for either testicle to be saved.

How does testicular torsion happen? The testicles, by necessity, are quite mobile, moving closer to or away from the body in response to heat or cold in order to maintain a constant temperature for the developing sperm. In some instances, however, a testicle may twist around its blood supply cord, trapping blood in the testicle and causing it to swell suddenly and massively as well as causing pain in the groin. A boy or a man may also experience nausea and vomiting.

This twisting may take place during strenuous activity or even during sleep. If this happens, don't just turn over and try to get back to sleep while waiting for the pain to pass. (The pain may pass, but only as the testicle dies—which can happen very quickly, within four to eight hours.)

Surgery for testicular torsion is quite simple. The testicle is untwisted and then fixed into place with a few stitches so that it will no longer be susceptible to torsion. If this surgery has been prompt enough to avoid any tissue damage to the testicle, fertility is generally not diminished. If the testicle has died, the surgeon may remove it and, at the same time, surgically anchor the surviving testicle so it will not be vulnerable to the same twisting.

Pain in the groin doesn't always signal testicular torsion. There are other common causes as well. One of these is *hernia*, which occurs when abdominal contents bulge through a spot in the abdominal wall. This can signal that the blood supply to that area has been reduced, which could be serious. Seek medical help immediately. Surgery is the usual method of treatment.

Swollen glands could be another cause of groin pain. Lymph glands in the groin region may become infected and swell painfully. Treatment with antibiotics will usually alleviate this problem.

Another cause for pain in the groin, which does *not* require medical attention, will happen when you have experienced sexual arousal and a prolonged erection without the release of semen—a condition commonly called "blue balls." This is caused by prolonged engorgement of blood in the penis and pubic area. It will go away without intervention—medical, your partner's, or your own—and with no harm done.

Ejaculation Problems

What if you get sexually excited, get an erection and everything, but then can't come? This has happened to me several times—once when I was masturbating and once when I was messing around with my girlfriend. Is this a sign that something serious is wrong with me?

Ryan K.

Inability to ejaculate during shared sex or masturbation is not unusual. It happens for a variety of reasons. Perhaps you were just not turned on enough to ejaculate. Maybe the setting or the other person wasn't right. Maybe you were feeling too self-conscious or guilty or pressured to perform. Inability to ejaculate can also be caused by the use of some commonly abused drugs (see Chapter 8).

Whatever the causes in your particular case, you may be reassured after discussing the matter with your physician. Chances are, especially if this happens only occasionally, you simply need to pay attention to what feels right for you and what doesn't in terms of partners, activities, location, and timing.

> The last two days, I've had pain in my penis and something that looks like milk comes out. I'm scared. I know it can't be anything sexually related because I haven't had sex, but what could it be?
>
> Marty S.

Marty's problem is seen frequently in adolescent males. His penis pain and milky discharge is probably caused by *retrograde ejaculation*, which occurs when an ejaculation (release of semen) is incomplete or prevented from happening. This may happen when a guy is masturbating, but reluctant, for any number of reasons, to ejaculate. So, as he feels ejaculation about to occur, he places a thumb over the head of his penis to prevent the ejaculate from escaping. Or he may be ready to ejaculate while kissing or petting with a partner, but the semen is held back by tight pants or, again, by a thumb over the opening of the penis.

In any case, the ejaculate may go backward into the prostate gland, causing engorgement and, at times, *prostatitis*, or infection of the prostate. In this condition, the symptoms may include pain felt at the base of the penis or in the testicles and a small amount of clear or milky discharge from the penis. (It should be noted, however, that prostatitis is not invariably linked to retrograde ejaculation or the sex practices just described.)

What can you do about retrograde ejaculation? Consult your physician. It may feel embarrassing, but doctors see this a lot and are likely to be very understanding and able to treat the condition. The best way to keep this problem from happening is to stop the practice of inhibiting ejaculation. However, if, unlike Marty, you are sexually active, a discharge from your penis may be a sign of a sexually transmitted disease; you need to be tested for that possibility as well.

> This is embarrassing, but I'm worried enough to tell you about it. See, last week I noticed blood in my come. (I noticed it while jerking off. I don't have real sex yet.) For the next two nights, blood was still in my semen. Now it has stopped, but I'm still worried. What's wrong with me?
>
> Dale C.

The condition that Dale describes, called *hematospermia*, is not uncommon in teenage boys. What happens is this: A very small blood vessel ruptures along the route which the semen travels—usually in the prostate gland or in the seminal vesicles. A tiny amount of blood is then mixed with the semen and may be evident for one or several ejaculations, which is why Dale noticed this for three nights and not again. The tiny break heals itself. This is quite common and not a sign of a serious problem.

> What causes "wet dreams"? I've had a few and it's fairly embarrassing.
>
> J. P.

"Wet dreams" (also called *nocturnal emissions*) are normal and involuntary (that is, you have no conscious control over them). These wet dreams are the release of semen during sleep and are most likely to happen in guys who don't masturbate much or have sex. These are not a sign that anything is wrong. It's just nature's way of releasing stored semen, which a man produces constantly.

■   ■   ■

GROWING FROM BOY TO MAN

While much has been said and written lately about the difficulty of growing up female, growing up male isn't exactly easy either. There are inevitable pressures from parents, peers, and society to look, act, or be a certain way. There can be a lot of self-inflicted pressure, too. Many guys have unusually high expectations of themselves and suffer when they fall short in some area or another. We'll be addressing self-esteem and other emotional issues in the next chapter, but just want to emphasize here that becoming a man is a journey unique, in many ways, to each individual.

Many men are take-charge, aggressive, strong, and tough; many equally masculine men are more low-key, gentle, and content to follow. Ideally, a man will have access to his full range of skills and feelings: expressing quiet, tender feelings as well as being decisive and assertive when necessary.

It's important to know, too, that healthy, masculine bodies come in all shapes and sizes. Taking good care of yourself—getting enough rest, good nutrition, and sufficient exercise; avoiding harmful habits such as smoking and drug use; doing monthly testicular self-exams; and seeing your physician for regular checkups—can help you get and stay in top form physically. You don't have to be a jock to be a real man. You don't have to be a leader or a sexual superman or dress or talk a certain way to be a real man. You are a real man just as you are: confident sometimes, scared sometimes; as likely to be shy and gentle as tough and assertive; straight or gay, athletic or not, tall or short. Being a real man comes down to just being you.

A MAN'S BODY

✔ Normal changes of puberty may begin as early as age 8 or as late as age 15 and finish between ages 14 and 18. Some very normal 13- or 14-year-old guys look like adult men, while their equally normal classmates still look like boys. The timing of puberty is unique and may be determined genetically.

✔ Monthly testicular self-exams are an important safeguard for your health, since testicular cancer is one of the most common cancers in young men between ages 15 and 35. When should you start these exams? When you're well into puberty—usually between ages 13 and 15.

✔ If you experience pain in your groin, see your doctor immediately! It could be something relatively minor (such as a sports injury) or it could be major (such as testicular torsion), where timely treatment is essential. Only your doctor can tell for sure whether your problem is major or minor. Don't take a chance on guessing wrong; call your physician!

✔ Masculine bodies come in all shapes and sizes. Keep in top form by developing healthy habits—getting plenty of rest, eating good food, getting exercise, avoiding harmful habits, and getting regular medical checkups.

CHAPTER FOUR

Feelings

I think something is the matter with me. I cry at the least little thing and feel down a lot, but I also enjoy lots of stuff, too, especially with my friends. Sometimes I hate my parents and think how I can't wait to be 18 and go away to college or get a place of my own and sometimes I love them so much I cry at the thought of ever leaving them. Do people go through this at my age (14) or is something wrong with me?

Taylor B.

Taylor's experience may sound quite familiar to you. Adolescence is, without a doubt, a time of feeling strongly and deeply the whole range of emotions. You may feel alternately bored and excited, depressed and elated, yearning for independence yet needing your parents. You may feel, as Taylor does, up and down a lot. Part of this may be due to the fact that you're going through a lot of changes: body changes, school changes (adjusting to junior high or high school or getting ready for college), changes in your family as you become more independent, and changes in your social life.

Some moodiness, too, can have physical causes. Scientists have discovered that some teen behavior can be linked to hormone levels. While we don't yet have definitive proof that hormones actually cause moodiness, it is quite possible that they play a role in up-and-down feelings, especially in the early teens when you are going through such dramatic physical changes.

Other strong feelings come from experiencing important changes and milestones for the first time. These aren't all Kodak or Hallmark moments like graduation or important birthdays. These are, in many instances, changes within and new realizations. For example, you're beginning to realize that your parents aren't perfect and that they don't have all the answers. (If you're tempted to say "Duh," just remember back to the time you thought they were perfect and all-knowing. There *was* such a time if you think about it!) You're starting to need and appreciate your friends more than ever and feel a need to be accepted by your peers. And you may well be having your first intense experiences with falling in love, which is certainly life-changing whether the love relationship lasts for a short time or a lifetime.

During this time of changing feelings and new experiences, you may find yourself loving and hating intensely, crying a lot, and feeling new fears about all kinds of things, including the fact that you're growing up. It's not at all unusual, in the midst of celebrating your growing competence and independence, to grieve a little for the past when life seemed so much simpler. As we grow, we experience losses: the loss of childhood innocence and sense of security and even the loss of a dream once we achieve it. In growing, of course, we gain a lot to replace these losses: the satisfaction of independence, the discovery of building new relationships with our parents and families, and the joy of reaching a goal and then finding new dreams to replace the ones we've realized—or decided to let go.

Keep in mind that growing up doesn't mean leaving the child part of yourself behind entirely. Each one of us, no matter how old we are, retains a part of the feelings and experiences of the child we once were. The child part of you can bring an openness, warmth, and special joy as you grow into a practical, responsible, mature adult. And you can keep the loving feelings you've had from and for your parents and others with you all your life. You can keep this love in warm memories and in the ways you pass it on to others.

FEELINGS ABOUT YOURSELF

I want to be the best I can be, but I'm not sure exactly who I am and I hate certain things about myself like my fat thighs and my bad temper. How can I be my best when I don't always like myself?

Hannah P.

Knowing what you value about yourself and what you'd like to change is all part of your vital journey of self-discovery. While you may share certain physical or emotional traits with a family member or two, no one on earth has exactly the same collection of traits that you do. Even if you're an identical twin, there will be personality and some life experience differences. What you do with your genetic legacy, how you develop or don't develop your special talents, how you choose to be, what values you take from your family and friends and which ones you reject all add up to a thoroughly unique you. The combination is, ultimately, largely your choice.

How do you begin to develop a sense of who you are?

- *Act—don't just react.* Make active choices on how you will behave. Reacting behavior can include rebellion or taking a different stance from your family just to be different from them. Becoming your own person means developing your own point of view without worrying whether it agrees or disagrees with the views of your parents. When you have a strong sense of self, you can even agree with your parents in many areas without feeling your independence or separateness threatened.

- *Make observations about yourself.* Stand back and look at what you choose to do and say, the routines of your life. Ask yourself questions such as:

  ✔ What would I like to see happen in my life? (And what can I do to make this happen?)
  ✔ When was the last time I really felt excited about something? What excites me or might excite me about my life?
  ✔ What flashes through my mind just before I go to sleep at night?
  ✔ When I'm free to choose, how do I spend my time? (If you spend most of your time in passive pursuits, like watching TV, you may not be too thrilled with life as it is right now. You can become more active toward change.)

- *Take inventory of your strengths and limitations, but don't let the latter get you down.* As you grow, you gain new insight not only into what you can do, but also into what your limitations are. Becoming aware of your limitations, possibly for the first time, can be a real shock. While you probably tend to be quite tolerant of faults you see in your friends, you may be your own worst critic. While it's important to be aware of your limitations as well as your strengths so that you can choose positive directions in your life, it's equally important not to overemphasize either. For example, you may be proud of your acting or singing talents, but fail to realize that hard work, ambition, and assertiveness are at least as important in building a career in show business. You can't just rely on your wonderful talent and sit passively waiting to be discovered. In the same way, if you dream of being a television news reporter but are so shy you can hardly speak up in class, you have a choice. You might decide that you want to pursue a career that is better suited to your personality as it is today—or you may decide to work to overcome your shyness (it *can* be done!) on the way to realizing your long-term dream. Some limitations can be overcome. Some can't. If you're tone-deaf and can't carry a tune, you're unlikely to become a famous singer no matter what your fantasies. But that limitation doesn't make your life worthless and doomed to a boring, meaningless existence. You have a lot of strengths and talents you may not have discovered yet, possibly because you got mired in one of the **Seven Self-Hate Traps**. Have you found yourself doing any of the following:

1. *Putting yourself down for making mistakes.* A mistake is a learning experience, not a tragic flaw. When you make a mistake, quit calling yourself stupid and start asking what you can learn from this experience.
2. *Letting feelings of inadequacy get between you and others.* If you're too afraid of rejection to risk saying hello and otherwise reaching out to others, life is going to be pretty lonely. If your own perceptions of your imperfections are holding you back from letting others know you, remember that it is the human part of you, the imperfect part, that others may find most likable. Think about it. We often love our friends most for their very human qualities, yet put ourselves down for being just as human. It

isn't fair. Give yourself a break. And don't deprive others of the pleasure of knowing you as you really are.

3. *Assuming that others are as aware of and as critical of your flaws as you are.* First, most people are so focused on their own concerns that they're not going to spend a lot of time thinking about what's right or wrong with you. Most people do tend to be fairly indifferent to each other until they get to know one another. If you feel others dislike or ignore you, you may be acting in a way that increases your invisibility or nondesirability. And you can start changing this right now. Make eye contact. Greet people warmly. Show an interest in what they're doing or feeling. You may find people's reactions to you changing.

   If you're self-conscious about a physical flaw and are sure others hate you because you're overweight or have acne or bad hair or because you're different in some way, keep in mind that in the real world people love other people for a wide variety of qualities. Being active, friendly, and kind; having a sense of humor; moving with confidence and grace (whatever your weight); and feeling at ease with yourself as you are can go a long way toward developing a positive self-image. Your self-acceptance can make you very attractive to others.

4. *Assuming that if you're not the best, you're nothing.* This mindset can stem from our cultural "Winning is everything!" philosophy. But it's wrong. You don't have to be No. 1 at everything (or anything!) to enjoy life. You can enjoy activities and hobbies or even professional pursuits without having to be the best at what you do. You don't have to be a great writer to keep a comforting and insightful journal. You don't have to be a great musician to love and enjoy music. You don't have to make the swimming team to enjoy swimming. Focus on

what brings joy into your life—and do it, whether you're good at it or not.

5. *Being prejudiced.* Studies show that people who tend to be prejudiced against certain racial or ethnic groups or certain religious or socioeconomic groups are likely to have low self-esteem and attempt to put others down to build themselves up. It can't be done. You can't build self-esteem on the basis of hate, intolerance, and scorn. This ugliness within will always prevent you from feeling good about yourself. Positive self-image grows from compassion, tolerance, and love; from being open and emotionally embracing; and from learning from others who are different from you.

6. *Calling yourself hurtful names.* Do you call yourself "dumb" or "stupid" or "nerd" or "fat and ugly" or even worse? Stop tormenting yourself when you make a mistake or discover a limitation. Stopping the hurtful labels can stop the painful feelings that go along with them. Treat yourself as gently as you would a good friend in the same situation.

7. *Being a perfectionist.* If you constantly expect perfection, you're in for a rough time. It's fine to have goals and dreams, but equally important to realize that you are a valuable person even though you're not perfect all the time. We all make mistakes. We all have moments when we say things we regret later. Being imperfect is a normal part of life. You don't need perfection, prizes, or great achievements to justify your existence. You need to embrace not only your wisdom and talents, but also the less perfect parts of yourself. All combine to make you the unique person you are. That doesn't mean that you'll seek to repeat mistakes or go around, as a matter of course, making comments that hurt people. You can choose to change certain aspects of your behavior. We're all constantly evolving and growing. But the most important

part of that growth is self-love and self-acceptance right here and now.

FEELINGS ABOUT YOUR PARENTS

I have a 15-year-old son and during an argument over curfew the other day, he said, "I hate you, Mom!" Five minutes later, he came back with tears in his eyes and said he didn't mean it. I tried to tell him that it's OK to feel hate at times for people you love. I'm not sure he really believed me. I do know that I have suffered greatly because no one ever told me when I was young that I could dislike or even hate my mother at times and so these furies were buried, only to engulf me in later life. I think this whole love-hate thing is important for kids to know about and to feel OK about.

A Loving Mom

While polls show that today's teens love and respect their parents more openly than other recent generations of teens, there still may be times when you have decidedly mixed feelings about your parents. You may love *and* hate them; yearn for independence yet need your parents very much. You may be struggling to find your own values while feeling influenced by theirs. You may come to the conclusion that growing up means rejecting the values of your parents as a way of declaring your independence and separateness.

Rebellion isn't inevitable, though conflict is likely at times as you and your parents—equally perplexed by the changes you're experiencing—adjust to your growing independence. Realizing that mixed feelings are normal can help. Respecting each other in the midst of all this can help, too. For example, you can respect and hear your parents' values without necessarily agreeing with them. And just because your parents may not see things your way doesn't mean they're being unfair. It may just mean that you're different people with differing points of view. To be truly separate and independent is to accept and recognize that each person is different.

If you realize this, you can be your own person, even in your parents' house, living by many of your parents' rules. It all depends, once again, on developing your own point of view, something that is not dependent one way or another on how your parents view things. When you have this sense of separateness, you may even feel free to agree with them at times, to make your own some of the values that they hold. That doesn't make you a dependent child. It makes you a growing young adult who has exercised his or her own choice. Just because a value or a choice happens to coincide with someone else's doesn't mean that it's not your own.

When you feel free to choose your own values—whether they coincide with those of your parents or not—you will be free to express more positive feelings around your family, whether you agree with them in all things or not. The stronger your sense of self, the more love you may feel for your parents. This often happens in the late teens and early twenties, when, after a few stormy years, you begin to see each other as *people*.

Good communication is based on seeing each other as people. Ideally, your parents will listen to you and care about your feelings. By listening to and caring about the two *people* behind the parental roles, you can help to increase understanding and acceptance of each other, even when you disagree. You can have very different viewpoints and live very different lives—and still love each other very much.

FEELINGS ABOUT YOUR CHANGING FAMILY

Why do parents think teenagers don't care about them divorcing? I'm hurting a lot about my parents' recent divorce even though I'm 14 and have friends and all. Something that makes it hard is that Dad has a girlfriend he expects me to like and accept—like instantly. Mom just started dating a guy who has a six-year-old son who is a brat and who came along with us to Six Flags last weekend and spoiled everything! How can I convince my parents to get back together again? Things weren't nearly as bad before (even though they did fight pretty much) as they are now.

Briana C.

It's very common, when parents are divorced or divorcing, to wish you could turn back time and live life as it used to be, because life with divorced parents and the new people they bring into your life is so complicated. Relationships, just like time, can't be turned back to replicate the past. (Even when divorced partners reunite, the relationship inevitably changes in some ways.) For most families this means adjusting to a lot of changes: being single parent–headed families or blended families with a sometimes awkward combination of stepparents, stepsiblings, and half-siblings.

You may find yourself torn between two warring parents you love very much—at a time when you need their united support as well as the security to begin to move toward independence in your own way and your own time. Maybe you suddenly have too much responsibility thrust upon you—as parents or stepparents assume you can handle more responsibility for caring for yourself or your siblings or stepsiblings than you feel you can manage. Maybe you're feeling that your family is changing so much, that it's so weird, so strange and complicated that love and unity aren't possible.

Maybe you're feeling incredible grief about the breakup of your everyday family—and upset that your parents don't seem as upset about it. It's important to know that many—though certainly not all—divorcing couples go through a lot of the grief process while making the decision to break up. For some, too, that final decision is a relief and a new beginning. For you, however, it can be a shock. You may be doing your grieving mostly after the fact. Grieving what you have lost is an important part of healing and going on with your life. People do this in a number of ways, some more obviously than others. But the process of grieving and letting go of what was is an important process.

Keep in mind that loving, though hurting, families can grow from all kinds of situations. It takes time and effort on everyone's part. It can help to talk with your parents about your feelings and what is comfortable for you and what isn't.

If, for example, a noncustodial parent expects you to spend every weekend with him or her and feels rejected if you don't, explain that you need time to spend with your friends and to have a social life, too, and that this doesn't mean that you don't want to be with him or her. Discuss possible compromises. Maybe your friends can join you and your parent for some activities. Maybe you can spend part of the weekend or every other weekend with your parent and then get together on a week-night for a dinner or special activity you both enjoy.

If a parent never spends any time with you alone (minus a girlfriend or boyfriend), let him or her know that you would treasure some time for just the two of you. (Keep it positive like this instead of sulking and complaining, "Why does *she* always have to come along?") Some parents assume you're at an age when time alone to talk doesn't matter as much to you—when, in fact, it can matter *more*. Some parents, too, get so caught up in a new relationship, eager to have you know and accept the new person, that they lose sight of the fact that you still need them to yourself sometimes. In these cases, it's up to you to tell them how you're feeling.

Accepting a new person in your parent or parents' life can be a complicated process: You may feel grief for your parents' lost relationship, guilt over liking this new person (even a little), jealousy over the place this person may have in your parent's life, and anger over issues that may exist between this new person and you—like the new stepfather who moves right in and starts giving commands or a stepmother who feels hurt if you don't call her "Mom." Talk with your parent or parents about the fact that you're trying to keep an open mind and open heart, but need time to adjust to all the changes. Ask for the time to accept this person in your own way and to develop your own relationship with him or her.

If you're in the midst of a blending family and it feels uncomfortable, it may help to know that this,

too, is not at all unusual and that it may take time—even a few years—before you all start to feel like a family. In the meantime, you may feel besieged by new responsibilities and expectations.

If you feel you're being overburdened with responsibility or that your needs are being ignored for everyone else's convenience, let your parent know how you're feeling without making angry accusations and see if you can work toward a compromise. For example, if you're expected to care for younger siblings or stepsiblings every afternoon and weekend nights, negotiate some free time for your own pursuits—maybe one or two afternoons off and certainly one weekend night free. If your parents have joint custody and you feel like you're spending your life living out of paper bags and commuting from one home to the other, work out an arrangement that would work better for you and present it to your parents. For example, if you spend part of each week with each parent, maybe you could arrange to spend alternate months with each. That might feel a little more settled for you.

Compromise and good communication can help you deal with a changing family. No matter what your family's lifestyle—whether your parents are single or remarried—you can feel part of a real and vital family, while growing toward independence, if you give love and unity the chance and the time to grow. Some families, it's true, are closer than others, but you can build shared respect, cooperation, peace, and some happy memories by keeping your mind and your heart open.

LOVE

My boyfriend Sean says he loves me a lot and I believe it, because he takes an interest in everything I do and even tells me what I should wear and is so jealous, he gets mad whenever I even talk to a guy at school. My friends say he's a jerk, but I think he really loves me. How can I convince them that this love is real so they'll be happy for me instead of criticizing Sean like they do?

Mandy Y.

It's impossible to set an age limit on ability to love. We love in different ways, according to the person and the situation, all of our lives. Valid and deep feelings have no age limits. However, the character of love may change, depending not so much on your chronological age as on your emotional maturity and feelings about yourself.

It really upsets me when my parents act like I don't know what I'm talking about when I say I love my boyfriend. They say I'm too immature to know what love is. I don't think that's fair. I'm almost 16 and am mature in a lot of ways. I think real love can happen at all ages. Am I right?

Lindsay B.

In the case of Mandy's boyfriend, Sean, love may be limited by his own insecurities and need to control her. In fact, Mandy's friends may see some trouble signs that she doesn't: A person who wants to control you in terms of limiting your access to friends and others, picking out your clothes, and generally ruling your life isn't doing this out of love but out of a need to control. These can be early signs of an abusive relationship that could escalate emotionally and even physically.

Some older people—often unfairly—label all young love as "infatuation." That isn't so. Some emotionally mature young people are quite capable of mature love and some older people are chronically infatuated. What's the difference between love and infatuation and between mature and immature love?

Infatuation means being "in love with love," when being in love is more important than loving and giving to someone. This happens in people of all ages who are emotionally immature. If love takes over your life and makes you unable to function in other areas because you're constantly fantasizing about the other person, you may be infatuated. If you feel a need to cling, if you feel a lot of insecurity in the relationship, if you're more concerned with getting than giving, you're likely to be infatuated. Immature people of all ages fall in

love with idealized images rather than people and when the real person doesn't live up to this vision, disillusionment quickly sets in.

How is mature love different?

- *Mature love is accepting.* You are aware of each other as independent people. You allow one another space to be yourselves and don't feel compelled to transform one another. You accept each other as you are and forgive what you are not, instead of criticizing and blaming each other.

- *Mature love is energizing.* It means that you have more energy to give in all aspects of your life: your studies, your friendships, your family relationships, and your special interests as well as your love relationship. All are enhanced by your good feelings, rather than ceasing to be important, overshadowed by your love.

- *Mature love can survive joy and pain.* You're strong enough and trust each other enough to be vulnerable, to cry as well as laugh together. You can risk being honest with each other and find the resources—together—to weather hard times, knowing that the true test of love is not just how you're there for each other in the good times, but how you make it through sad, lonely, or difficult times in your relationship.

- *Mature love means that there is more to your relationship than physical attraction. You are, first and always, best friends.* You can get just as excited talking and sharing feelings as you can about sex. You treat each other as dear friends, not letting old expectations about what it means to be in love come between you.

- *Mature love is enhanced by time.* You know that, as you grow as individuals and as a couple, your relationship will only get better, so who needs to rush anything? Real love takes time and growth. It's worth working and waiting for.

- *Mature love means neither instant fulfillment nor diminishment of who you are.* You have a solid sense of yourself as a distinct individual. You feel that your partner is wonderful, but realize that you're special, too. You have the security of knowing that if, for some reason, your love for each other would die, *you* could survive.

The shock and sorrow of losing a love is familiar to all of us. What do you do when the worst happens?

Perhaps the healthiest response is to go with your pain and grief and work it through. Let it happen. Rage. Scream. Cry. Write in your journal. Let all the pain and anger out in nondestructive ways. Destructive ways of coping such as anesthetizing yourself with drugs, alcohol, frantic activities, an instant involvement with someone else, overeating, or ceasing to function in other areas of your life will only make you feel worse. It's important to feel the pain in order to grow past your grief. Forgiveness, which will be possible in time, is also an important part of healing. Forgiving the person you lost frees you to love again.

The freedom that comes with forgiveness can let joy into your life again, not only in terms of being ready to take the risk of loving again, but also finding yourself again and realizing how you have grown as the result of loving and losing a love. Then you can celebrate what was good in the relationship and let go, little by little, of the pain.

Sad and wistful moments may come—even over a period of years—when you hear a certain song on the radio or smell a hint of that special perfume she wore or aftershave he used or when you see a spectacular sight your lost love would have enjoyed. But, if you have grown with your grief, your sadness will be mixed with joy—joy not only because you survived the loss of a special love, but also joy in the fact that you were able to love then and will, someday, love again.

■ ■ ■

ANGER

I get really mad at some things people at school say or do and I've been in trouble for fighting. It's scary to fight at my school because, even though we're in a fairly nice area, there are gangs and you never know if someone has a knife or gun or if their friends will get you later on. What can I do when people are acting like shitheads so they'll leave me alone and not get myself in trouble?

Kyle H.

Of all the emotions, anger is the one most often denied, unexpressed, or harmfully expressed. Unexpressed anger can seep out in strange ways. You might fly into a rage at someone over some minor annoyance or take your anger out on an innocent person. You might turn on yourself with destructive habits such as driving recklessly or taking chances you shouldn't or eating or drinking too much. You may get depressed. Many mental health experts believe that depression is often anger turned inward. Unexpressed anger may turn on you in physical ways—with stomachaches or headaches.

Can it harm you to pretend you're not angry when you really are? My mom insists that I be nice to everyone all the time and she always acts like everything is just great even when it's not. The only way I can tell that she's upset is that she gets quiet. But she'll never admit to being mad. Sometimes I yell when I'm angry and then feel awful for doing it. But I can't help it! How can I handle anger better without being like my mom?

Madison M.

Expressing anger can have its risks, too, in this age of increasing violence in schools. Fights can escalate to life-threatening encounters. Gangs are a presence nationwide, in rural and suburban schools as well as inner-city schools. It isn't safe these days to tell someone off or get into a fight at school no matter how intensely angry you are.

So how can you deal with anger in a way that will help deal with these feelings without making the situation worse?

- *Report how you feel rather than attacking the person who makes you angry.* This can defuse dangerous situations—whether it's a peer ragging on you or a parent with an opinion that differs considerably from yours. It's better to say, "I feel angry about what you just said," instead of, "You're a jerk!" or "You always say that! You don't understand me at all!"

- *When you can't express your feelings directly, look for constructive ways to deal with anger.* If, to protect yourself at school, you've needed to ignore taunts that sting or if a parent has said, "I said no and I don't want to hear anything more about it," expressing your anger directly isn't possible. So what can you do? You can ventilate anger safely in another way. Some suggestions:

✔ Get physical! Exercise can be a great anger release. Play tennis or any sport with hitting. Or run until you're exhausted.

✔ Take a long walk to let off steam and to notice beautiful and/or interesting things along the way.

✔ Pound your bed pillows and scream into them to discharge some of that angry energy.

✔ Write a letter expressing exactly how you feel. Then tear it up.

✔ Try some hard physical work—such as scrubbing a bathroom or a floor, gardening, or mowing the lawn. You'll get rid of angry tension and accomplish something else useful, too!

✔ Cry. Crying can be very therapeutic for men as well as women.

✔ Talk about your feelings with someone who will listen and help you work your feelings through (without telling the world).

These are just suggestions. You may find your own best ways to deal with anger. Just remember: Don't let it simmer. Unexpressed anger can cause painful depression and physical symptoms. It can also block out happy feelings. Working through your anger will help to clear the air for joy.

SHYNESS

I miss out on a lot because I'm so shy. How can I be more normal when meeting people so I can have friends and fun like everyone else?

Scott J.

People describe themselves as shy for a variety of reasons. Some are socially isolated and have trouble talking with anyone they don't know well. Others are shy with the opposite sex only. Some are fine in social situations but get weak in the knees at the thought of speaking in public.

Why are you shy? Some researchers are exploring the possibility that a tendency toward shyness can be inherited, just like blue eyes or red hair. Some experts feel that shyness can also have its roots in childhood experiences. Maybe your parents expected a lot of you. If you have been held to impossibly high standards by your parents, your extended family, or even just yourself, you may find yourself afraid to try new things or meet new people. You may feel that if you're not the best or the wittiest or the life of the party, you're a social failure. Not true at all, of course. You can reach out in small ways, in your own way, and make an important difference in your life.

How can you begin to conquer shyness?

- *Learn to see risk taking in a different way.* Maybe fear of making a mistake keeps you tongue-tied. All of us make mistakes, say the wrong thing, or face rejection at times. That's just part of life. It can be a valuable learning experience. Viewing possible mistakes as learning opportunities may ease your fears. It may also help to keep in mind that risk taking doesn't have to be major. Start small by reaching out in ways that make you least uncomfortable and build up to the scarier challenges.

- *Take your conversational cues from listening to others.* You don't have to be brilliant or witty to have a good conversation with someone else. Listen and ask questions. Laugh. Comment on what another has said. These are all ways to show signs of life in a conversation or in a relationship. If you can get away from your own fear for a time and get interested in what another has to say, you may surprise yourself.

- *Set a goal and a deadline.* You might say hello to five people this week. Just "Hello." Start small. This will help you get in contact with others and build your confidence little by little.

- *Don't expect the world to change when you take the first step.* It takes time for others to get past indifference to the point of wanting to know you. It takes time for you to get to know and feel comfortable with others. Don't overburden yourself or others with high expectations. You can still be friendly no matter how others respond to you at first. And change will happen gradually. Be patient with yourself and with others—and don't stop trying to reach out just because you don't see instant, dramatic results.

- *Accept yourself as a normal and unique person.* As such, you'll make mistakes at times. At worst, you'll make a mistake and learn from it. At best, you'll learn and feel the joy of connecting with others, so the risks you take by reaching out aren't so terrifying. Knowing this can give you a new sense of power and control in your own life.

■ ■ ■

BOREDOM

I live in this horrible small town where nothing ever happens and life gets really boring. What can I do to stop being so bored with life?

Rick G.

Boredom, which can be closely tied to depression, can come from a variety of causes. Some of these causes are: nonparticipation in life due to lack of confidence or motivation; fear and a sense of hopelessness because goals and dreams seem so far away; the inability to make your own fun and joy in life when your general environment isn't especially stimulating.

What can you do if you're bored all the time?

- *Explore reasons you may be bored right now:* How long has this been going on? When did it start? What is behind it? What feelings are you not expressing? What goals and dreams seem impossibly far away? (Maybe if you're living too much in a fantasy future, the present time can't possibly measure up.)

- *Remember that if you're bored, you're boring!* Psychologist and author Dr. Sol Gordon often tells teens this—and it's true! He goes on to list the five most boring things you can do (and these add to your own boredom and boringness): running yourself down, telling your friends how rotten you are, telling people you're horny, bragging about things everyone knows you haven't really done, and watching TV for more than an hour and a half a day. Avoid boring behavior and you may take an important step away from boredom!

- *While planning the future, don't forget to live now.* Give yourself intermediate goals. Planning for a bright, fascinating future may combat boredom, but making these future fantasies the only source of your excitement may make the here and now even more boring than it has to be. Think of the least boring thing to do—and do it. Do volunteer work. Spend time with someone who is lonely. Get a part-time job. Take a course just for fun at a local college. Read something new and challenging. Keep thinking of things you can do now that will help you find joy and purpose in living right now. Action of any kind can break the cycle of boredom.

- *Be open to new experiences and vow to learn one new thing every day.* Learning something new every day—a word, a fact, a skill—can help you feel in touch with the world and grow in exciting new ways. Be open to new experiences, new people, and differing opinions and ways of seeing the world. Curiosity, joy, and diversity in your life will help you retain the best qualities of youthful exuberance and curiosity as you grow up.

- *Make a list of things you love in life.* Just thinking of things to include can help lift you out of boredom and the blahs. If you can't think of anything right now, think of what you used to enjoy or could still enjoy if you'd let yourself. The more you think about what you love in life, the more you will rediscover the joy and excitement of simply being alive.

FEELINGS AND CYBERSPACE

My parents are bugging me because I spend so much time on the Internet, but they're too dumb about computers to understand how great it is. I especially enjoy chat groups. These have really helped me because I'm gay and just came out to my family but haven't told anyone at school, so chat groups are a safe way to talk about my feelings with guys who are older and more experienced and who can help me in a way my family can't. How can I make my parents understand?

Jon P.

Surfing the Internet can be a fascinating, rewarding, and wonderfully educational experience for people of all ages. As in all good things, however, moderation is in order. If you find that you're hooked on the Net to the exclusion of time with friends and family, time for study, time for other hobbies and interests, and time for healthy exercise, your life may be a bit out of balance.

It's also important to know, too, that while chat groups can be interesting and helpful, you need to exercise caution. There are people who victimize the young and vulnerable or the gullible of all ages via the Net. Be very careful to protect your identity. Don't agree to meet an adult who befriends you in a chat room. The situation may be entirely harmless or potentially risky, and you may have no way of knowing which. In Jon's case, the chat groups may be useful to a point, but when he's ready to talk face to face about his coming out, it could be much more to his advantage to find and join a support group for gay teens or for him and his family to become involved in a group such as PFLAG (see the appendix) than to risk direct contact with any of his chat room buddies.

In summary, the same rules of common sense—moderation in all things and the importance of protecting oneself from con artists and predatory strangers—apply to new technology as much as traditional socializing.

STRESS

I feel so stressed out, I dread getting up in the morning. It's like I'm on this treadmill of school, community service, work, homework, and all the time feeling the pressure to make good grades so I can get into a top college and later get a good job. I don't seem to have time just to be young and enjoy life. My friends feel the same way. What can we do? Doing less isn't really an option right now.

Elizabeth A.

A lot of pressures come with being an adolescent. There may be pressures from your parents to measure up to their expectations of you. There may be pressures from your teachers and from your peers.

The greatest pressures, however, tend to come from within. There are the pressures that come with change, trying to reconcile in your own mind the fact that you seem to both love and hate your parents; that you love, yet compete with your friends; and that while you're trying to be part of the crowd, you're also trying to become your own person and define your own values. You're trying to find out who you are and make important decisions that may influence who you will become. You begin to see, with new clarity, your limitations as well as your possibilities.

Sometimes it may seem as if your life is in a period of suspension. All you seem to do is wait for the things you want. You're hungry for independence, yet may be a bit afraid of it and, in any event, you're still dependent on your parents in many ways. And your parents may have trouble interpreting your drive for independence as a positive part of your growth rather than as a personal rejection. There may be times when demands seem to be coming from all sides: from parents and teachers to do well in school so you can get into a good college; from friends to be there for them; from your family to assume your share of household responsibilities; from employers to perform on the job; and from yourself, most of all, to be the person you want to be.

What can you do when stress is getting to you in a major way?

- *Be aware.* Keep a stress diary, pinpointing when you feel stressed and what precipitated these feelings. Be very specific about the sources of stress in your life. Which of these can be changed? Which can't? Which can you do something about right now?

  Making a mental priority list of things you can do to reduce stress now can help. It's not useful to get stressed out about doing well on your SATs a year from now, but it may be helpful right now to keep up in your classes. Taking your life stresses in moderate doses, focusing on what you can deal with or change right now, can also cut down on feelings of helplessness. Nothing is more nerve-racking than a whole list of worries that you can't do anything about. Concentrate on what you can handle now. You can make a difference. You *do* have control over your life in many ways.

- *Set realistic goals.* Examine your goals and ask yourself two questions:

  1. Is this a possible, attainable goal for me?
  2. Do I *really* want it?

  For example, if you hate science and it has always been your worst subject, medical school may not be a realistic goal for your future. Another example: If you aspire to be popular, keep in mind that it's impossible to be liked by everyone; even if you could, you might find yourself giving up important parts of yourself, aspects of your personality, or personal preferences to fit in with other people's expectations—and that can be very stressful.

  Another part of realistic goal setting is starting small, one challenge at a time. If you always try to take on a bunch of challenges at once, you may be paralyzed with anxiety and frustration. One at a time, however, your problems can be resolved and/or your goals met.

- *Put your stresses in perspective.* It's easy to put stress on yourself by saying things like, "If I don't pass this test, that's IT!" *IT*—your worst-case scenario—may be uncomfortable, inconvenient, embarrassing, or even devastating, but it *isn't* the end of the world or even life as you know it. The world is full of happy and successful people who didn't get into their first-choice colleges—and who subsequently had great experiences at their second- or third-choice schools. Ask yourself, even as you're envisioning the possible scenarios for whatever stressful event is happening, how profoundly this will affect your life next year or ten years from now. This doesn't minimize the impact of stress and pain right now, but knowing that this won't be forever or doom you to a life of unhappiness and failure may take some of the heat off. Whatever happens, you'll get through it and the stressful time will pass.

- *Realize that you and only you can change your life.* Only you can choose to be nervous or to alleviate some of your stress. Taking responsibility for your own nervousness makes it possible for you to do something about it. For example, you can say, "I get nervous when I'm with strangers," instead of, "Strangers make me nervous." You, not they, are in control. And you can work to change this uncomfortable feeling within when you're with people you don't know well.

- *Be good to yourself.* Eat a healthy diet and cut down drastically on or even eliminate junk food and beverages that contain caffeine (such as coffee, tea, and colas). These beverages can make you even more nervous and irritable. Be sure to get enough sleep every night. Take a warm bath or shower just before going to bed and try to go to bed at the same time every day whenever possible.

- *Make time for fun.* Enjoying hobbies, relaxing times, friends, meditation, a long walk, or other exercise (exercise is a *great* stress reducer) can help you manage stress and tension. Laugh heartily and often. Cultivating a sense of humor about your situation helps you put things in perspective. But there is also a physical benefit to laughter. Blood flow to the brain increases when we laugh, and we release hormones called endorphins that help us feel better and reduce the levels of stress hormones in our blood.

- *Take action on your own behalf.* This may mean making a decision—even a small one—instead of staying mired in stressful indecisiveness. It may mean taking a stand and letting people know what you want and how you feel.

Write about your feelings in your journal. Call a friend. Do whatever it takes to help yourself to *actively* face down your stress.

- *Find your stress-busting pleasures and DO them!* Seek out and do whatever relaxes you—listening to or making music, taking a warm bath or shower, or going swimming (some people find water very relaxing). Take a walk and notice the beauty all around you. Close your eyes and travel back in time to a moment when you felt very relaxed. Breathe deeply and let that feeling of deep contentment and relaxation come back to you.

- *Reach out to others.* It's a real temptation when you're feeling stressed out to isolate yourself, but don't do it. Share your feelings with others you trust. This can help you feel less alone and may also help you test reality. If conflict with another is causing you stress, talk to that other person or persons and work things out as much as you can so you don't have to worry about it anymore. If you're feeling stressed out about everything in your life, enlist the aid of a friend, parent, teacher, school counselor, or professional psychotherapist in sorting all of these out and exploring your choices.

No matter how impossible or hopeless a situation seems to be, there *is* hope and there *are* choices. And no matter how alone you feel right now, there are people in your life who care and who want very much to help you. All you need to do is reach out to them.

DEFIANCE AND SELF-DEFEATING BEHAVIOR

I hate my life right now. My dad left my mom for another woman and my mom yells at ME all the time and I never see Dad anymore. I hate both of them and am getting back at them by skipping school and not doing my homework. They always put pressure on me to make good grades so I could go to a top college and my grades have been very good, but now I'm getting C's and D's in most of my classes and may even get an F in algebra (I hate the teacher because he reminds me of my dad). When my mom finds out about this, she will go ballistic, which would be worth it to me, and maybe my dad won't even care. I think I should feel great about getting them back, but I still feel miserable. What can I do?

Steve T.

Defiant, self-defeating behavior usually comes from a lot of stress and anger in your life. You may feel backed into a corner by circumstances and feel like lashing out—even if it hurts you most of all. As Steve is discovering, you may be able to get to a parent or someone else who cares about you by doing things that are harmful mostly to yourself. The person may recognize this behavior as a cry for help and positive attention—or he or she may not, acting in punishing rather than nurturing ways.

What can you do if you find yourself in this situation or one very similar?

- *Recognize that the person you're hurting most is yourself.* You may upset your parents by self-defeating behavior, but it hurts you—immediately or long-term—most of all. Your parents won't feel the consequences of your actions nearly as much as you do. So if you get back at education-conscious people by messing up at school, you're the one who may have fewer options in the future. If you get back at weight- or health-conscious parents by gaining weight, you're the one who will have to live with the social stigma (however unfair that is) and the health risks of being overweight. If you lash back at puritanical parents with wild behavior that is shocking even to you (if you stop and really think about it), you're the one taking the potentially life-changing or even life-threatening risks. Instead, expressing your anger in words to a parent or parents can save you a lot of heartbreak.
- *There are better ways to let your parents know that you're angry or unhappy with them.* Talk to them. Write them a note or talk with a trusted adult relative, friend, or teacher who can help you express what you're feeling to your parents.
- *Encourage your parents to seek family counseling where all of you can express what you're feeling in a safe environment with a professional who can help you sort out and resolve your situation.* Even though it can be very hard for adults as well as teens to seek professional help, it can be well worth the effort. It isn't an admission that you're crazy or a horrible family or incompetent people. It *can* be a sign that you love each other (deep down) and are committed, as a family, to making things work better for everyone. It's well worth a try.

FEELINGS ABOUT THE "ISMS"

I'm 16 and am an African American living in a mostly white suburb. I have friends at school but sometimes I feel lonely and angry because they can't understand how things are for me at times. My parents, who are well off because my dad is an attorney and my mom is a teacher, bought me a used BMW for my birthday and I couldn't tell you how many times the police follow me or stop me when I'm driving just because it's a nice car and I'm black and they think I stole it. And some of my friends' parents don't treat me like just a normal friend. Either they ignore me or they act overly nice if you know what I mean. And lots of people at school, especially girls, if they didn't know me, would cross the street or not get into an elevator if they were to encounter me as a stranger but no one wants to admit the little bit (or more) of racism they have inside. Everybody always says I should be grateful for the good life I have. I AM glad to be growing up in my family and having what I do, but there are times I wish I could just relax with people who really understand what it still means to be black in this country no matter who you are or how much money or other stuff you have.

Alex J.

People at school make fun of me because I'm fat and ugly. I weigh 200 pounds, wear glasses, and have bad skin. People tease me all the time about how I look and I cry every day at school and then come home and eat. I hate getting up and going to school in the morning. My parents tell me not to pay any attention to the teasing, but that's impossible! What can I do to make them stop or to feel better?

Courtney B.

"Isms" such as racism, sexism, or "lookism" are hurtful not only to the people being singled out for discrimination or ridicule, but to us all. These ways of thinking and acting diminish and divide us. Often, those who are most prejudiced against others have very little going for them personally, low self-esteem, or limited life experience outside their own ideologies. Of course, that doesn't excuse any of their hurtful attitudes and behavior, but may put some of it into perspective for everyone else. Some people try to build themselves up by tearing others down—instead of looking within to see how to improve their own lives.

What can you do if you're feeling besieged by an "ism"?

- *Look for ways to educate others.* Especially for someone who is a racial minority, this may seem a wearisome, never-ending task. But you don't have to be alone in your efforts. Enlist the aid of a teacher or an organization at your school. Perhaps the school could sponsor awareness days or intercultural workshops or other events that will raise people's levels of consciousness about others who are different in some way.
- *Let others know how you feel.* We aren't necessarily suggesting that Alex bare his soul to the police, but when you see signs of unfair assumptions, racism, or sexism in people you know, let them know how this affects you. Many people don't realize how ingrained the "isms" are in our society and how we all have pieces of these buried within. When people begin to hear what they're saying or assuming, and understand how this affects someone they know in a direct way, they may be motivated to change. It's important for others to know that hurtful teasing, thoughtless comments, or racist assumptions are *not* OK with you. Or, if you have simply misunderstood each other, this can be a chance to clear things up instead of living with hurt.
- *Find safe places of solace.* If you're being teased or excluded or discriminated against, you're likely to have feelings that you don't feel safe sharing with the perpetrators or with others you're not sure will understand. Think about people with whom you feel safe to be yourself: family, close friends, a special teacher, a counselor, a church group, or a special-interest group. It's important to be able to express your hurt and anger to someone or some group who can listen with understanding and compassion and help you sort out what you're feeling and the best way—for you—to resolve these feelings.
- *Make a truce with your world—and with yourself.* The pain of being different in some way and being the target of an "ism" can make you bitter—or it can make you stronger and wiser. Life isn't fair a lot of the time. Racism, sexism, and "lookism" unfairly hurt and sometimes limit the potential of many good, talented, and deserving people.

Accepting the fact that this unfairness exists does not mean saying it's OK or accepting limits on yourself. It means that you decide to make a difference in your own life, by not letting bitterness and despair kill your spirit. You can use your pain and your anger in positive ways—to strengthen your resolve to have a happy, productive life despite its inherent unfairness. It means making an effort in your own way, your own style, to try to change patterns of thinking that perpetuate those life-limiting "isms."

PHYSICAL, EMOTIONAL, AND SEXUAL ABUSE

My parents are always hitting me and telling me they wished I was never born—mostly when they're drunk. Even when she's sober, my mom is always criticizing how I look (she thinks I'm ugly) and my dad yells at me for never doing anything—schoolwork, housework—as good as he thinks I should. I hate my life. What can I do?

J. J.

Abuse at the hands of family members, especially parents, can be a devastating experience, and each type of abuse—physical, emotional, sexual—has its own singular kind of pain. You may fear for your safety and even your life. You may feel guilt, sometimes blaming yourself for your family's problems, sometimes feeling confused about conflicting feelings of love and hate for the person who is abusing you. You may feel isolated and alone, feeling so different and so certain that no one else shares your situation. You may be terrified that friends and others at school will find out—and, at the same time, long for help and support from others. You may be afraid to tell anyone for fear you will be blamed or not believed or that your family will be torn apart. You may feel angry, frightened, and used. You may also feel special—for being singled out for attention by a parent. You may feel shame, yet strong family loyalty.

My dad has been forcing me to have sex with him several times a month since I was 10 (I'm now 13). I tried telling my mother hundreds of times, but she says she doesn't want to know what she calls my "dirty little lies." I feel like I'm walking around with compartments in my mind. At school, I'm friendly and outgoing. With my mom, I'm angry and upset. With my dad, I'm just numb. Does this mean I'm going crazy?

M. T.

How can you deal with these feelings and begin to heal?

- *Realize that you're not alone.* The pain of isolation can increase the pain of abuse. It's important to know that you're not alone. There are more people than you could ever imagine who have experienced some form of abuse at home. It doesn't make you—or your family—uniquely horrible. It *is* a sign of significant family problems, but help is available. However complicated and painful your situation is, it is *not* hopeless.

- *Realize that you're not to blame.* Even if your behavior hasn't been beyond reproach—and you've done things such as talking back to a parent or defying rules—this still doesn't justify a beating or consistent emotional abuse. Even if you've had sexual fantasies about a family member or even flirted a bit, this is not a reason or justification for incest. It's the adult's responsibility to use his or her power in a positive way—whether it's in admonishing you or punishing you for inappropriate behavior or whether it's steering your relationship clear of overt sexual activities.

So abuse, whether physical, sexual, or emotional, is a sign of a problem with the adult. A healthy parent will punish in ways that do not crush the spirit. He or she will encourage better judgment or behavior the next time. Abuse is attacking, not teaching. It harms the body and the soul. Deep down, you can feel and know the difference.

- *Take a step to get help for yourself and your family.* Abuse represents family problems that are too serious and complex to be handled or resolved within the family. Professional help is vital. But it may feel too threatening or totally impossible to discuss this option with your parents. If this is something you can't discuss with them, ask for help yourself by talking with a teacher, school counselor, clergyperson, or hotline for emergency help. It takes a lot of courage to make this step. It's important to know that some professionals such as teachers or counselors are bound by law to report abuse of minors. It *is* possible that social and legal agencies may intervene. But it's important to remember, too, that the abuse isn't likely to stop until others step in to help. Your first priority must be to protect yourself and stop the abuse. That may mean living outside your family setting for a time—or it may not. It may certainly mean counseling for you and your parents and, perhaps, other involved family members. There are no quick or easy solutions, but there can be an end to your abuse and, eventually, to your pain.

■ *Healing means making a choice to survive and to live for you—not for them.* While some people live lives scarred by pain and bitterness as a result of their early abuse, others survive horrible home situations to live happy, productive adult lives. You can, too. Your courage in facing your present crisis and in resolving your feelings with the help of therapy can have a very positive impact on your life in years to come.

The healing process can be long and painful. You may go through a period of grief for a childhood of pain, for a family so troubled. You may feel a combination of anger and great sadness. In order to be free, you need to resolve these feelings and then grow past this traumatic time. If possible, you might think about forgiving your parents sometime in the future. This doesn't mean that they were right. It's more for *you* than for them. Prolonged feelings of anger and revenge can keep you tied to the past. Forgiving your parents sets you free to value yourself and live for you—not them. In time, with forgiveness and supportive therapy, you will find new freedom to be yourself, to realize and celebrate your separateness and uniqueness, to reach out to others, to trust and to love.

DATE RAPE

I'm still shaking. I went out with this really popular guy last weekend and on our way home from this party, after we'd both had too much to drink, he parked on this golf course and forced me to have sex with him. He said he knew I wanted it even when I told him "No!" because I wouldn't have dressed so sexy or danced so close if I hadn't wanted it. But I didn't! I was a virgin and now I feel just terrible. I wanted my first time to be wonderful, not like this. I can't stop crying, but when my parents ask what's wrong, I can't tell them.

Brandi W.

Date rape is a terrible reality for many teens these days. Some are confused about what it really means. Others don't take it seriously, thinking that it really isn't rape if it happens on a date or between two people who know each other well.

Actually, rape is rape. It is forcing someone to have sex when they don't want to. It often happens when a boy won't take no for an answer and physically overpowers his date. But a girl who nags and threatens a boy into having sex when he doesn't want to may also be guilty of a form of date rape.

Date rape is about not respecting another person's right to say no and to control his or her own body. It is more about power than sex and more about control than caring.

How can you avoid getting into this situation?

■ *Be selective about your dates.* If a guy thinks he's a divine gift to women and that his feelings and desires always come first, avoid him—no matter how cute or popular he is. Guys who see women as objects rather than as equal people and who give you the impression that your feelings and opinions aren't important can be big trouble.

■ *Don't drink—particularly to excess—on a date.* Alcohol can play a major role in date rape, not only in terms of making some men more aggressive, but also in lowering both people's inhibitions and decreasing one's ability to stand up for oneself or see warning signs before the situation becomes a crisis.

- *Question assumptions.* Some people believe that if a woman flirts with a man or agrees to be alone with him somewhere, this means she wants sex. While a woman does need to exercise good judgment and avoid risky situations, a man has no right to force a woman to have sex. Paying for a date does not include the right to another's body. Nothing—even marriage—gives another person the right to control the body and the choices of an individual.

If You Are Raped

- *Tell someone who can help.* Talk over your feelings with someone you can trust, who will listen and be supportive. Call your local rape crisis line (check your phone directory or call Information). Talking with an experienced counselor can help you feel calmer as you review your options: to keep the incident private and work out your feelings, or to file charges against your attacker. A professional counselor can also help you work through your feelings of anger, grief, shock, and betrayal. The counselor may direct or guide you through a hospital examination and treatment if you need medical attention or decide you want to file charges.
- *Don't blame yourself.* The person had no right to force you to have sex. In the future, there may be some steps you can take to avoid getting into a similar situation. But rape is *never* acceptable, tolerable behavior. It isn't cute or funny or macho. It's violent, abusive, and illegal.

DEPRESSION

I've been feeling really bad. At first, I thought it was depression over my parents' divorce, but things are better now and I still don't feel right. I have no energy. I get irritated with my mom AND with my friends(!) for no good reason. My grades in school are falling because I just can't concentrate. What's wrong with me?

Caitlin O.

When people talk about depression, they can mean many different things. Crying and feeling down after the death of someone you love (whether a person or a pet) is grief. Feeling down after a romantic breakup or not making a team could signal a depressed mood. A clinical depression is much more complex—perhaps initially springing from an identifiable event, but quite often not. For some, depression can be a lifelong illness that comes and goes in a recurring cycle.

Depression is, in short, often used as a catch-all phrase to describe a variety of symptoms. It is often the result of a complex mix of social, psychological, and/or physical factors that can trigger sadness, hopelessness, feelings of inferiority, powerlessness, and helplessness.

Grief is a natural response to loss. A depressed mood is usually a relatively brief period (a few days or a few weeks) of feeling sad over a specific event. Clinical depression, on the other hand, is more persistent and severe.

There are several types of clinical depression as described by the American Psychiatric Association in the *DSM-IV*, a diagnostic guide published in 1994 for physicians, psychologists, and other mental health professionals. The types of clinical depression include the following:

Major Depressive Disorder, Single Episode or Recurrent

To be diagnosed with major depressive disorder, you must have suffered from *five or more* of the following specific symptoms for more than two weeks in a way that interferes with your daily life. These symptoms include the following:

- Depressed or irritable mood most of the day, nearly every day.

- Loss of interest or pleasure in activities you have previously enjoyed.
- Significant weight loss (without dieting) or weight gain (a change of more than 5 percent of body weight in one month); diminished or increased appetite.
- Insomnia (difficulty sleeping) or hypersomnia (sleeping too much) nearly every day.
- Feelings of restlessness or being slowed down.
- Feelings of fatigue and loss of energy nearly every day.
- Feelings of worthlessness or excessive or inappropriate guilt on a daily basis.
- Diminished ability to think or concentrate or persistent indecisiveness nearly every day.
- Recurrent thoughts of death (not just fear of dying); thoughts of suicide with or without a specific plan and/or suicide attempts.

How long does major depressive disorder last? Some people have one episode in a lifetime and never repeat this experience. Others have a number of depressive episodes (separated by at least two months in which the person does not have symptoms of a major depression).

Dysthymic Disorder

Teenagers with dysthymic disorder experience depressive symptoms that are long-lasting (for at least one year without having been symptom-free for longer than two months at a time), but this depression may not be quite as life-interrupting as major depressive disorder. Teens with dysthymic disorder may go through all the motions of everyday life and do all the things they are supposed to do, but without ever feeling free of depression for long. The symptoms, which must be present for most of the day, nearly every day, for a year or more, include the following:

- Poor appetite or overeating.
- Sleep problems—sleeping too much or insomnia.

- Low energy level and fatigue.
- Low self-esteem.
- Poor concentration or difficulty making decisions.
- Feelings of hopelessness.

If you have dysthymic disorder, you may be cranky and irritable most days as well as being depressed. You may have trouble making friends with peers or talking to adults. You also tend to be a pessimist about life in general.

Bipolar Disorder

Teens with bipolar disorder have mood swings that go quite beyond the usual changeable moods of adolescence. If you have bipolar disorder, you will have moods alternating between highly energetic (*manic*)—during which time you sleep very little, talk a lot, have a surplus of energy, and feel wonderful about yourself—and major depression.

A chronic form of bipolar disorder is called *cyclothymia*. Here the teen has bipolar episodes for at least a year without more than a two-month respite from symptoms (either manic or depressive).

What can you do if you're feeling depressed? It depends on the kind of depression you have.

If You're Grieving a Loss

- *Let your feelings happen.* You may be feeling a confusing combination of feelings. You may feel angry one minute and profoundly sad the next. You may cry or be unable to cry. There is no right way to grieve—only *your* way. It's important to know, too, that tears can mean courage, not weakness. It takes courage to fully experience your pain and work it through.
- *Share your feelings with others.* This might be family or friends or an understanding adult, such as a teacher or clergyperson. Or it could mean joining a support group for teens who

have experienced loss. Having a chance to talk and be truly understood and hearing that others share many of your feelings and experiences can be a huge step toward healing.

- *Realize that the grief process can mean zigzagging emotionally between pain and healing.* Getting through the grief process takes time. You may have periods of feeling OK and then find yourself experiencing a wave of grief again. You're not going crazy. It's a normal part of the grief process. Just remember that the pain-free moments, the times of laughter and enjoyment of life between your waves of grief, will give you strength as you work through your pain.

If You're in a Depressed Mood

- *Change the pace of your life.* Go for a walk. Listen to upbeat music. Act as if you weren't feeling depressed and do things you would do if not depressed. Your dark mood may lift!

- *Resist the drug or alcohol "cure."* Don't try to deaden your pain with alcohol or drugs. This just postpones and sometimes even *prevents* life-affirming solutions.

- *Get daily exercise.* Even if you have to force yourself, do some kind of exercise every day. Studies have found that regular exercise and general physical fitness can help combat depression and anxiety.

- *Release feelings in ways that feel safe.* Sometimes unexpressed anger is an important part of a depressed mood. Try releasing angry feelings by pounding pillows, crying, writing in a journal, or talking with friends.

- *Keep a journal or diary.* Studies have found that keeping a journal can help alleviate stress and depression by helping you express in writing the feelings you have difficulty expressing any other way. You may also come to understand these feelings—and yourself—better by keeping a journal.

- *Give yourself something to look forward to every day.* This doesn't have to be something major, just something pleasurable to you: time spent on an interest or hobby, taking time to notice beauty around you, meditation, listening to music you enjoy, reading for pleasure, talking with someone you like or love, or taking a soothing bath. The point of this whole exercise is to give you a reason to anticipate rather than dread each new day.

If Your Depressed Mood Persists

- *Talk with your parents about seeking professional help.* If you can't talk to your parents about this, talk with someone who can help you get through to them—a relative, a teacher, or a trusted adult friend. Getting help from a mental health professional—a psychiatrist (M.D.), a psychologist (Ph.D. or Psy.D.), or a psychotherapist (MFT or LCSW)—doesn't mean you're crazy. It can be an important step toward healing when there doesn't seem to be anything you, on your own, or those around you can do to make a positive difference.

- *Be open to help beyond talk therapy.* Much of the time, talking with a therapist (as well as with family and friends) can help a lot in sorting out your feelings. But there are times when you need more help than that. Some major depressive episodes may be severe enough to warrant the use of anti-depressive medication. And if you have bipolar disorder, medication can help to even out your mood swings. It isn't a matter of taking a pill so life will be perfect. But many health professionals now believe that some depression has chemical origins and that medication can restore your body's chemical balance and make you better able to cope with the ups and downs of life as well as making better use of therapy. Medications aren't appropriate for everyone who is depressed, but they can be real lifesavers for some.

With supportive therapy and, possibly, appropriate anti-depressant drugs prescribed by a psychiatrist, you can begin to leave the darkness and pain behind and rediscover hope.

SUICIDAL FEELINGS

I don't know why I'm writing this except to say maybe I'm looking for a reason not to kill myself. I think of dying every day because living is just too awful. I have parents who are fighting over their divorce, my best friend at school won't speak to me anymore, and now that I'm 14 and in high school, I'm nothing. I didn't make the soccer team and my grades aren't as good as they were. I mean, what's the point? I used to enjoy my life, but now I just want to die. Help!

Megan M.

Many teens feel as Megan does: depressed and despairing about life and looking for a way out of their pain. What many don't realize is they may not want to die as much as *to live differently*. But when you're feeling depressed and hopeless, it's hard to see how life might be different. Many teens like Megan cling to a tiny spark of hope and seek help. Tragically, many others do not.

Suicide is the third leading cause of death in adolescents. While boys are more likely to kill themselves, girls are more likely to attempt suicide. Among various ethnic groups, Native American teens are more likely to kill themselves than other ethnicities, and Latino males and females are more likely to attempt suicide. (Statistics from the National Adolescent Health Information Center reveal that 34 percent of Latina high school students considered suicide in 1993, and nearly 20 percent of these young women attempted it.) While white teens traditionally have had higher rates of completed suicides and suicide attempts, young African Americans are catching up—with a 114 percent increase in reported deaths by suicide over the past eighteen years. Some feel this is due to more middle-class African Americans losing ties with church and family. Others believe that better access to weapons and the increased willingness of families to disclose death by suicide may account for the statistics.

Beyond statistics, however, every single loss of a young life to suicide is a tragedy. When a young person dies in this way, the people who knew him or her ask each other, "Why?" Most often, there is no one answer to this. Some suicidal teens experience not one critical event, but a series of stressors in the areas of family, friends, school, and other important areas of their lives. Mix a combination of stressors, depression, and perhaps some substance abuse (which can make depression worse) and you can have a recipe for disaster. Suicide may begin to seem like the logical or only solution.

If you have a friend or loved one in trouble, be alert for signs of suicidal feelings or behavior. Don't dismiss them as bids for attention or conditions that will pass. It may not be possible for a severely depressed teen to "just forget it" or "snap out of it." And if someone is seeking attention via suicidal threats or plans, this is a definite cry for help.

Some of the signs that your friend may be suicidal are the following:

- Severe depression that lasts months or years.
- Sudden elation or a burst of energy after a prolonged depression. (It's quite common for a suicidal young person to find the energy to commit suicide after the most immobilizing part of the depression begins to lift.)
- Talking about dying or committing suicide. This is especially serious if he or she has a plan of action.
- Giving away possessions, especially prized ones.
- Sudden withdrawal from friends and family.

What can you do if someone you love is showing some or all of these signs?

- *Take all comments about death and suicide seriously.* Ask your friend directly whether he or she has thought of suicide or has a method in mind. The more thought and planning that has gone into this, the more immediate the crisis. Instead of dismissing such comments as attention-seeking tactics or a passing mood, urge your friend to get help.

- *Show that you care.* Let your friend talk while you listen. Let your friend know that he or she matters to you. Emphasize that, no matter how hopeless life can seem, it can change. Even the worst pain and hurt imaginable diminish with time—even though that might seem impossible right now.

- *Urge your friend to seek immediate help.* Get him or her in touch with a suicide hotline or with an adult who can make a difference: a parent, a counselor, a teacher.

- *If your friend won't seek help, get help for him or her.* Your friend may be furious, but his or her life may well be at stake. Don't let yourself be part of a tragic conspiracy of silence. It's better to risk a friend's wrath than be mourning his or her death. This is a secret you *must* not keep! Tell one or both of your parents or your friend's parents. If that isn't possible, tell some other adult who can help. It's worth risking a friendship to save that person's life!

If You Are Feeling Suicidal

- *Ask yourself whether you really want to die—or to live differently.* Life *can* be different. As long as there is life, there is hope. Some things that seem unchangeable now will change in time. Even serious depression doesn't last forever. No matter how appalling your life circumstances, help is available if you tell someone, if you reach out. While there are no easy or instant solutions to life's major problems, there *are* alternatives to the anguish you're feeling right now. You can—and you will—feel better.

- *Real-life suicide is not tragically glamorous the way it may be depicted on TV or in the movies.* Suicide is an ugly act. There is no glamour or beauty in it at all. Many of your classmates, friends, and acquaintances might feel sad at the moment, but will go on with their lives, maybe even forgetting you. Those who truly love you will be devastated and their lives will never be the same. To society, you'll be another statistic. And *you* will no longer be. That's the saddest, most tragic fact of all.

- *Remember that people care—and reach out for help.* Ask those close to you for help. Tell them what you're feeling. If that just doesn't seem possible right now, call your local suicide hotline *or* **Boys Town National Hotline** (offering help to girls as well as boys!): (800) 448-3000. The hearing impaired can call (800) 448-1833. This hotline is free and totally confidential. You will find someone to listen, to offer counseling, and to direct you to help in your own area. You *can* change your life and your feelings. There *is* help, no matter how alone you're feeling right now. And there *is* hope.

FEELINGS AND YOUR HEALTH

Is it true that your feelings can make you sick? If you never feel anything, does that mean you'll live longer and be healthy? How can you go through your life and never feel anything? (My dad never seems to feel anything and he has colds all the time.)

Matthew Z.

Feelings can cause physical reactions as well as lifestyle choices that can influence our health. Some people, for example, drink or smoke or overeat when they're tense or stressed out; all of these can contribute to health risks.

Of course, it's not possible to go through life without feeling. We suspect that Matthew's dad may feel a lot, but can't express these feelings.

Keeping his feelings bottled up inside may indeed be making him more vulnerable to illness.

What have researchers found out about the role feelings play in health?

- Hostility can be a factor in heart disease. In fact, a Duke University study found that teens with hostile attitudes may develop high cholesterol levels while growing up, with high blood pressure and heart disease possibly shortening their lives.
- Sharing feelings with friends, family, or a diary can strengthen the immune system.
- Optimists have better physical health than pessimists, mostly because they handle stress better. This gives them a longer life expectancy and stronger immune systems.
- Depression can be a factor in disease. Various studies have shown that depression can weaken immunity and, long-term, can make a person more likely to develop cancer.
- Loneliness can kill. Studies at the University of Michigan and Ohio State University found that loneliness impairs the immune system and that those with few friends have higher death rates.

So what can you do to deal with feelings and maximize your health?

- *Make and keep connections with others.* We all need love and trust in our lives. This love can come from a variety of people—from friends and family as well as from lovers. You will also find that when you're kind and warm toward others, you'll feel better yourself. Cultivate a positive attitude toward people in general. Most people are interesting if you give them a chance. They want to be fair and kind—and they can teach you important lessons. Be open to others.
- *Cultivate a sense of humor.* Humor puts life in perspective and takes the edge off your pain. It will also attract others to you and will make it easier to live with yourself. Laughter is a wonderful safeguard for both mental and physical health!
- *Accept the fact that you will have pain, disappointments, and setbacks.* These are all part of life. Let yourself experience and learn from the inevitable pain in your life instead of trying to avoid it at all costs.
- *Tell yourself—and really believe—that you're in charge of your own life.* You can make your own life, your own good luck, your own choices, and your own love. Whatever your circumstances, you don't have to be a helpless victim. You can do more than you ever imagined. You can overcome terrible pain and loss if necessary. You can lose a special love and survive to love again. You can have a worthwhile, happy life without being a genius or a great beauty or super-talented. You just need to be the best you know how to be. You need to accept and learn to live with your feelings, your strengths, and your limitations (without letting any of these overwhelm you). You can choose to be in charge of your life. And, if you choose, this life can be full and rewarding with an abundance of love and growth and joy.

QUICK FACTS FOR PARENTS

- Depression is not unusual in teens. It can vary from a depressed mood over a particular loss, a life situation, or a series of stresses to a clinical depression that may require professional help and possible medication. A depressed mood lifts, while clinical depression endures longer than a few weeks and significantly interferes with life. It's important to know that a depressed teen may seem angry and irritable rather than sad.

- Suicide is the third leading cause of death among adolescents. Girls are more likely to attempt suicide, while boys are more likely to complete a suicide. While white males are still the most frequent suicide victims, certain ethnic groups—especially Native Americans—have alarmingly high suicide rates.

- Danger signs of a potential suicide include the following:

  ✔ Severe depression or a sudden improvement in mood after a severe depression.

  ✔ A substance abuse problem, especially if coupled with depression and feelings of hopelessness.

  ✔ Expressing feelings of hopelessness.

  ✔ Talking about suicide, **especially if he or she mentions a preferred method.**

  ✔ Previous suicide attempts.

- **Any talk of suicide should be taken seriously.** Show your caring by seeking professional help for your child immediately! Ask your family doctor for a referral or call a local suicide hotline or the Boys Town National Hotline: **(800) 448-3000.**

Eating for Good Health

My health ed teacher at school said something about what you do as a teenager can make a difference in how healthy you are later in life. Are there some basic things I can do to stay healthy without spending a lot of time at it? The reason I'm asking is that I don't have a lot of free time between school and work and time with my friends. Some books and articles I've seen about healthy eating have all these complicated recipes that my mom doesn't want to make and I don't have time to make. What can you do if you want to be healthy but don't have a lot of free time?

Sarah H.

It's true that what you do now—how you eat, how you exercise (or not) can have a lifelong impact. A large part of this is developing healthy habits now that, if continued, can make a long, active, healthy life possible.

There seems to be a correlation between health and happiness. It's hard to be happy if you're not feeling well. And, if you're feeling unhappy with yourself, you may tend to neglect your body and thus get caught up in a spiral of bad feelings, both mental and physical. If, on the other hand, you feel well physically, you're likely to do better in all aspects of your life. Your body *is* you and it's vital that you build a strong, healthy body to go along with your active, healthy mind.

Seven Steps to Lifelong Good Health

1. Eat a healthy, balanced diet.
2. Get regular exercise.
3. Maintain a healthy weight for your height and build. If you're overweight, pay attention to what you eat (making health-minded choices), and get moving with a regular exercise plan.
4. Don't smoke or take drugs.
5. Get regular medical checkups and inoculations as required, and visit your dentist at least once a year.
6. Get involved in work and/or a cause you believe in or activities that help you feel good about yourself and of service to others.
7. Build strong friendships and love relationships. Those who form warm, loving bonds with others tend to live longer, healthier, happier lives.

ARE YOU WHAT YOU EAT?

Yes! What you eat has a huge impact, not only on your physical health and appearance, but also on your emotions.

As you can see from the following Food Guide Pyramid illustration, a balanced diet requires a variety of foods in four different categories. And as you will see from the charts after that, the vitamins and minerals required for optimal health also come from a variety of foods.

Food Guide Pyramid

- Filling up with empty calories: sugary snacks, soft drinks, potato chips and crackers.
- Eating on the run with a high-fat fast-food diet. With a steady diet of fast food and/or high-calorie snacks, you can take in a lot of calories and gain weight and *still* be malnourished because you're not getting the nutrients you need.
- Dieting so stringently—often skipping meals or eating only a few varieties of food items—that important nutrients are missing from the daily food intake.

Three of the most common problem eating patterns among teens are the following:

How do you build a balanced diet? Does it mean that you have to eat stuff you hate or never go to a fast-food place with your friends again? Balance doesn't mean deprivation or never having fast food or candy. It means paying attention to what you're

6 VITAMINS YOU NEED FOR A HEALTHY BODY

Vitamin	How It Helps	Where to Get It
Vitamin A	Growth, healthy skin, teeth, gums, eyes, digestive and urinary tract	Milk, butter, margarine, carrots, liver, eggs, fruit, dark green and yellow vegetables
Vitamin B-1 (thiamine)	Converts carbohydrates into energy. Promotes healthy eyes, skin, body tissues	Meat, fish, poultry, rice, whole-grain breads and cereals, fruits, vegetables
Vitamin B-2 (riboflavin)	Smooth skin, clear vision	Dairy products, enriched bread, cereal, eggs, poultry, fish, meat
Vitamin B-6 (pyridoxine)	Healthy skin, red blood cells, and nervous system	Vegetables, cereal, lean meat, milk
Vitamin B-12	Healthy nervous system; also safeguards against certain types of anemia	Eggs, liver, meat, milk
Vitamin C	Healthy teeth, gums, bones, and capillaries	Citrus fruits, cantaloupes, berries, tomatoes, green peppers, broccoli
Vitamin D	Helps body use calcium and phosphorus in building strong bones and teeth	Fortified milk, liver, eggs, and fish, especially salmon
Vitamin E	Theory is that this prevents abnormal breakdown of fat in body tissues and aids absorption of nutrients	Seeds, nuts, soybeans, wheat germ, leafy vegetables, whole-grain cereals
Niacin	Converts food to energy and aids production of certain hormones	Halibut, tuna, poultry, milk, eggs, whole grains, peanut butter, fruits, and vegetables
Folic acid	Helps red blood cell formation and safeguards against anemia	Asparagus, broccoli, spinach, lima beans, liver
Pantothenic acid	Helps metabolize carbohydrates and fats	Broccoli, nuts, eggs

MINERALS YOU NEED FOR A HEALTHY BODY

Mineral	How It Helps	Where to Get It
Calcium	Healthy teeth, bones, muscles; also helps blood clot normally	Green leafy vegetables, shellfish, milk products such as yogurt and cheese
Phosphorus	Helps get energy to body's cells	Meats, cheese, milk
Fluoride	Helps build and maintain strong, healthy teeth and bones	Lettuce, onions, soybeans, and specially treated water
Potassium	Growth, a strong heart, and healthy nervous system; also helps regulate water balance in the body	Bananas, orange juice, leafy vegetables, dried fruits, lean meats
Iodine	Essential aid to the thyroid gland in regulating energy and metabolism	Seafood, iodized salt
Iron	Increases resistance to disease and prevents some forms of anemia	Dried fruits (especially raisins), whole-grain breads, cereals, liver, eggs, lean meat

eating and making sure that you're getting the vitamins and minerals you need.

The Food Guide Pyramid suggests the optimal balance of a diet that emphasizes fruits and vegetables, grains, cereal, pasta, lean meats, and dairy products (or their nondairy equivalents). Within the basic food groups, you have many choices. For example:

- Milk products such as yogurt, low-fat cheese, or cottage cheese may be more to your taste than plain milk. Or you may choose to use milk in soups, casseroles, or puddings.
- You don't have to eat plain, recognizable eggs if you don't like them. Eggs can be ingredients in casseroles, soufflés, omelets, custards, and other dishes.
- If you hate vegetables, try new varieties or the same variety in different form. If, for example you find canned green beans totally disgusting, try steaming some fresh green beans with a touch of herbs. It's a whole different taste. Steaming fresh or frozen vegetables with subtle seasonings can make a big difference. A little cinnamon sprinkled on yellow squash can transform it into a delicious snack or side dish. A touch of lemon or apple cider vinegar can bring new zest to broccoli. If you still hate veg-

etables, try them in a stew or soup or stir-fried Chinese dish.
- Cut down on red meat, substituting chicken, turkey, fish, seafood, and tofu. There are many wonderful ways to prepare these—from salads to hot entrées.

If you're a vegetarian or thinking of becoming one, balance in your diet is vital, too. While vegetarians generally are less likely to suffer from heart disease or obesity (which are often linked with overconsumption of animal protein and fat), you still need to keep a balance of fruits, vegetables, and proteins in your diet and not overdo it with sugars and starches.

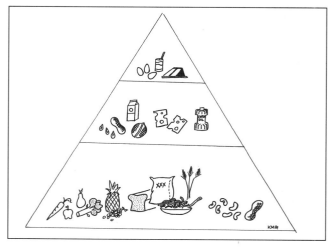

Vegetarian Food Pyramid

⑧

CUTTING DOWN ON DIET HEALTH HAZARDS

Food Hazards	How These Are Hazardous	Foods to Avoid or Cut Back	Good Food Substitutes
Soft drinks/caffeine	Can add to stomach acidity Can add empty calories Caffeine can contribute to sleep disorders, heart rhythm disturbances	Sugary soft drinks Colas (no more than two a day *at most!*) Coffee Bottled iced tea with sugar	WATER is #1! (Drink at least eight glasses a day!) Fruit juice Vegetable juice Herbal tea Green tea
Sugar	A factor in obesity, heart disease, diabetes, hypoglycemia Contributes to tooth decay Personality and behavior problems	Sugary soft drinks Candy, cake, cookies Ice cream Convenience foods (packaged meals or fast food may have lots of sugar)	Fruit Fresh foods that you prepare or that you get from a restaurant salad bar
Salt	Can be factor in high blood pressure Can increase miseries of PMS water retention	Canned soups and vegetables Frozen convenience foods Snacks such as potato and corn chips Fast food (even milkshakes have high salt content)	Lemon juice or herbal seasonings as salt substitute Fresh meals you make yourself *or* soups and frozen entrees that are low-sodium (check labels!)
Fat	Contributes to obesity, heart disease (which can start in adolescence!), and certain cancers	Fried foods Bacon, sausage, and spareribs Butter, margarine, fatty dressings Snacks such as donuts, chips, or rich nuts (such as macadamia nuts)	Lean meats and fish that are baked or broiled Low-fat or nonfat dairy products (including low-fat yogurt or nonfat sour cream as a potato topping) Low-fat or nonfat salad dressings

Teens need to be particularly careful to get sufficient nutrients for their growing bodies. Protein-rich legumes (beans), milk, eggs, cheese, tofu, and perhaps fish and seafood can help a lot. In these growing years, you need protein and calcium, so nutrition experts tend to discourage teens from following a strict vegetarian diet.

Before beginning a new way of eating, make up a week-long menu and check it out with your physician, your school nurse, or a nutritionist to make sure that such a diet will be sufficiently balanced to meet your nutritional needs.

IMPROVING YOUR EATING HABITS (PAINLESSLY!)

Here are some of the best ways to start:

■ Cut down on (or cut out) foods that are hazardous to your health.

■ Find ways to incorporate good eating habits into your busy daily routine—even if you find yourself at a fast-food place with your friends.

Making healthy food choices helps you look and feel better today—and establish good eating habits that will give you lifetime benefits. In these years, many of your long-term food habits and preferences are being formed. At age 30 or older, you may not be able to eat the way you do today without piling on weight. It may be much more difficult to change your eating habits—and, certainly, to lose weight—as you approach middle age. So start now! Even if healthy food tastes weird and lame, stick with it for a few weeks or months and you may be amazed to see how your tastes change. You may find that those old sugar- and fat-laden treats don't taste nearly as good as they used to.

Growing up with healthful eating habits—salads, vegetables, seafood, fish, turkey, chicken, beans, and tofu—will help you maintain your

⑨ GOOD FOOD ON THE RUN

YES! It's possible to enjoy fast food with your friends if you're savvy about substitutions!

Instead of . . .	Try This!
High-fat burgers and sandwiches; potato salad, French fries, onion rings	Salad bars (greens, fruit, veggies; no creamy salads—e.g. potato, macaroni, ambrosia) with low-fat, nonfat, or minimum amount of dressing
Cheeseburger	Hamburger
Fried chicken or fish sandwich or chicken nuggets	Chicken breast sandwich or chicken fajita pita
Fried fish sticks	Seafood salad
Fried tacos and burritos	Soft tacos and burritos
Meat pizza	Vegetarian pizza
Milkshake	Plain or chocolate low-fat or nonfat milk
Cola	Water with lemon slices or iced tea (with no sugar)

weight and your health now and throughout adulthood.

REACHING AND MAINTAINING YOUR BEST WEIGHT

If You Feel You're Underweight

I'm 14 and skinny and everyone teases me about it. Some of my friends are jealous because I eat whatever I want and never gain weight, but other people make fun of me. What can I do?

J. K.

While underweight teens may be the envy of their classmates, being skinny and unable to gain weight can be as serious and emotionally painful a problem for someone faced with this situation as being overweight may be to another teen.

What can you do? First, check with your physician to see if you are, in fact, underweight. If he or she agrees that you are:

■ *Consider your age, state of physical development, and body type.* The growth spurt in early adolescence burns a lot of calories. As your growth rate slows down a bit, you may start to

fill out. Some people, of course, have a naturally lean, angular (*ectomorphic*) body type. Many models and actresses fall into this category—which is why so many women who have different, more rounded body types, get so frustrated in their futile attempts to diet their way down to similar slenderness.

■ *Work out with weights for greater muscle definition.* This can give a lean body a few more curves. Both men and women work out with weights in health clubs, at school, and at home these days—and this form of working out can help you look and feel stronger.

■ *Keep a diary of everything you eat for at least a week.* Note your eating habits. Do you eat three well-balanced meals a day, or do you snack a little here and there and skip meals a lot? Do you have trouble eating when you're nervous or upset? Are you extremely active or so busy that you often find you don't have time to eat? Are you a nibbler who tastes food, but who never finishes anything? In your food diary, note how much (or how little) you actually eat. It could give you some important clues.

■ *Change behavior that keeps you too skinny.* Never skip a meal. Even if you're upset, try eating regular meals. Your body needs essential nutrients no matter what you're feeling.

And a well-nourished body can give you extra strength to deal with a crisis.

- *Eat more nutritious snacks.* Trying to gain weight on candy and other junk food does more harm than good. Instead, pamper your body with snacks such as granola, bread and peanut butter, milk products, and fruits and vegetables.

- *If you're only a little underweight, consider counting your blessings.* A slender body that is nevertheless well-nourished can be a healthy, attractive one. Find a fashion style that works for you and dress to accentuate your best features. As time goes by and your calorie needs decrease, you may tend to put on weight anyway. You may want to start a little low and thus reach (and then maintain) the average weight for your height after your growing years are over.

- *If you're active, don't stop!* Regular exercise is a health *must* for everyone. If you're set on gaining weight, simply increase your calorie intake, but do keep exercising!

Diet Danger: Too Thin on Purpose

Some young people, usually girls, fit into a different category of underweight. These are teens who suffer from dieting-connected disorders, most notably anorexia nervosa and bulimia.

Because these disorders have psychological as well as biological aspects, we will be discussing them in greater detail in Chapter 9, "Mind over Body", but we'll mention both briefly here. Both disorders often begin when teens who are normal weight or slightly overweight start a diet regimen to become fashionably slender. Unlike many young people who go on and off diets regularly, these teens are unable to stop dieting and develop bizarre rituals to avoid gaining weight. A teenager with bulimia usually indulges in alternate binging and purging, eating too much and then getting rid of the food by vomiting and taking laxatives. She may also diet stringently between binges. Most bulimics don't get seriously underweight, but there are serious health risks associated with the binge-purge behavior characteristic of this disorder.

Teens with anorexia nervosa, however, diet and exercise compulsively, sometimes starving themselves down to skeletal proportions and risking a number of life-threatening complications. Although these girls are often alarmingly thin—sometimes weighing only 50 or 60 pounds—they have a distorted body image, seeing their emaciated bodies as fat or just right and so are very resistant to efforts to help them gain weight.

If You Feel You're Overweight

How can you tell if you're overweight? I feel fat even though my parents say I look fine. All of my friends are on diets even though some are much thinner than me. I'm into sports and am pretty health conscious. I don't want to be like a skinny model, but I want to be a healthy weight. How can I tell if I am?

Cherise A.

Whether a teen is normal weight, slightly overweight, or obese, weight is a major concern among teens—especially teen girls—today. Unfortunately, it's quite common for girls to be dissatisfied with their bodies—overweight or not—and to start dieting at a very young age. When scientists at the University of California at San Francisco studied dieting behavior in young girls, surveying 500 girls ages 9 to 18, they found that while 58 percent of the girls considered themselves too fat, only 15 percent were actually overweight. Nevertheless, some 50 percent of 9-year-olds, 80 percent of 11- to 12-year-olds, 70 percent of 12- to 16-year-olds, and 90 percent of 17-year-olds were dieting to lose weight. These findings, and others like them, concern medical professionals for several reasons:

- *Low-calorie diets can interfere with adolescent growth and development.* You need 2,500 to 3,000 calories a day during the prime years of physical development in order to experience your full growth and development and to have healthy bones. Too few calories can stunt growth.

- *Early dieting can put you on the road to a lifetime of yo-yo weight fluctuations.* When you diet, you change your metabolism. Your body learns to get by on fewer calories and you gain weight more rapidly after you stop dieting. Trying to reach some impossible standard of thinness in your youth can set you up for a lifetime of struggling with your weight.

- *Intense focusing on body weight and dieting at a young age can make you feel worse about yourself.* When your body and your life are changing, it's quite common to feel insecure at times. But if you are constantly comparing yourself to famous models or actresses (whose body types may be genetically quite different from yours), you're setting up standards that may not be attainable for you. While you might like to look like a model, not looking like one doesn't mean that you're a failure, ugly, or without any redeeming value as a person. You have your own strengths and talents and unique beauty. Obsessing about what you aren't or can't be and dieting to reach a goal that might not be healthy or even attainable usually doesn't do much for your weight and it can do great harm emotionally to the special person you're struggling to become.

I'm pretty fat—like about 160 pounds and I'm only 5'1". I was going to go to a doctor and get diet pills, but then the good ones got banned or something. Would stuff they call herbal PhenFen work? I'm desperate!

Kimberlee J.

Before you compare yourself too much to others—models, actresses, or even your friends—there are several important facts you need to know:

1. *People have genetically determined body types.* *Ectomorphs* are thin and angular. Many models and actresses are born with such bodies. *Mesomorphs*, on the other hand, are muscular with broad shoulders and slim hips. *Endomorphs* tend to be rounder and have more body fat and softer curves. So if you're an endomorph, you may be at your ideal weight, yet look heavier than a friend of the same weight who has the ectomorph body type. Genes are important. You're not likely to be slender and willowy if you come from a family of short, stocky people. Studies of people who were adopted as children have found that their weight and body shape more closely matches those of their biological rather than their adoptive parents. This doesn't mean that if you have obese parents, you're doomed to a lifetime of obesity. It may mean that you have to watch what you eat and exercise regularly in order to maintain a healthy body weight.

 Certain ethnic groups may be more likely to have higher percentages of overweight people. This may be a combination of genetics, eating habits, and cultural preferences. (Not all cultures venerate thinness as the ultimate in beauty and virtue!) For example, in a study of percentages of overweight children and adolescents by ethnicity recently released by the Centers for Disease Control, the percentage of overweight teenage males was 11.6 percent for whites, 12.5 percent for African Americans, and 15 percent for Latinos. Their overweight female counterparts comprised these percentages across ethnic lines: 9.6 percent for whites, 16.3 percent for African Americans, and 14 percent for Latinos.

2. *Females quite normally have a higher percentage of body fat as they mature during puberty and, over a lifetime, more body fat than males.* As we saw in Chapter 2, adolescent girls need a certain percentage of body fat for the changes of puberty to even happen. And while both boys and girls gain weight during puberty, boys put

on more muscle tissue while girls put on more fat—usually going from about 8 percent body fat in the pre-puberty years to 21 to 22 percent body fat after the changes of puberty. Striving for much less than that can be harmful. Unfortunately, the media ideal has been to keep women looking like pre-pubescent children. Think about the implications of that. At a time when you're struggling to assert your independence and become your own person, do you *really* want a childlike body?

3. *Before deciding that you're too fat, you need to understand what that means:*

   ✔ *Overweight* means that you weigh more than other people of your sex, height, and body build.
   ✔ *Obese* means that you carry too much fat on your body. It is usually used to describe someone who is more than 20 percent over his or her ideal weight.

An athlete may be overweight, but not overfat, carrying that extra weight in muscle mass. On the other hand, a normal-weight couch potato may have too much body fat due to lack of physical exercise.

How can you tell if your weight may be a problem?

- *See if you can pinch an inch.* Pinch a fold of skin on one side of your waist or on your upper arm. If this fold measures an inch or more, you may have too much body fat.
- *Check your BMI.* BMI stands for *body mass index.* This is a ratio of height to weight. You can determine your BMI by dividing your weight (in pounds) by your height squared (in inches). Multiply the result by 705. Ideally, your BMI should be between 19 and 22 if you want to be healthy and avoid developing heart disease. Those whose BMIs are 25 have a 30

percent higher risk of heart disease, while those with BMI of 26 or higher have an 80 percent increased risk of heart disease as well as a higher risk of developing cancer than those with lower BMIs. Those with a BMI over 30 are at risk for much more immediate health problems.

For example, a girl who is 5'4" (64 inches) would have a BMI of 20 at 116 pounds, 25 at 145 pounds and 30 at 174 pounds. If you want to calculate your own BMI but are feeling a bit mathematically challenged, consult chart 10:

- *Consult your physician.* He or she can plot your weight to see if it's in line with your height, body build, and stage of development. If your doctor finds that you're just a little overweight—ten pounds or less—stepping up your activity level (maybe taking a walk after school instead of watching TV) or starting a new sport or an aerobic exercise program may be all you need to do.

SENSIBLE WEIGHT LOSS

It is better to make slight changes in your lifestyle and eating habits and to lose weight gradually than to go on and off strict diets, losing and regaining the same ten pounds over and over again. By taking your time, you'll have a better chance of reaching and maintaining your best weight.

If you and your doctor determine that your weight problem is serious, you need to take several steps:

FINDING YOUR BMI (BODY MASS INDEX)

Height						Body Weight							
4'10"	91	96	100	105	110	115	119	124	129	134	138	143	148
4'11"	94	99	104	109	114	119	124	128	133	138	143	148	153
5'0"	97	102	107	112	118	123	128	133	138	143	148	153	158
5'1"	100	106	111	116	122	127	132	137	143	148	153	158	164
5'2"	104	109	115	120	126	131	136	142	147	153	158	164	169
5'3"	107	113	118	124	130	135	141	146	152	158	163	169	175
5'4"	110	116	122	128	134	140	145	151	157	163	169	174	180
5'5"	114	120	126	132	138	144	150	156	162	168	174	180	186
5'6"	118	124	130	136	142	148	155	161	167	173	179	186	192
5'7"	121	127	134	140	146	153	159	166	172	178	185	191	197
5'8"	125	131	138	144	151	158	164	171	177	184	190	197	203
5'9"	128	135	142	149	155	162	169	176	182	189	196	203	209
5'10"	132	139	146	153	160	167	174	181	188	195	202	207	215
5'11"	136	143	150	157	165	172	179	186	193	200	208	215	222
6'0"	140	147	154	162	169	177	184	191	199	206	213	221	228
BMI	19	20	21	22	23	24	25	26	27	28	29	30	31

Step One: Examine Your Eating Habits and Behavior

■ *I eat when I'm upset, angry, nervous, or bored or to reward myself.*

Action Plan

1. Find ways to deal with your feelings that do not involve food.
2. Make a list of healthy pleasurable activities you can engage in to reward or comfort yourself.
3. Find more constructive solutions to anger or stress—such as talking, meditating, or exercising.

■ *I skip meals (especially breakfast).* (**Note:** Meal skippers are, as a group, more likely to be obese. This is *not* a good way to control your weight!)

Action Plan

1. Don't skip meals. Eating regular meals is a major step forward in controlling your weight because you never get starved and then lose control and load up on food (and calories) late in the day.
2. Always eat a nutritious breakfast. No time? Get up half an hour earlier. Or grab something portable, such as low-fat yogurt and a piece of fruit.
3. Try the following balance: hearty breakfast, reasonable lunch, and light, early dinner with no big evening snacks. Your weight-loss progress may surprise you!

■ *I'm really busy and don't have time to fix fancy meals and my mom won't make special diet stuff for me. I usually grab . . . whatever.*

Action Plan

1. Eat what your family eats—only watch your portions. Drink a large glass of water half an hour before your meal; this will help you to eat less.
2. Read labels on convenience foods. Many are full of sodium, which doesn't exactly help your weight loss even if the food is low in fat or calories.
3. If you're eating on the run, carry healthy, portable meals and snacks: fresh fruit, raw vegetables, a piece of whole-grain bread, rice cakes, low-fat cheese, yogurt, or a healthy sandwich with vegetables and/or lean meat.
4. If you and your friends are into fast food, refer to Chart 9 to start making some calorie-saving, healthwise choices!

■ *My fat protects me from social situations I find scary.* (**Note:** Fat can be a protective shield against expressing your sexuality or dealing with pressures to be sexual or even to date another person. It's not uncommon for those with a history of sexual trauma to find solace in food rather than risking relationships.)

Action Plan

1. Explore and find ways to solve your fears— write in your journal. Talk with people you trust.
2. If you have trauma in your past, consider getting help from a professional psychotherapist to deal with these troubling feelings.
3. Understand that you can make active choices that protect you without using weight as a shield. You can stand up for yourself and still have friends. You can say no to sex and still have a social life. You can learn to handle pressures and stress. When you use fat to protect you from these, you may also miss a lot of fun.

■ *I watch TV a lot and never exercise.* (**Note:** If you want to control your weight and build a healthy lifestyle, you *must* exercise regularly.)

Action Plan

1. Start moving in small but significant ways: Walk instead of riding or driving whenever you can. Take stairs instead of elevators and escalators. Volunteer to walk the dog.
2. Rediscover old pleasures: Get that old bike out of the garage and ride it; swim laps; walk with friends or family or by yourself (this can be a time to think, plan, and dream).
3. Learn a new sport you enjoy—or find one you hate the least and give it a try. You may be pleasantly surprised.
4. Realize that even very moderate exercise can bring wonderful benefits. You don't have to jog five miles a day, seven days a week to improve your fitness (in fact, we'd advise against such a grueling regimen, especially for a beginner!). A half-hour walk three to five times a week will make a positive difference in your life and your health—especially if, until now, you've been immobilized in front of the television set most afternoons or evenings.

■ *I am rebelling against someone.* (**Note:** It's quite common for someone whose parents are really into thinness and/or popularity, looks, and so on to rebel by getting fat. A Harvard research project showed that the obese women studied tended to have mothers who pushed them to succeed at everything and who equated thinness as a moral virtue and being fat as the worst possible fate.)

Action Plan

1. There are other ways to be unique and to stand up to your parents. You don't have to fight them with your body—in a way that hurts you.

2. Work on asserting yourself more often. Tell your parents what you think and how you're feeling.

3. Express your uniqueness through conversation, creative hobbies, journal writing, or other activities you enjoy.

4. If your family conflicts feel impossible to resolve, ask your parents about the possibility of family therapy so that you all can learn to communicate better and work better together as a family.

Step Two: Be a Smart Diet Consumer!

Many people seek miracles to lose weight: magic pills, instant diets that let you eat all you want while the pounds melt off, and weight loss while you sleep. If it sounds too good to be true, it probably is. In search of weight-loss miracles, too many people endanger both their bank accounts and their health.

Learn to be skeptical of outrageous claims. Face it: You can't melt off body fat overnight or lose 20 pounds in 72 hours or have a lasting weight loss with no effort on your part.

- *Fact: There are no miracles.* Avoid quick fixes and magic pills. They don't work—and aren't good for you. A slow, steady weight loss—no more than two pounds per week—is best for your health, and the best way to achieve it is with a well-balanced diet and exercise plan.

- *Fact: Old-style diets don't work.* Dieting, especially dieting without exercise, doesn't help you lose weight and keep it off. You may lose weight initially, but are likely to regain it quickly. The deprivation of an old-style diet can trigger binge eating. The body will also adapt to lower calorie levels and begin to store fat

and maintain weight at progressively lower calorie intakes. Dieting keeps you on the lose-gain weight roller coaster.

- *Fact: Weight control takes effort and sensible action.*

1. Plan well-balanced food choices that do not eliminate any of the basic food groups.

2. Follow a regular exercise program.

3. Make the commitment to eat well and exercise and just hang in there long-term to see the positive results. (No instant magic, but lots of long-term rewards!)

4. Consult your physician for diet and exercise tips. You might also want to consider the plan shown in Chart 11.

11

GUIDELINES FOR HEALTHY WEIGHT LOSS

Courtesy of Dept. of Nutritional Services, Kaiser Permanente Medical Group, San Francisco

Food Group	Daily Servings	One-Serving Examples
Protein	2	2 eggs
		2–3 oz. poultry, fish, meat
		3–4 oz. tuna
		1 cup beans/lentils
		4 Tbsp. peanut butter
Milk products	4	1 cup yogurt
		2 cups cottage cheese
		1 cup milk
		2 slices cheese
Breads and starches	4	½ cup hot cereal
		¾ cup dry cereal
		1 slice bread
		1 tortilla
		½ hamburger bun
		½ cup rice, noodles, pasta
Fruits and vegetables	4	1 whole fruit
		½ cup fruit juice
		1 cup vegetables

Step Three: If You Can't Do It Alone, Seek Help

You can get help from family, friends, or diet programs such as Weight Watchers, TOPS, or Shapedown. You can also get help from your physician. In fact, you need to consult with your doctor before you start any weight-loss program, especially if it will go on for an extended period of time. You and your physician can determine together the best way for you to lose weight and the minimum number of calories your body needs to lose fat and still be well nourished. You may also find psychotherapy useful if your eating patterns or weight gain have roots in psychological stressors or conflicts.

Step Four: Start Living a Full and Healthy Life Today

You don't have to wait until you're slim to do this. Living fully doesn't have to depend on the shape of your body. There is a lot more to looking good than having a certain body shape or wearing a specific dress or jeans size. And there is much more to value about yourself than your looks. Good health (the result, at least in part, of good nutrition and regular exercise), energy, and a positive outlook on life can make you wonderfully and uniquely attractive.

You *can* have a full and happy life—whatever your weight, whatever your shape. Being enthusiastic is attractive. Being smart is attractive. Being compassionate gives you a very special beauty. You can be the best possible you—starting today—no matter what you weigh.

Making good health (rather than a certain weight) your top priority will help you build a rewarding new lifestyle—starting today!

EATING FOR A GOOD HEALTH

✔ Seven steps to good health are eating a balanced, healthy diet; getting regular exercise; maintaining a healthy weight; not smoking or doing drugs; having regular medical and dental checkups; getting involved in work or activities you love; and developing strong friendships and love relationships.

✔ Some painless ways to cut down or eliminate hazardous foods are drinking mineral water or fruit juice instead of sodas and coffee; trying herbal seasonings instead of salt; eating more fresh fruit and fewer sweet baked goods; eating chicken, fish, and tofu instead of red meat; and choosing fast-food salads, baked potatoes, and nonfried chicken sandwiches instead of burgers.

✔ Weight control tip: Make slight changes in your lifestyle and lose weight gradually. That way you have a better chance of reaching and maintaining your best weight. Strict diets and fad diets are out! They're especially unhealthy for growing teens.

CHAPTER SIX

Exercising for Good Health

I'm overweight and my doctor says I have to exercise as well as eat less to lose the weight. The problem is, I HATE exercise! Is it really something I have to do?

Cory Y.

When you're busy, don't have a lot of money to spend, and/or are embarrassed about your body, it's hard to imagine even doing, let alone enjoying, exercise. If you're a couch potato, you're in the majority. Recent studies have found that preteens and teens today are less fit than ever before. Tightened school budgets that all too often eliminate daily physical education classes are a major factor. So, too, are some of the favorite pursuits of today's teens: watching TV, playing computer games, surfing the Net.

I used to be active as a little kid, but the last few years, I've been so busy with school, dates, and activities that I've stopped exercising much. What can I do that would help me get back in shape and yet not take a lot of time and money?

Megan M.

But if you're active, or open to the idea of becoming more active, you can reap enormous benefits that can far outweigh any investment of time or risk of initial embarrassment about your body or your beginner status in a sport. Exercise is important for everyone: young, old, overweight, underweight, and all those in between.

What's the best kind of exercise program?

YOUR BEST EXERCISE PLAN

1. *Aerobic exercise.* This strengthens your heart and lungs. It includes fast walking, biking, running, swimming, dancing, aerobic dancing, and rowing. You need to exercise for at least 20 minutes three times per week. Aerobic exercise also helps build bones and aids digestion, helping you make the best possible use of vitamins and minerals. It's essential to your good health!
2. *Strengthening exercise.* This helps build muscle and bone mass and tones your muscles. It might include weight lifting, working out on gym equipment, or doing exercises at home such as pushups, abdominal crunches, sit-ups, or leg lifts.
3. *Stretching exercise.* This might be yoga, ballet barre exercises, or simple stretches at home that help you be more flexible.

Exercise can have many additional benefits, beyond helping you lose weight and keep it off and being an important part of building a healthy, strong, flexible body that will serve you well for years to come.

- *Exercise can safeguard your mental health.* Studies show that being physically active increases your self-esteem, improves your body image, and decreases your risk of serious depression. Exercise also helps prevent or reduce anxiety. It can be a great stress reducer and mood enhancer.
- *Exercise can help prevent catastrophic diseases.* It not only protects your heart and lungs, but also can be a factor in preventing certain forms of cancer. For example, studies have found that women who are physically active as teens and young adults significantly reduce their lifetime risk of breast cancer (as well as osteoporosis, the painful and debilitating loss of bone that cripples many women in their later years).

What are the best forms of aerobic exercise? It depends. To reap the benefits of such exercises, you must do them at least three times a week—and four times would be even better. Look at the following list of suggested aerobic activities and ask yourself which one(s) you would like best (or hate least) and would be likely to do on a regular basis. In building physical fitness, consistency is very important.

- *Brisk* walking
- Jogging or running
- Cross-country skiing
- Bicycling—regular or stationary bicycle
- Lap swimming
- Racquetball, handball, squash—if played vigorously
- Jumping rope
- Dancing—including aerobic dance
- Ice skating or roller skating—if vigorous and continuous

Other factors besides immediate preferences may influence your choice of activity. For example:

- *If you're significantly overweight:* Jogging or running may not be a good idea until your weight is closer to normal. Instead, you might try sports such as walking, cycling, and/or swimming.
- *If you want to exercise in private:* Stationary cycling, jumping rope, using one of the new stepping/climbing home exercisers, or exercising to any of a number of excellent aerobic tapes, CDs, or videotapes may be fun for you. Walking can also be a nonthreatening form of public exercise.
- *If you have trouble with motivation:* Join an exercise class at your local Y or youth club, or find a friend or family member with whom you can exercise regularly. A vigorous walk every day with a special friend or family member can be a great way to get fit and to share some special talking time together too!
- *If you're in very poor physical condition:* Stick to walking and swimming—at least at first.

FOR A SUCCESSFUL START TO YOUR ACTIVE NEW LIFE

- *Check with your physician.* This is especially important if you have an underlying medical problem, but can be helpful, too, in discovering the safest kind of exercise for you. A complete sports physical is especially important if you're going out for team sports, competitive sports such as gymnastics, *or* physically demanding activities such as cheerleading, serious ballet, or other dance training.

  Why does this need to be a complete physical? Because where you are in your adolescent development can make a major difference in your bone and muscle growth. A physician needs to determine your physical readiness to take on such challenges and help you plan for an exercise training and nutritional regimen that will maximize your good health and fitness and help you avoid serious injuries.

Your physician may not always tell you what you or your parents want most to hear. For example, if you're tall, but have not developed the muscle mass and strength to match, you may not be ready just yet to compete with more developed peers in a contact sport such as football. Taking time to let your strength build and your body develop may mean a better sports experience later on and a healthier, injury-free body throughout your participation in team sports.

Also, with a thorough sports physical, your physician may be able to spot potential problems and refer you to an orthopedic specialist or physical trainer before a little problem becomes a big one that may threaten your continuing with a sport or continuing to be healthy and fit.

Especially if you're active in a sport that has stringent weight demands—such as wrestling, running, gymnastics, ice skating, or ballet— you need to get regular checkups and advice from your doctor on proper nutrition, eating habits, and health guidelines in general so that you will not lose your good health while pursuing your active interests.

Developing a cooperative relationship with your doctor can mean that you have a special advisor on your team! If injuries happen, it's important to seek medical care right away and to follow your doctor's guidelines for healing before returning to full participation in your sport. Though injury-caused waiting times can be frustrating, taking time to heal properly from a strain, sprain, fracture, or contusion can mean a longer and happier sports experience.

If you have a special medical condition such as diabetes, asthma, or epilepsy, it is very important that you check with your doctor before starting a new sport or stepping up your activity level. Chances are, your medical condition will not keep you from doing what you want to do. However, it's vital, for your maximum benefit, that your condition be well con-trolled. If you have diabetes, you and your doctor need to discuss what additional nutritional needs you may have when you increase your activity level. If you have asthma, a minor adjustment in medication may be necessary when you become more active. And if you have a seizure disorder, your physician will probably advise you against diving, equestrian, or rock-climbing activities (even if your seizures are well controlled by medication) while encouraging other sports activities.

- *Start slow and set realistic goals.* If you've been sedentary for years, you won't become a marathon runner in a week. Instead, you might start your exercise training with brisk walking, followed by several weeks of walking and jogging before you try running full time. Remember: running isn't for everyone. Taking a 30- to-45-minute walk every day may be better for *you*. Do what you like most—but don't try too much, too soon. That's how injuries— and discouragement—happen.

- *Don't torture yourself.* If you make your exercise regimen torture, you'll become a fitness dropout. Make it as easy as possible to do what you need to do. Exercise at a time of day when it is both convenient and comfortable. Avoid the heat of the day and drink liquids as you need them. It's not only OK, but helpful, to drink water while you exercise. And, while you need to exercise vigorously three to four times a week to get maximum benefits, working out more often than that can actually be detrimental to your body. If you allow your muscles 48 hours between workouts to heal, you'll be less prone to injury.

- *Try a fun exercise combination.* This is especially important if you're the type of person who, like many of us, needs to exercise every day in order to keep motivation high. Cut the risk of injury (and boredom) by alternating your activities. Three or four days a week, you might walk or swim or cycle. The other days, you might work out with weights—either with

12

HEALTHY EXERCISE

Exercise	Common Injuries	Prevention
Jogging	Shin splints, strain of Achilles tendon, foot and knee pain	Wear good running shoes with proper cushioning. Warm up and cool down. Run on softer surfaces such as soft track and asphalt rather than concrete. Use proper running technique—flat-foot or heel-toe rather than running on toes.
Walking	Plantar fascitis, blisters	Use proper warm-up and cool-down. Wear good walking shoes with proper cushioning and support. If previously inactive, don't try too far too soon.
In-line Skating	Wrist fractures, facial lacerations, elbow or lower leg fractures, wrist or ankle sprains	Wear protective padding every time! Learn proper techniques for stopping. Keep speed under control especially if you're a beginner.
Bicycling	Head injuries, knee injuries	Wear a protective helmet every time you ride. Change gears—and take stress off your knees.
Snowboarding	Wrist and ankle sprains and fractures, head injuries	GET INSTRUCTION before hitting the slope. Even one lesson will decrease chances of injury. Use proper equipment—helmet and wrist pads.
Skiing	Head injuries, broken bones	Wear a helmet! Use common sense–recklessness on the slope can be deadly. Get good training and be physically fit. If you're tired, stop skiing. Most injuries happen when the skier is fatigued.
Dance/cheerleading	Knee, ankle, and back injuries	Do proper warm-up. Use correct technique. Wear correct, well-fitting shoes. Allow rehab/recovery for injuries before full activity again.
Surfing	Head and spine injuries for body surfers; various injuries from being hit by surfboard for board surfers	BODY SURFERS: Avoid crowded beaches. Do not surf unless waves are breaking in deep water. Arch body with head back while riding wave. When leaving wave, roll to one side—*do not somersault.* BOARD SURFERS: Surf with a companion and try to stay with your board. If you wipe out in deep water, try to fall behind the board, diving deep and staying under for a while. When you come to the surface, protect your head with your arms. For shallow water wipeout, try to fall flat, feet or buttocks first.
Swimming	Middle ear infection if you swim with a cold; swimmer's ear.	Don't swim if you have a cold. Staying out for a few days is better than having to be dry-docked for six weeks with a painful ear infection. Keep your ears clean and dry. If your physician suggests it, use alcohol-based eardrops.
Tennis	Tennis elbow	Best prevention is playing well: power for swings should come from the shoulder, with the forearm used only for control. Try a two-handed backhand. Wear a band just below your elbow to keep the muscles of the forearm from squeezing bone ends.

free weights or on a Universal machine or Nautilus equipment—to exercise a different group of muscles and build upper body strength. Or run or walk outside when the weather is nice and save your indoor cycling, rowing, climbing, or cross-country simulation for days when the climate is less hospitable.

■ *Exercise vigorously enough to reach your target heart rate.* In order to realize the benefits of aerobics, you must sustain the exercise for 20 to 30 minutes and your heart rate must get up to its target level.

ANABOLIC STEROIDS
AND OTHER SPORTS SUPPLEMENTS

- *Anabolic steroids are bad news.* Taking anabolic steroids to build muscle mass or, supposedly, strength, is dangerous—whether you're male or female. These synthetic hormones have *not* been shown to increase strength, though they may increase muscle bulk somewhat. But athletes who build muscles by taking such substances may pay a terrible price: serious liver damage or disease, jaundice, and/or cancer. These drugs can also adversely affect blood cholesterol level. In males, there may be some decrease in size of the testicles and possible infertility. In females, masculine body hair patterns, thinning of the hair on the head, deepening of the voice, and clitoral enlargement may be irreversible even after the use of steroids is discontinued. Also, for those who are still growing while they are taking anabolic steroids, there is the risk of permanent short stature as the hormones cause the long bones to fuse prematurely. Some synthetic hormones, popularly referred to as "brake drugs," have been used in some countries to delay growth and puberty in female gymnasts. Such drugs carry the same risks as other steroids and, furthermore, in closing off the long bones to prevent growth, cause some body distortion and spinal curvature as other parts of the body continue to grow.

- *Don't take amphetamines to enhance sports performance.* Some athletes have used amphetamines to increase endurance, but these drugs, too, exact a price: They mask fatigue limits and may make you risk injury.

- *Say "no" to creatine.* This popular sports nutrition supplement can cause muscle cramping and gastrointestinal problems. Since its long-term impact on athletes is not known at this time, it is best to avoid using this supplement until experts have a better idea of how it helps or hurts not only sports performance, but also long-term health.

- *Be cautious about herbal supplements.* There has been some concern about herbal supplements such as ephedrine. Ephedrine is closely related to the stimulant methamphetamine and can lead to high blood pressure, heart attacks, seizures, and strokes in active young people trying to boost athletic performance. This substance may be found in such products as Herbal Ecstasy and Ripped Fuel.

In sum, these drugs are *never* advisable for athletes. Real strength, skill, and endurance are built only by hard work and commitment.

13 **RX FOR SPORTS INJURIES: RICE**

R = Rest! Stop what you're doing and rest the injured body part.

I = Ice. Apply ice immediately to reduce swelling and internal bleeding. Continue ice treatment for first 24 hours. Crushed ice in plastic bags works best.

C = Compression with an elastic bandage also helps reduce bleeding into the tissues.

E = Elevation. Keeping injured body part elevated may help to reduce swelling.

How do you know what your target level is? Your target heart rate is 70 to 85 percent of your maximum suggested heart rate of 220 minus your age. Generally, someone under 20 years of age would have a maximum heart rate of 200 with a target heart rate range of 140 to 170. To test your heart rate, take your pulse at your wrist or at your neck for six seconds.

Then multiply that number by 10. Ideally, your 6-second heart rate should be between 23 and 28. Multiplied by six, this would put you between 138 to 168 heartbeats per minute—your target heart rate.

■ *Remember the value of warm-ups and cooldowns.* You need to do stretching exercises before any kind of aerobic sport—including

14 **COMMON SPORTS INJURIES**

Injury	What Is It?	Symptoms	Treatment
Strain	Injury to muscle or tendon	Mild aching, stiffness or pain and swelling	RICE
Sprain	Injury to ligaments	Pain, swelling, more pain on movement	RICE—but if severe, see a physician to make sure there is no fracture.
Muscle cramps	Cramping of muscle due to lack of potassium and insufficient warm-up	Pain in affected muscle	Moist heat, pressure and massage of affected area, then slow stretching.
Patellar tendinitis	Inflammation of the patellar (knee) tendon	Pain	As long as the pain is mild, you can keep exercising. If it gets worse, see a physician.
Tennis elbow	Tendinitis in the elbow	Pain	RICE—then see a sports trainer for tips on strengthening injured muscles. See your coach for improvement of technique.
Shin splints	Injured muscles as the result of muscle imbalance: calf muscle much stronger than shin muscle	Pain in front of lower leg	Strengthen shin muscles (running up stairs is a good exercise) and stretch calf muscles by leaning against a wall and stretching the muscles slowly (NO bouncing!).
Plantar fascitis	Tear of fascia covering muscles at bottom of foot	Pain just under heel bone or on bottom of foot	Rest. Then make sure your shoes have proper support.
Achilles tendinitis	Inflammation of Achilles tendon—caused by tight muscles	Pain in area of Achilles tendon (back of ankle/heel)	Stop exercising for several days until the pain stops. Then do slow, gentle stretches to help stretch out the muscles.
Blisters	Caused by friction of ill-fitting shoes	Pain and appearance of blister	Cover with sterile bandage. To prevent: make sure your shoes fit well and are specific to your sport. Also keep your feet dry with foot powder.
Stress fractures	Cracks on the surface area of bones	Pain—especially when you press on the injured area from above or below	Rest so the fracture can heal. Temporarily switch to a non-weight-bearing exercise such as swimming or cycling.

swimming or stationary bicycling or even walking. It's also necessary to allow time to cool down gradually as well. Abrupt starts and stops can lead to injuries or dizziness and other negative feelings during or after exercise. If you warm up, exercise, and cool down properly, this activity should make you feel better and full of new energy instead of worse and more fatigued.

■ *Do what you most enjoy (or hate the least!).* Going into a new exercise program with positive feelings is a must! If the activity is at least somewhat enjoyable, you're more likely to stick with it and make exercise an important part of your life.

EXERCISING FOR—AND IN—GOOD HEALTH

If you're a sports lover or an insecure beginner who has a penchant for getting hurt regularly, this may be a sign that you need to be careful. How can you boost your sports performance without injury?

■ *Warm up properly—and every time!* Failure to warm up properly is a major cause of sports injuries.

■ *Start slowly and build your strength.* Too much too soon causes injuries. Don't go for peak performance your first time out.

■ *Know and admit when you've had enough.* Most sports injuries happen when people are tired and the reflexes, coordination, and judgment slack off.

■ *If you're injured, rest and recover—don't quit!* As you become more physically fit and expert in a sport or activity, you're less likely to be injured. Don't quit. Just rest and recover. Then work to strengthen the affected muscles as you ease back into full activity.

Remember that the better shape you're in, the less likely you will be to suffer injuries—and the more likely you'll be to stay healthy, active, and attractive all your life!

EXERCISING FOR GOOD HEALTH

✔ You need regular aerobic exercise at least three times a week for 30 minutes or longer each time.

✔ Check with your doctor before starting an exercise regimen. Regular sports physicals are especially important if you're in a highly demanding sport such as gymnastics, running, figure skating, or ballet.

✔ A good warm-up and cool-down, the proper equipment, good technique, and common sense are the best safeguards you have against sports injuries.

✔ If you're injured, rest and recover—don't quit the sport!

CHAPTER SEVEN

Good Health and Good Looks

I feel ugly. I hate my zits. My nails break all the time and my hair is gross. I wear dorky glasses because my parents won't let me get contacts. I HATE HOW I LOOK!!! Help!

Michelle A.

This girl at school won't go out with me because she only likes guys who remind her of Leonardo DiCaprio. I can't possibly look like him (and I wouldn't want to . . . can't stand that guy!) and I guess I'm pretty average-looking, but how could I look my best so some girl (maybe not this one) will like me enough to hang around with me?

Austin H.

The secret to being attractive is to feel as good as possible about your strengths and all you have to offer as a person—right now. Then, because you deserve tender loving care, you need to take good care of your body. Good looks come from good health. Head-to-toe attractiveness starts out with a good diet and exercise program. Eating protein, for example, can help your skin stay smooth and your hair grow strong and shiny. Vitamin A, (acquired via diet, *not* extra supplements), is great for healthy skin, and the B vitamins help you have healthy hair.

Cleanliness is important, too. A daily bath or shower—plus extra face cleansings if you, like most young people, have oily skin—helps clear away dirt, oil, and dead cells, preventing the accumulation of bacteria on your skin that can cause body odor.

However, sometimes looking your best is a bit more of a challenge and takes a little more care than just the basics.

HEALTHY SKIN

Skin, not surprisingly, is a number-one concern among teens; acne is the most common skin problem that young people seem to have.

Acne

A recent survey on adolescents and acne that was commissioned by the American Medical Association found that most teens (83 percent of those surveyed) were very concerned about skin appearance and acne, with about a third of these teens saying that they thought zits were the first thing people noticed about them. Some 18 percent reported depression about acne. But only 16 percent had sought help from a doctor, with most (67 percent) using over-the-counter medications that weren't especially effective.

To find appropriate help—or to help yourself—you need to understand how acne happens, its stages, and the best treatments for each stage. You also need to know the truth behind common myths about acne, such as "You'll outgrow it," "Just give up chocolate," or "Just keep clean. Acne comes from dirt." The fact is, untreated severe acne can scar you for life, both physically and, perhaps, emotionally. There is no conclusive evidence that chocolate or any other foods trigger acne. And acne does not come from dirt, though a good cleansing routine can help keep excess oils from accumulating.

So why do some people have severe acne and others have little or none at all?

Heredity, which determines your skin type along with other important characteristics, can have a lot to do with whether or not you have acne. The condition of adolescence, however, seems to be a major factor, too. At this time, there are many changes going on in your body: growth spurts, physical maturation, and a surge—and possible imbalance—of hormones. These hormones—progesterone in girls and testosterone in guys—become part of your lifelong body chemistry. So acne can flare up at any time later in life, too. But it seems most common in adolescence. Acne may be a problem for you for a short time—a year or so—or for a number of years.

How do your hormones trigger acne?

As hormone levels increase, the oil, or sebaceous, glands (which are quite numerous on your face, shoulders, chest, and back) become more active, producing a fatty substance called *sebum*. This sebum travels from the gland to the pore (opening of the skin) and produces the oily skin so common in teens. If this passageway becomes blocked with sebum, the first step of acne—blackheads—may develop. Blackheads are black, *not* from dirt, but from oxidation of sebum and skin pigments in the pore.

If these blackheads are not removed, the sebum continues to fill in the duct of the gland, pressure will build, and bacteria may invade the area. The resulting infection may cause red papules and pustules (filled with pus), which we most often call *zits* or *pimples*. In more serious cases of acne, these may progress to cysts and subsequent scarring.

Can washing your face and other affected areas help prevent acne progression?

It certainly can. Removing oil from the skin surface and keeping pores open through cleansing with ordinary or antibacterial soap two or three times daily is the first step. Frequent shampoos—to keep oily, greasy hair from adding oil to the affected areas—may also be helpful. In mild cases of acne, some over-the-counter acne lotions and creams may aid drying of the skin.

If you're female and wear makeup, be very careful about the makeup you use. Oil-based makeup will only clog your pores more. However, a non-oily and/or medicated makeup that may even have astringent qualities can be helpful.

If you're troubled by acne on your back, a shower once or twice daily with antibacterial and abrasive soap, using a back brush to scrub the back thoroughly, may help, too.

If you have blackheads, a pulverized soap may help to remove the blackheads and open the pores, but do be careful! These soaps are abrasive to the skin, so don't use them more than once or twice a day. Wash your face in hot water and rinse with cold water to help close the pores again. You may even wish to swab your skin with an alcohol-soaked pad after washing to help remove the last trace of oil and dirt. Used in moderation, alcohol is a good astringent. If your skin starts to feel dry, however, you may be using too much, depleting your skin's natural oils.

Washing isn't always enough, however, since sebum and blackheads start below the skin surface. Blackheads may be removed with a device called a *comedo extractor*. When used correctly, this device can be very effective in removing blackheads (also called *comedones*). When applied over the blackhead, this device exerts uniform pressure, expelling the blackhead and thus removing the oil duct blockage. This extractor works well and does not leave scarring, which might happen if you pick at a blackhead with your fingertips. Although the area around the blackhead may be a little red (from the pressure) right after removal, this will fade quickly.

Your physician may use a comedo extractor to remove blackheads for you, or you can learn to do it yourself. You can buy a comedo extractor at a surgical supply store (easy to find in most large cities) or, in some instances, at a drugstore or pharmacy.

We'd like to emphasize that a comedo extractor is useful for *blackheads only!* When the blackhead becomes infected and turns into the classic red bump we usually call a pimple, the comedo extractor will do more harm than good. At this stage, exerting pressure could damage the skin and cause scarring. So don't use this device for pimples *and* don't pick at or squeeze your pimples in any way!

Several conditions may aggravate acne. *Fluctuating hormone levels*, present just before a woman's menstrual period, cause increased oil production and the chance of an acne flare-up. *Stress*, which may be present before an important event, may also be a predisposing factor. While there is no absolute scientific proof that this is so, such ill-timed pimple attacks are seen by many doctors and suffered by many teens. While sunlight combined with dry heat may help to dry out oily skin, *hot, humid weather*—like that in Hawaii or Florida or in most of the United States during the summer—can aggravate acne. *Salt water* may also aggravate acne. If you're a beach lover, but find that you seem to break out more after a dip in the sea, try washing your face and showering with fresh water right after you finish swimming.

As you may have noticed from looking around at your friends as well as from your own experience, acne can range from mild to severe. Where are you in this scenario—and what can you do about it? The following chart may help.

As you can see from the chart, there are several ways your physician can work with you to control stubborn or severe acne. The following are among the most current treatments:

Prescription Gels and Lotions

These include a particularly effective benzoyl peroxide gel and various antibiotic lotions that combat acne by suppressing follicle bacteria. In the past, acne patients often took antibiotic pills (for example, tetracycline) to help clear up acne lesions. While many still do take oral medications, topical antibiotics, which penetrate to the follicles,

15
STAGES AND TREATMENT OF ACNE

Stage	Symptom	Recommended Treatment
One	Blackheads	• Wash once a day with pulverized soap. • Over-the-counter or prescription medications containing benzoyl peroxide 5–10% once a day. • Comedo extractor (buy from pharmacy). Use on blackheads *only*.
Two	Blackheads and pimples	• See your physician. • Use benzoyl peroxide 5 or 10% twice a day. • Prescription topical antibiotics twice a day. • Retin-A if your acne is severe or resistant.
Three	Pustules	• Benzoyl peroxide 10% twice a day OR benzoyl peroxide 10% in morning and Retin-A 0.05 at night (if physician recommends this regimen). • Oral antibiotics such as tetracycline (used only if there is no response to topical medication). • Birth control pills (females only; also only if not responsive to topical forms of treatment).
Four	Severe, cystic acne	• Try all of the above. • Discuss use of Accutane and possible referral to a pediatric dermatologist with your physician. *Please note*: Accutane should only be taken when acne does not respond to any other form of treatment. If you take Accutane and are female, you *must* avoid pregnancy while taking this drug, as it can cause severe birth defects.

have become quite popular in the past few years. The most widely used include clindamycin lotions (called Cleocin T) and an erythromycin lotion.

Retin-A, a vitamin A acid, has been used as an effective topical medication, but its use lately has become somewhat controversial since many physicians have found that it can cause a lot of skin irritation. If you use Retin-A, be sure to wash your face first with a very gentle cleanser, then wait about half an hour before you apply Retin-A. Spread it evenly over your face, avoiding areas right around the eyes, nose, and corners of the mouth. *Don't* be tempted to spot-treat blemishes with it. Extra Retin-A won't make the zits go away sooner; it could simply irritate your skin. Be sure to pamper your skin during treatment, wearing a sunscreen and a moisturizer to protect your face from the elements.

Oral Medications

The most common of these is tetracycline. This can be used alone or in combination with topical medications. However, because of possible side effects from oral medication, this is generally used only when a person's acne does not respond to treatment with topical antibiotics.

If you're female and your acne doesn't respond to any of the above treatments, your physician may prescribe birth control pills, which have been approved by the FDA to treat acne as well as to prevent pregnancy. Hormones, as we have seen, *do* exert a strong influence on acne. The hormone estrogen, which birth control pills have always contained, seems to suppress oil gland secretions and, in the process, may help to control acne.

For those with *severe, cystic* acne that has resisted other forms of treatment, there is an oral prescription drug called Accutane (13-*cis*-retinoic acid). This powerful drug should be used only in severe cases and then only under the direct supervision of a dermatologist.

Accutane treatment, which involves taking a pill daily, lasts eight weeks, followed by an eight-week rest period and then continuation of the drug for

another eight weeks, if necessary. Studies indicate that many patients continue to improve after the medication has been stopped.

The drug does have side effects—most commonly, severe drying and chapping of the lips. This occurred in most patients tested. A smaller number also experienced some rise in their cholesterol levels. And there have been some recent cases of teens on Accutane who have episodes of depression, psychosis, or suicidal behavior. (If you're taking this medication and begin to feel depressed, let your doctor know right away.) More significantly, medical experts say that the drug cannot be given to a woman who is pregnant or who has a possibility of becoming pregnant during the treatment, since 13-*cis*-RA is in a class of chemicals known to cause quite devastating birth defects.

If you and your doctor feel that this drug treatment is your best alternative *and* you are sexually active, it is crucially important that you use TWO *very* reliable birth control methods during your course of treatment.

Eczema

I'm a 15-year-old girl who has bad eczema. I've had this for a long time. How can I get rid of it?

Desperate

Eczema is a chronic skin allergy and, like many allergies, there is no sure cure; however, there are ways to control it. Treatment with steroid creams to control the inflammation and itching may help a lot, but this is available by prescription only, so check with your physician.

Psoriasis

I have these awful patches that hurt and itch and have white scales on them. My mom thinks it's psoriasis and made a doctor's appointment for me. My friends think it's gross and won't be around me. How soon can I get rid of this?

Jessica S.

Psoriasis is a very common chronic skin disorder that usually first appears between ages 15 and 35. It is caused by too-rapid skin cell growth. Cells build up on the skin surface with resulting swelling, redness, scaliness, and discomfort (either pain or itching). It's like having hyperactive skin! Parts of the body most likely to be affected are the hands, feet, knees, elbows, and scalp.

Psoriasis is not contagious, nor is it necessarily an inherited condition. While one in three people with psoriasis do have a family history of it, many more do not. And while this condition is not curable, medication can control it and clear it up for varying amounts of time. Your physician will work with you to determine what treatment regimen will be best for you. If you have just a few lesions, he or she might suggest using moisturizers and, possibly, a prescription topical medication, such as low- to medium-potency steroids for a short period of time. (Long-term use of steroids is not suggested due to possible side effects.) There are other types of topical prescription medications—such as vitamin D-3 (not the same as vitamin D sold over the counter), coal tar, or, in severe cases, anthralin.

Your physician may also suggest light treatments—from natural sunlight to ultraviolet light (UVB) treatments—which can bring some relief. In severe cases, a short treatment of UVB combined with an oral medication may be used.

The emotional impact of this disorder can be at least as painful as the lesions. You may feel very much alone at times. It's important to share your feelings with those who love you—and you may also find reassurance via a pen pal match with another teen with psoriasis. If you're interested in getting a pen pal (or special information about this disorder), write to the National Psoriasis Foundation, 6600 S.W. 92nd Ave., Suite 300, Portland, OR 97223-7195 or call (800) 723-9166.

Warts

What causes warts? Are they contagious? My boyfriend has a wart on his hand and I'm almost afraid to hold hands with him.

Shelly

Warts are caused by a virus and come in many varieties. Some, like venereal warts, which occur around the genitals, are quite contagious. Others, such as those occurring on the arms, legs, hands, and feet, are usually not contagious. There is a great deal of speculation about how one gets these warts. We do know that warts are caused by a virus—not by frogs, as the old myth goes—but beyond that, we have very little conclusive evidence about what exactly causes this virus to happen in some people.

Some warts on the hand can be treated at home with topical application of an over-the-counter preparation such as Compound W. This type of treatment usually requires persistence and repeated applications, however, so don't get discouraged if your warts don't disappear on the first try.

If your warts seem immune to nonprescription preparations, your physician may be able to help in several ways. He or she may remove the warts via electrocautery (burning off the warts with electrical heat), topical application of certain prescription medications, liquid nitrogen (which turns warts white, "freezing" them and causing them to die and eventually fall off), or even a systemic approach, using vaccines to remove and prevent recurrence of the warts.

Another kind of wart is something else altogether: the *plantar wart*. This type of wart, usually found on the sole of the foot, is not raised like most other warts, but burrows deep into the skin. This wart, which may be very painful, is also caused by a virus, which may be picked up by a minor break in the skin at places like gym shower rooms.

Plantar warts should *not* be treated with home remedies. If the wart is not particularly painful and does not appear to be multiplying, some physicians prefer to leave it alone. These warts will often disappear in a month or so when the body begins to reject the wart. However, if the wart is painful and/or starts to multiply, the physician may remove it with liquid nitrogen or by treatment with an acid solution.

Moles

I have several moles on my neck and chest. Are they dangerous in any way? Should I have them removed?

Don R.

Moles, medically termed *nevi*, are very common in all age groups. Basically, a mole is an area of the skin where there is a heavy concentration of the skin pigment *melanin*. Generally, moles are harmless, though in some instances and locations, they may be cosmetically unappealing.

If you have a mole that begins to enlarge or change in color, however, this is reason for concern. This could be a symptom of a rare but serious condition called *malignant melanoma*, a cancer that can kill young people as well as older ones—and can do so rather quickly without prompt treatment. So if you notice any changes in a mole, do see your doctor.

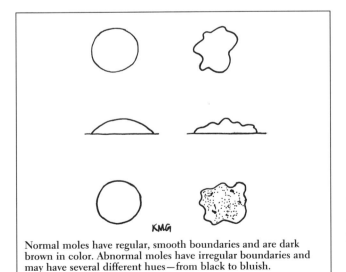

Normal moles have regular, smooth boundaries and are dark brown in color. Abnormal moles have irregular boundaries and may have several different hues—from black to bluish.

Moles—Normal and Abnormal

If you elect to have your moles removed for cosmetic or other reasons, see a dermatologist or a plastic surgeon.

A Sun-Lover's Guide to Protecting Your Skin

I practically live on the beach in the summer and love to get deep tans. I've read some stuff, though, about too much tanning making you wrinkle like a prune before you're even old and that you might even get skin cancer. I hate to think about giving up my tans. Is any of this stuff true?

Mary B.

Yes—unfortunately, it *is* true that your skin can age prematurely or that you can get skin cancer, often at quite a young age, by overexposure to the sun. Malignant melanoma, the deadliest form of skin cancer, was diagnosed in some 40,000 people in 1997 (the last year in which statistics were available) and there were 7,300 deaths from the disease.

Those most at risk for sun-related skin cancer (or skin damage) are:

- Those with fair skin and light hair and eye color.
- Those with a family history of melanoma.
- Those with unusual or changing moles on the skin.
- Those with painful or blistering sunburns in childhood or during adolescence.
- Those who spend their recreational time outdoors.

If you, like many young people, practically live outdoors in the summer, here are some common-sense tips that may help minimize skin damage from the sun:

- *Use a sunscreen.* This applies to everyone, especially to those with fair complexions. Use a sunscreen with the highest sun protection factor you can find. Look for a "broad spectrum" sunscreen that helps to block both ultraviolet A and B (UVA and UVB) radiation.

Apply your sunscreen before going outside. Once you are out, perspiration may dilute the sunscreen and prevent some of the sun-blocking ingredients from penetrating your skin. Reapply the sunscreen occasionally while you are out.

- *Protect your lips.* Use a special lip sunscreen that applies like lipstick.
- *Realize that sunscreen can't do it all.* It offers protection, but it doesn't make you free to roast yourself for six hours in the midday sun in search of a perfect tan.
- *Shun the sun in high-intensity hours.* Avoid direct sunbathing or prolonged sun exposure between the hours of 10 A.M. and 2 P.M., when the sun's rays are most powerful and direct. If you must be in the sun at this time, wear sunscreen and protective clothing. Take refuge under a beach umbrella or in the shade of a tree.

    If you're swimming, remember that water is no protection. It admits the sun's rays, too. In fact, wet skin is more receptive to ultraviolet rays than dry skin, so apply a sunscreen before swimming *and* after you get out of the pool or the surf.
- *Take care to protect the most vulnerable parts of your body.* Your nose, ears, lips, knees, and shoulders are more exposed and will burn faster than other parts of your body, so give these extra protection. Be sure to apply sunscreen, too, to the areas often forgotten (until a painful sunburn reminds you!): your ankles, the tops of your feet, the tops of your ears, and the back of your neck.
- *Dress for maximum protection.* Don't use a sheer, gauzy cover-up when you're at the beach. Ultraviolet rays penetrate these fabrics easily. A long-sleeved, dark-colored shirt or coverup is better. Best of all would be clothing that is specifically made to block harmful rays: tightly woven fabrics that have specific SPF ratings (and are sold in sporting-goods stores or in specialty catalogs). Also, wear a hat with a four-inch brim to give your nose (the most common site for skin cancer) some extra protection.
- *Remember that weather is no protection.* You can burn as easily on a cloudy day as a sunny one, so use that sunscreen even when clouds or haze hover over the beach!
- *Your ethnicity doesn't make you immune to sun damage.* Black or other dark skin can burn, though not as easily as lighter skin. While whites have 20 times greater risk of getting skin cancer than do African Americans, *everyone* needs to be cautious and use sunscreen.

If all of this sounds a tad sun-phobic (not to mention totally geeky), remember that we're talking to you from a health-oriented (rather than fun- and fashion-oriented) point of view. However, protecting yourself doesn't mean that you have to become a creature of the night, forgoing any fun in the sun or any kind of cool clothing. Just be as careful as you can.

Why are we going on so about skin cancer? Because studies have found that malignant melanoma has its origins in these early years. What happens to your skin *now*, when you're in your teens, can have a major impact on your health in later years—or maybe even a few years down the road. (Sandi, a close high school friend of Kathy's, was a blue-eyed, blond sun-lover who spent all her free time at the beach in search of the perfect tan. She developed malignant melanoma when she was in her early twenties and, despite extensive medical treatment, died while still a young woman.)

Other, less serious types of skin cancer can result from prolonged sun exposure over a lifetime. These are more easily treated than melanoma and have a lower fatality rate (1 percent compared to about 25 percent among those with melanoma). But for optimal health and peace of mind, it simply makes sense to try avoiding such problems altogether.

Prolonged sun exposure can also make you look old long before your time. Damage to the elastic fibers of the skin by overexposure to the sun can cause wrinkles. These fibers, which keep the skin soft and elastic, cannot function well if damaged; this may lead to wrinkled, saggy, leathery skin at a fairly early age. You may find yourself at 35 looking like you're 70!

I'd like to get a sun lamp with a timer for safety. Could it still hurt my skin? I really would like to have a year-round tan.

Sunny

We do not recommend either sun lamps or tanning salons. The risks to your skin are simply too great. Tanned skin is, essentially, damaged skin and, as we pointed out earlier, can make you look old and leathery well before your time. In the more immediate future, sun lamps can give you a nasty burn if you spend too much time under them (usually by falling asleep and forgetting to set or not hearing the timer).

We recommend that, for your best health and lifetime good looks, you avoid tans both of the indoor and outdoor variety!

HEALTHY FEET, NAILS, AND HAIR

Feet

Some of the most common foot problems, their causes and treatments are listed in the following chart.

16 TLC FOR COMMON FOOT PROBLEMS

Problem	Cause	TLC Solution
Blisters	Rubbing, friction	• Buy shoes that fit. • Wear socks (preferably synthetics). • Put Vaseline or a sports lotion on area likely to rub or blister.
Bunions	Ill-fitting shoes; can also be hereditary	• Buy shoes that fit comfortably. Avoid narrow, tapered styles. • Use orthotic inserts in your shoes. • If bunions are painful, use ice and elevation to alleviate pain and swelling.
Corns	Ill-fitting shoes; can also be hereditary	• Buy well-fitting, comfortable shoes. • Soak and moisturize your feet daily. • Use over-the-counter corn pads (such as Dr. Scholl's OneStep). • If you have diabetes, discuss foot care with your doctor before using any over-the-counter corn pads.
Fungus (athlete's foot)	Going barefoot in moist, warm environments such as gym showers or pool decks	• Avoid going barefoot in public showers and on poolsides. Use shower sandals or other shoes designed for use in water. • Treat with over-the-counter antifungal powder or cream. • See your doctor for prescription treatments if the above doesn't help.
Hammertoes	Hereditary; can also be caused by shoes that put pressure on toes (too small, very high heels, ballet toe shoes, etc.)	• Wear shoes that fit comfortably and do not put pressure on toes. • See your doctor about surgery if your case is severe.
Ingrown toenails	Too much clipping and/or tight shoes	• Soak and dry feet, use only toenail clippers, and file nails straight across. • Use antibacterial ointment to avoid nail fungus infection. • Wear sandals with open toes whenever you can. • See your doctor if the problem is severe.
Toenail fungus	Injury to nail and/or too much clipping	• If over-the-counter antifungal medications don't work, see your physician for prescription oral medications.
Smelly feet	Heredity; wearing shoes without socks; wearing nylon stockings for long hours	• Wash and dry your feet thoroughly at least once a day. • Wear socks (preferably synthetic). • Use deodorant foot powder or cream or deodorant spray on feet. • Soak feet in warm tea.

Three Rules for Happy Feet

1. Wear shoes that fit your foot comfortably. Shop for shoes in the afternoon, when your feet tend to be bigger.
2. Bathe and powder your feet every day.
3. Use common sense. Avoid certain types of shoes: very high heels or platform shoes, which can cause ankle-spraining (or ankle-breaking) injuries; flats without adequate arch supports; and tight-fitting boots that may restrict blood circulation in your legs. Your best bet: comfortable, well-fitting shoes with a slight heel.

Nails

My fingernails are flaky and chip easily. Would drinking gelatin help? I want to have pretty nails like everyone else.

Bethany

If your nails are brittle and chip a lot, analyze your habits. Do you have nervous mannerisms, such as drumming them, or picking or biting them? All of these can retard nail growth and cause chips, spots, and pits in the nail. So can a fungal infection or poor circulation. If there seems to be a skin infection involved, you may want to visit your doctor for treatment. If there is no infection involved, you might try soaking your nails in a combination of water and gelatin for temporary hardening—or use one of the nail hardeners-lacquers available at your local drug or department store.

I've been using artificial fingernails over my own nails, but I've noticed lately that my own nails are getting separated from the skin and really look gross. What's wrong?

Jill

You may have *onycholysis*, a condition usually caused by a fungal or bacterial infection or by an allergic reaction to the glue used on fingernails. Stop using the artificial nails (and the glue) immediately and see your doctor. Usually, removing the cause of infection will cure the problem and the nails will grow back.

Hair

I have oily hair and like to wash it every day. My mother objects because she thinks I'll lose all my hair. I have acne, too, so feel it's especially important to keep my hair clean. Am I right?

Chrissy

It's a good idea to wash oily hair every day if desired, not only to keep from aggravating any acne that may be present on the face or back, but also to stimulate the scalp. This stimulation, in combination with a mild shampoo, may actually enhance hair growth by stimulating the hair follicles and the scalp's natural oils.

Recently when I shampoo my hair, I lose more hair than usual. Is something horrible wrong with me?

Worried

It's normal to lose some amount of hair every day. Hair follicles have distinct cycles, involving active growth of hair followed by shrinkage of the follicle and then rest. After producing hair for several years, a follicle may shed its hair and rest for a few months. This is occurring on a constant basis with the countless hair follicles on your head.

Some factors can trigger some of the hair follicles to take an unscheduled rest and shed hair: bodily upsets such as stringent dieting (as with anorexia nervosa) or severe illness; certain anti-cancer drugs; infection of the scalp (which can be caused by allergies to a hair product such as shampoo, conditioner, or a hair-coloring agent); and hormonal changes brought about by thyroid abnormalities, some birth control pills, or pregnancy.

My hair is dull and looks faded. How can I make it look shiny?

Carla A.

There are a number of reasons for dull-looking hair. A buildup of dirt or hair products (like conditioner or hair spray) on the hair can make it look dull. So can a residue of shampoo if you don't rinse your hair thoroughly after washing it. Frequent shampoos—possibly with a protein shampoo product—may help make your hair shine.

As we have discussed, your diet is extremely important to your looks. Dull hair may be an indication that you lack vitamin B-12 and could use some more lean meats, fish, eggs, milk, and liver to start feeling—and looking—your best.

HEALTHY EYES

Your eyes, too, can be a reflection of your general health. A specially trained physician may be able to see symptoms of diabetes, liver disease, or high blood pressure—to name a few disorders—while examining your eyes. Your vision may also have a huge impact on how you do in school. If you suffer from headaches after reading or find it hard to keep your place while studying, you should get your eyes checked. But whether or not you experience any troublesome symptoms, periodic eye examinations are advisable.

Who are the professionals who do eye exams? An *ophthalmologist* is an M.D.—a physician—whose specialty is diagnosing and treating diseases and defects of the eye. He or she performs surgery when necessary. An *optometrist* is not a physician, but has a Doctor of Optometry degree (O.D.) and is highly trained and licensed by the state to diagnose eye problems and diseases. He or she may prescribe glasses, contacts, or other optical aids. An *optician* is the technician who grinds lenses, fits them into frames, and then adjusts these frames to each individual.

If you go to an ophthalmologist, he or she may refer you to an optometrist or an optician for glasses or, if you desire, contact lenses.

■ ■ ■

Contacts

I wear glasses now, but would really like contacts. My girlfriend says that the new soft contacts are great. Are they really good? Are they better to have than hard contacts?

Tom

There are many different types of contacts available now: hard lenses, gas-permeable hard lenses (these let more oxygen reach the eye than traditional hard lenses), hard/soft combination lenses (still very new, these have a hard middle and are soft around the edges, and can be a bit difficult to handle), and soft lenses (more comfortable, in general, than hard lenses, but less durable; they may not give adequate vision correction to all forms of vision defects). In the soft-lens category, there are, besides the lenses you take out and put in every day, extended-wear contacts (which, supposedly, you can leave in for up to two weeks at a time, but which for best care of your eyes and the lenses should be removed once or twice a week for cleaning). There are also colored lenses that can make even very dark eyes a different color—and correct your vision at the same time!

How safe are extended wear contacts—the ones you can wear for two weeks at a time? They sound great!

Jamie T.

There is no one kind of contact lens that is right for everyone. Check with your doctor to see which type may be right for you and your special vision problem.

My best friend and I both wear contacts. She wets hers by putting them in her mouth. She says it's perfectly OK to do. But I heard it's not good. Who's right?

Amy L.

Amy is right. Placing your lenses in your mouth may spread infection. It is also not advisable to clean your lenses in tap water, according to a new warning from the American Academy of Ophthalmologists. Cleaning your lenses in tap water puts you at risk of getting an eye infection called *acanthamoeba keratitis*, which can cause blindness. Distilled water isn't completely sterile and shouldn't be used either. Clean your lenses in sterile saline solution *only!*

Other practices to be avoided: rubbing your eyes with contacts in, wearing them too long or, if you don't have extended-wear lenses, sleeping with your contacts in place. If you're careless, your eyes could suffer serious irritations.

Eye Surgery

I've heard about an operation that stops nearsightedness and makes your vision normal without glasses or contacts. I'm really interested. Could you tell me more about this?

Brian K.

There are several laser surgeries including LASIK and PRK (Photo Refractive Keratotomy). Both treatments involve using a laser on the cornea to remove and then refold layers of corneal tissue to get the corrective angle.

However, these procedures are generally not recommended until early adulthood. The minimum age at which a physician will consider accepting a patient for this treatment is usually 21. These procedures are also quite expensive, running about $4,000 total for both eyes.

At this point, we would recommend putting up with your glasses or contacts for a few years more until you're 21 or until more is known about the long-term advantages or disadvantages of these procedures.

Caring for Your Eyes

I have normal, good eyesight, but my eyes get bloodshot and water sometimes. Why does this happen?

Alex G.

Bloodshot, tearing eyes can be the result of several possibilities—allergies, eye strain, and pollution being the most likely. Washing the eyes with water may help. If you have a chronic problem involving allergies, an eye preparation such as Visine may help. However, if the problem is severe or chronic, see a physician.

Is it true that you're not supposed to wash just under your eyes? Someone told me that and I just can't believe it. Why should that be true?

Bev W.

It's *half* true. The skin around the eye is very delicate, should not be scrubbed, and needs to be moisturized regularly. However, you can clean the area and remove eye makeup with a cleansing cream or a special makeup remover made just for the delicate eye area.

For some time, the white parts of my eyes have had a slight yellowish color. Could this be serious?

Worried

A condition like this—called *icterus*—may or may not be serious, but it's certainly worth checking with your physician. Icterus may be a sign of a liver disease, such as infectious hepatitis. Then, too, it may mean nothing. There are some entirely healthy people who may have slightly icteric eyes. However, only your physician can tell whether this condition is normal for you or whether it is a symptom of a serious health problem.

HEALTHY TEETH AND GUMS

Help! I have bad breath and nothing, even mouthwash, does any good! What's the matter with me anyway?

Embarrassed

What causes bad breath? Persistent bad breath can be a symptom of indigestion or one of a number of diseases. However, it is often caused by decaying teeth and/or a gum problem.

Many people, young and old alike, worry about bad breath and the social problems it may cause, and try to mask the symptom rather than to cure the underlying causes by seeking dental help.

Your teeth and gums are an intrinsic part of your total health. Too many young people seem to be ignoring this fact. Among the statistics compiled by the American Dental Association, one in particular stands out: Fifty percent of young people age 15 and younger have *never* been to a dentist.

Your dental health is an important part of your total health and can be an important barometer of your body's health—or lack of it. Decayed teeth and tender gums can serve as early warning signals that what you're doing—especially what you may be eating—is not good for your body. And dental problems are widespread among young people. The ages of 13 to 16 are particularly cavity-prone years.

Teens in this age group can be especially likely to get cavities because these are busy years: You're always on the go, often eating on the run. You may not be taking time to clean your teeth properly. Also, you may be eating a lot of junk food or convenience food that may be laced with sugar. Neglect plus sugar can equal a buildup of *plaque* on the teeth.

What *is* plaque? It is a film of harmful oral bacteria that forms on the teeth. Combined with sugar, certain bacteria in the plaque form acids that attack tooth enamel, leading to decay and, even worse, to gum disease. Although you can remove some of this plaque by brushing and flossing your teeth twice daily, regular visits to a dentist for a more thorough cleaning are essential to remove plaque from the hard-to-reach areas on your teeth. Too often, people put off going to a dentist until an emergency—such as a toothache—hits. But good preventive care can keep such painful emergencies from happening.

Although tooth decay is extremely common in young people (it is estimated that by age 17, the average young American has nine decayed, filled, or missing teeth), the possibility of gum disease causes the most concern among dentists. Gum disease, also called *periodontal disease*, is what usually makes people lose their teeth later on in life. A third of all Americans have no natural teeth left at all by age 60. Sixty may seem a long way away, but the damage can start now.

The damage caused by gum disease may not be just to your teeth, but also to your health in general. Researchers have found a link between gum disease and serious conditions such as heart disease, heart valve damage, stroke, and, in mothers who have gum disease, a greater possibility of giving birth to a premature baby.

Periodontal (Gum) Disease and Its Prevention

I have had a problem with my gums bleeding when I brush my teeth for a couple of months now. Is this serious or not? If it matters, I'm 14.

Allen

Periodontal disease—or advanced gum disease—is seen most often in adults, but teenagers can show signs of the early stage, called *gingivitis*.

During a visit to my dentist, I found out I had gum disease. My parents think that sounds strange, since they say that usually happens to older people. Can someone who is 15 have gum disease?

Lisa R.

What is this and why does it happen? Irritating poisons and enzymes, produced by the bacteria that grow in plaque, invade the area below the gum line and can cause your gums to become inflamed and to bleed slightly during brushing. This "pink toothbrush" symptom is the most common sign of gingivitis. Other symptoms are gums that are swollen and inflamed.

What happens in more advanced gum disease? The plaque on the teeth, extending below the gum line,

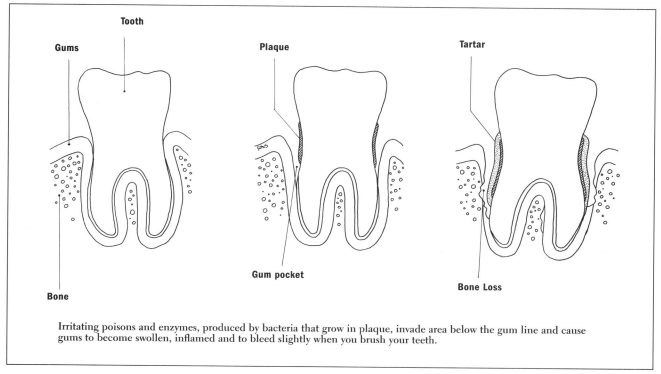

Irritating poisons and enzymes, produced by bacteria that grow in plaque, invade area below the gum line and cause gums to become swollen, inflamed and to bleed slightly when you brush your teeth.

Gingivitis

starts to harden, building up into a substance called *calculus*. This causes even more irritation of the gums, and eventually the gums begin to separate from the teeth. Bacteria begin to fill the spaces in between and attack the gums and the bone structure that supports the teeth, causing the teeth to loosen and, possibly, to be lost.

Four Steps to Healthy Teeth and Gums

1. *Visit your dentist at least once a year.* Twice a year for a professional cleaning and checkup is even better during these cavity-prone years.

2. *Brush your teeth at least twice a day.* Most dentists recommend brushing at least twice a day (and rinsing your mouth after eating in between). Use a soft-bristled toothbrush, and check it carefully for signs of wear. A toothbrush full of loose and bent bristles isn't going to do you much good. Plan to replace yours every one to three months.

   In brushing your teeth, it's important to be thorough, covering the teeth and the gum line with a gentle, circular motion, and to follow up the brushing with dental floss, to reach the cavity-prone areas between the teeth where your toothbrush can't reach.

3. *Floss every day.* Flossing between your teeth is important, too. Lots of teens think that they don't have time to do this, but it's so easy. Just do it while you watch TV or listen to music. If you're not sure how to do it properly, just look at the illustration on page 96. Note that flossing involves not only cleaning between your teeth, but also up to the gum line. This removes food and plaque that may be forming at the base of your teeth.

4. *Eat a good, healthy diet.* That means lots of fruits and vegetables instead of sugary and sticky carbohydrate snacks. When you eat candy or granola or some other tooth-unfriendly snack, brush your teeth (or at least thoroughly rinse your mouth) as soon as possible. Better still, learn to like salads and raw vegetables. Carry strips of bell peppers, carrots, and celery sticks with you to school. You *can* acquire a taste for these (really!).

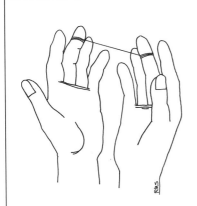

1. Grasp the floss firmly in both hands.

2. Use it between all your teeth (those hard-to-reach ones need it a lot!).

3. Be sure to work the floss into the gum line to get rid of plaque where it really starts to cause trouble.

Flossing Technique

Bleaching, Bonding, Invisible Braces, and Other Dental Innovations

I'm real depressed. My dentist says I ought to have braces but I'm scared that this will interfere with my modeling career. I do modeling for a local department store several times a year and hope to get into some ads. I think braces would really hold me back. I heard about invisible braces and would like to know more about these. Are they for real?

Kerry A.

Recent advances in dentistry are giving hope to many people who have stained or chipped teeth or who can't face the idea of having metal braces. While some of these recent options aren't for everyone, they can be very helpful to many young people concerned about the appearance of their teeth.

My teeth are all stained because of tetracycline. Is there any way a dentist could make these stains less obvious or get rid of them completely? I heard about something called bleaching and wonder if that would work well for someone like me. What do you think?

Denise

I recently chipped my tooth playing football and it looks awful. My mom has been so mad because she thinks I'll need a crown or cap or something and that's real expensive. I haven't seen a dentist yet. Is there a way to fix my tooth that wouldn't cost so much?

Brad

■ *Bleaching.* This dental treatment can remove or lighten a variety of stains on the teeth. It is particularly effective in removing stains from cigarettes, coffee, or excess drinking-water fluoride, but somewhat less so in improving the appearance of teeth stained by tetracycline, which causes stains to develop within the tooth rather than just on the surface. However, light tetracycline stains can be improved. Bleaching is a painless procedure that involves several visits to the dentist. First, the tooth is coated with hydrogen peroxide and another solution that aids penetration of the tooth by this bleach. Then a heating instrument starts the chemical reaction that penetrates and bleaches the tooth. The most dramatic improvement will probably be noticeable after the second treatment and the benefits of bleaching may last from one year to a lifetime. There are a number of dentists who point out that bleaching is not appropriate in *every* case of stained teeth; check with your dentist to review all the options available to you.

- *Bonding.* This treatment is also sometimes used instead of capping to improve the appearance of teeth that have been chipped or broken, are stained or cracked, or have gaps. This treatment is fast, requires no drilling or anesthetic, and is less expensive than crowns/caps. In this procedure, diluted phosphoric acid is applied to the tooth. This etches tiny pores into the tooth enamel. Then a sealer—a coat of liquid plastic—is applied. The next coat is a paste made up of plastic and very finely ground glass, silica, or quartz. This paste, which is tinted to match the natural color of the tooth, is put on in very thin layers and then molded to whatever shape is needed. Each layer is hardened and bonded by a 40-second exposure to visible or ultraviolet light waves; then, when all the layers have been applied and hardened, the newly constructed tooth is finely contoured and polished. The cosmetic results can be dramatic, but there are limitations. Bonding can't be used on the chewing surfaces of the back teeth and lasts only about half as long as conventional capping (about 5 to 10 years versus 10 to 20 years).
- *Invisible Braces.* Those who cringe at the thought of being called "Metal Mouth" may find some hope in recent advances that make braces more or less invisible. In one technique, clear plastic braces are bonded onto the surface of the teeth and held together with a single metal wire. To the casual observer, these braces are almost unnoticeable.

There is also a new orthodontics technique pioneered by Dr. Craven Kurz in Beverly Hills, California. Here, braces are attached to the *backs* of the teeth and are unnoticeable to others. This new technique is becoming popular, especially among teens and adults, but there are drawbacks. These braces are more expensive than conventional braces—costing an average of $4,000 to $5,000 over a two-to-three-year course of treatment versus $2,500 for conventional braces. Also, these braces can cause speech difficulties and trouble chewing food until the tongue adjusts to their presence. Still, as more orthodontists offer this alternative, it could be a reassuring, workable option for many young people.

I'm 14 and hate going to the dentist because I have a lot of cavities. The shot of novocaine is just the worst and the drilling just makes me crazy! I hate it! What can I do? I don't want to have awful teeth, but I almost get sick from nervousness about going to the dentist. Help!

Pam A.

There is also hope for those who, like Pam, are upset by shots and dental drills. More dentists these days are using painless electronic anesthesia and lasers to reduce or eliminate that nerve-racking drilling! These techniques are expected to be the dentistry of the future in the next 10 to 20 years. In the meantime, some dentists are already using these new techniques.

Usually, with lasers, the work on the tooth is so quick that the pain doesn't have a chance to register, so that novocaine is not necessary. Lasers are quickly replacing old dental equipment, including drills. However, currently lasers can be used to remove decay from a tooth, but have difficulty getting through the tough enamel outer layer of the tooth, so a little drilling may still be necessary for a while. (But it's definitely on its way out!)

Electronic anesthesia, which is painless and does not expose you to the risk of electric shock, happens when the dentist places two small electrodes, held in place by adhesive sponges in the patient's mouth. This low electrical current blocks the brain's pain response and can be controlled by the patient during the dental procedure with the use of a hand-held device. There is no numbness later and this new anesthesia can be used by those allergic to conventional local anesthetics. However, it cannot be used by those with seizure disorders or who are pregnant.

If you're interested in finding a dentist in your area who uses electronic anesthesia, call the Center for Dental Information at (609) 921-8622. To find a dentist who gives laser treatment, call American Dental Laser at (313) 540-6450.

SPECIAL HELP FOR GOOD LOOKS

Plastic Surgery

Although a healthy, well-nourished, and exercised body is a great start toward a more attractive you, it may not always be quite enough. What you may want most of all, perhaps, whether you're male or female, is to be attractive and be accepted by others.

You may have a feature that you feel keeps you from looking your best: a large nose, a receding chin, ears that stick out, or skin pitted with acne scars. You may be plagued with excess body or facial hair. You may wonder about the safety of ear piercing or the safety and effectiveness of cosmetics and beauty aids. You may be willing to settle for something less than stunning beauty. You may just want to look, essentially, like everyone else, minus an embarrassing flaw or two.

People see so-called flaws in a variety of ways. Many contend that flaws add to your character, your individuality. Many people aren't bothered at all by a prominent nose, for example. Others, plagued by self-consciousness and shame, find that for them a physical defect, however slight to others, is a major problem.

Help is available. Plastic surgery is the answer for some. Special cosmetics may be fine for others. However, it's important for all of us to realize the limitations of these beauty aids. They may help you look better, but how you feel about yourself and how you choose to live your life go far beyond these procedures. Even though the results, in some cases, can look miraculous, it's important to realize two things about plastic surgery:

- *Plastic surgery can change a physical feature. That's all. It is* not *guaranteed to change your whole life for the better.* Plastic surgery to reduce the size and shape of your nose, for example, will do just that. It is not guaranteed to turn your life around, make you the most popular person in school, or drastically alter who you really are. It may help you feel better about your appearance, but it will not guarantee instant self-esteem or an immediate sense of self-worth.
- *Plastic surgery is* surgery, *not magic. It has its risks, discomforts, and considerable costs. It is not a decision to be made lightly.* We're discussing it in this book *only* because we've had so many letters and questions about it and feel that we owe you some honest answers. And we honestly feel that plastic surgery has its limitations in terms of its ability to enhance your life and your own singular beauty.

The most beauty-enhancing quality one can have is self-acceptance. If you think that life is worthless unless you're a C cup or have a cute little nose, instead of the smaller breasts or larger nose you were born with, then you need to do a lot of thinking and working on improving your feelings about yourself.

Think for a moment:

- Beyond the physical, what are your best qualities? Aren't these the qualities that make your best friends, the ones who really count in your life, like you?
- What aspects of yourself make you feel glad to be you? Think about it. You're special and beautiful in your own way whether or not you decide to have cosmetic surgery. A surgeon's knife can make certain physical changes. But

it can't change the person you've grown to become.

Special beauty help, combined with your growing sense of the worthwhile person you have always been, may add a great deal to the good feelings you already have.

Plastic surgery can be a great help to someone whose life has been adversely affected by a defect. It can also be a tragedy when practiced by an incompetent, inexperienced surgeon or when a patient is not given adequate screening to determine whether he or she will be able to have cosmetic surgery without undue physical or psychological side effects.

These two concerns often go together. The inexperienced surgeon, whose technique may be faulty, may *also* accept patients who have physical or emotional problems that preclude the possibility of successful cosmetic plastic surgery—patients that a more knowledgeable surgeon will advise *not* to have such surgery.

How can such incompetence happen? Any profession has its share of incompetent people, of course, but in the area of cosmetic plastic surgery, there is an added complication. The problem is that *any* licensed physician may do surgery, including plastic surgery, even if he or she has not had any specialty training.

Major surgery, of course, is usually done in a hospital, and hospitals generally don't grant surgical privileges to physicians without specialized surgical training beyond medical school. Therefore, it would be highly unlikely to find a physician without specialized training doing open-heart surgery.

Plastic surgery, however, is often done in an office or clinic setting. So physicians are not necessarily dependent upon hospital affiliation and may simply set up their own operating rooms in their own offices or clinics. (This is not to say, of course, that all plastic surgeons who do office or clinic surgery are incompetent. Many are well qualified and may also have hospital affiliations.)

If you're like most people, you probably want the best surgeon you can find. So how do you find a qualified, well-trained plastic surgeon?

1. Instead of looking for ads in the paper or in the Yellow Pages of your telephone directory, ask your family doctor for a recommendation or check with your county medical society.
2. Check the physician's credentials, making sure that he or she is a *board-certified plastic surgeon.* Most competent, experienced physicians who have specialties are board certified in that specialty. Make sure that the plastic surgeon you choose is board certified in *plastic surgery.* You can find out whether a surgeon is board certified by calling the American Board of Medical Specialties at (800) 776-2378.
3. Choose a doctor who is affiliated with an accredited hospital. Even if the procedure that you're contemplating may not involve a hospital stay, it's important that your doctor have a hospital affiliation—both as a measure of competence and in case of an emergency.

A competent, experienced plastic surgeon selects his or her patients with care. As we said earlier, some people are not good candidates for cosmetic plastic surgery. For some this may involve physical reasons: a tendency toward excessive bleeding or clotting difficulties, anemia, or diabetes. Those who suffer from asthma or other respiratory disorders may be advised not to have surgery that may involve general anesthesia. For others, psychological factors may make the plastic surgeon hesitate or refuse to operate at all.

Even if cosmetic plastic surgery is not a miracle, it can help improve your appearance, sometimes dramatically. There are a number of different procedures. The ones that teens have asked us most about are rhinoplasty (nose surgery), mammoplasty (breast enlargement or reduction), liposuction, and tattoo removal. The following chart will give you an idea of what each of these procedures involves and what it costs.

COMMON PLASTIC SURGERY PROCEDURES TEENS SEEK

Procedure	What Happens	Discomfort Zone	Cost	Other
Rhinoplasty (nose job)	Doctor (in outpatient clinic or in hospital) does surgery to change shape of and/or reduce size of nose. Local anesthetic most often used.	Some pain, swelling, and discomfort (from surgical packing in nose). Nose is splinted for several days. Eyes may be blackened for some days. Some swelling and bruising for 3–4 weeks. Complete healing may take six months.	Varies: $4,000 to $7,500 by a private doctor, or $1,350 to $3,000 at a special clinic.	Best age for this is 16–17 for girls and later teens for boys. This is when nasal bone growth is complete and the face is more adult.
Mammoplasty (breast enhancement)	Doctor makes incision just below each breast and inserts implant (usually saline) through incision to enlarge the size of breasts.	Procedure done at clinic or hospital with general anesthesia. Some pain, swelling, and discomfort after surgery. There are possible health risks involved in use of silicone breast implants.	$6,000 to $8,000 by a private doctor, or $1,400 to $5,800 at a special clinic.	We do not recommend this for teens, especially those whose breasts are still developing. Breasts continue to grow through the adult years. Push-up bras work great, too!
Mammoplasty (breast reduction)	This is major surgery done under general anesthetic and usually only in cases of extreme physical discomfort. Skin and excess breast tissue are removed. It usually involves several days in the hospital.	Considerable pain and discomfort. Sutures and bandages usually in place for several days. While general recovery is 3 weeks, woman must be careful to wear a well-fitting bra for several months. There may be significant scarring on the underside of the breast.	Varies to more than $9,000 with all costs.	This is major surgery that should only be done in cases of extreme necessity.
Liposuction	This is usually done in the "tumescent" form, which involves injecting a saline (salt water) solution mixed with lidocaine (a local anesthetic) and epinephrine (a drug that prevents blood loss) into the fat and then using a vacuum device inserted into small incisions to extract the fat.	The "tumescent" presurgical injection speeds recovery and limits the amount of swelling and pain during that time. While this is usually done as an outpatient procedure, recovery isn't without discomfort. Patients usually "drain" saline solution from their incisions for a day or two. There may be pain for a week or so. Support garments in affected areas must be worn for varying times: a chin strap (for double chin liposuction) for five days; a support girdle (for saddlebag hips and thighs) for 2–3 weeks. If liposuction is in calves and ankles, support hose worn for 6 weeks. Swelling may last up to three months, with scars fading after a year or two.	$4,000 minimum by a private doctor, or $1,000 to $3,000 in a special clinic.	This is not a magic solution to obesity. Only a small amount of fat can be removed at one time with relative safety. This is suitable mainly for stubborn fat deposits that have not responded to diet and exercise such as thighs with saddlebags, a double chin, or fat deposits around knees or ankles.
Tattoo Removal	Doctor uses laser to remove tattoo. This may require several laser sessions.	This procedure is painful and may need to be repeated several times.	$800 to $1,600	Results vary: black ink is easy to remove, while green ink is difficult to remove; homemade tattoos are often more difficult to remove than a tattoo done by a professional.

Special discounted plastic surgery is available at five special clinics (offering training to surgical residents supervised by experienced surgeons) nationwide. These are located at Manhattan Eye, Ear and Throat Hospital and New York Eye and Ear Infirmary Clinic in New York City; University of Pennsylvania; University of Texas Southwestern Medical Center in Dallas; and University of Southern California in Los Angeles.

Cosmetics

I try all kinds of cosmetics, but it never looks as good on me as it does on the models. I feel cheated. I try to buy good stuff but can't afford really expensive makeup. Would it be worth it to save up my money and get the most expensive? Is the quality that much better?

Janine G.

Cosmetics play a big part in many of our lives. We spend billions of dollars each year on soaps, shampoos, deodorants, perfumes, aftershave lotions, makeup, and moisturizers—among many other items. All too often, these products disappoint us, failing to live up to the promises of the ads. They may even cause more problems for us, triggering allergic reactions, irritations, or, in some cases, infections. They may also put a strain on our pocketbooks. As costs—and consumer expectations—rise, it's vital to choose cosmetics with care.

I notice that ingredients are now listed on cosmetics. Why? Most of it doesn't mean that much to me and most things seem to have pretty much the same ingredients.

Georgia B.

In an attempt to protect your health and your cash, the Food and Drug Administration (FDA) now requires cosmetics companies to list the ingredients on product labels in descending order, with the major ingredient at the top of the list. If you read labels carefully, you may find that there is little, if any, difference between a cheaper brand and a more expensive cosmetics line. In the latter case, you may be paying for a famous name and, perhaps, for more elaborate packaging.

The new labels can be health protectors, too, since if you do have an adverse reaction to a product, you and your doctor may be able to determine, possibly, which substances may be involved and which ones you might avoid in the future.

What are some of the ingredients you're likely to find on a cosmetics label?

- *Solvents*—primarily water and alcohol—are liquids in which solid substances are dissolved. Purified water may make up a large percentage of some cosmetics; generally, this is one of the cheapest and safest cosmetic ingredients. In fact, it may be better for your skin if you use a cosmetic with a high water content rather than one with a high oil content. This may be particularly true of makeup bases. In some cases, the cheaper brands, which tend to contain more water, may actually be better for you. Alcohol is a frequent ingredient in astringents, perfumes, and aftershave lotions.
- *Emollients*—such as mineral oil, lanolin, and glycerin—make the skin feel smooth, either by preventing loss of moisture from the skin surface or by getting moisture from the air. These are found particularly in moisturizers and hand and body lotions.
- *Emulsifiers*—such as sodium lauryl sulfate—are a component of lotions and keep water and oil ingredients from separating, and *stabilizers*—such as sodium citrate—work with the emulsifiers.
- *Preservatives*—such as parabens—keep harmful bacteria from growing in cosmetics.

A number of teens claim to like the natural look in cosmetics and express a desire to shun products with artificial preservatives. Most cosmetics, however, even those claiming to be "natural," contain preservatives. There is an important reason for this. Growth of bacteria in cosmetics, particularly in eye makeup, may endanger your health.

I'm not sure, but I think I may be allergic to makeup. I started using a new lipstick and got a blister on my lips. Could this be an allergy?

Paula W.

It could be an allergy or it could simply be a skin reaction, an irritation caused by a particular product. *Contact dermatitis*, as this is called, is usually confined to the site of contact; irritations, rather than allergies, account for most common adverse reactions to cosmetics. Such a reaction does not mean that you have to give up cosmetics. You may find that you can use another product that contains a different concentration of the irritating ingredients with no adverse reaction at all.

Identifying the source of irritation isn't always easy. Cosmetics may not be at fault, in some instances. You may, for example, have an adverse reaction to the metal in earrings or hairpins. However, some common ingredients are more likely than others to cause irritation. A study by the FDA found that the highest rate of adverse reactions was found in deodorants and antiperspirants, hair sprays, hair colorings, bubble bath, mascara, moisturizers, eye creams, and chemical hair removers. So if you suffer from an irritation and use one or several of these products, you might examine the possibility that this may be a likely source of your problem.

You may keep a troublesome irritation from happening on a large scale by trying a preliminary patch test, recommended particularly in the instructions for hair-coloring products, permanents, and chemical hair removers. If you're plagued with allergies, do a patch test on any product you're thinking of using, preferably before you buy it. Many stores have demonstrator samples available for such testing.

Are hypoallergenic cosmetics better than regular ones for any type of skin? Are they guaranteed not to cause problems? Just how good are they?

Pamela J.

"Hypoallergenic" on the label of a particular cosmetic means that it is less likely to cause adverse reactions. The Food and Drug Administration now requires all cosmetics manufacturers using the term *hypoallergenic* to run numerous tests proving that these products really are less likely to cause allergic or irritation reactions than are competing products.

If you have a history of allergies or irritations, it's a good idea to pick a hypoallergenic product. These days, a number of choices are available in all price ranges. However, it's important to note that while hypoallergenic products may be less likely to irritate your skin, they will not clear up or cure existing skin problems such as acne.

I've heard that mascara may be dangerous. How come? Also, my girl friend says that you should never share eye makeup with anyone else. Is she right or is she just being selfish?

Sue Y.

It's true that mascara and other eye makeup has been under close scrutiny by the FDA. The problem is that possible contamination of the cosmetic through normal use may trigger physical symptoms—some serious—in the user.

While most eye makeup is pure at the time of purchase, skin bacteria can reach the makeup in a number of ways—for example, when you put your finger in any eye-shadow container or touch a mascara wand to your eyelid. This bacteria may grow in the cosmetic and become dangerous to the eye, causing red eyes, sties, inflamed lids, or, at worst, an eye infection that if unchecked may lead to blindness. This kind of infection might happen, for example, if your hand were to slip while you were applying mascara and the cornea of your eye were scratched by the contaminated mascara wand.

A number of reports of corneal infection and ulcerations due to use of contaminated cosmetics have reached the FDA, which is now strongly recommending that all manufacturers use special preservatives, particularly in eye makeup, to prevent the growth of such microorganisms.

There are several steps that you, too, can take to safeguard your eyes:

- Don't lend or borrow eye makeup.
- Be sure that the makeup you use contains a preservative. (Check the label!)
- Don't keep mascara too long. Preservatives may begin to lose their effectiveness after three or four months. Replace your mascara after that time, even if you have plenty still left.
- When you buy new mascara, *always* discard the old brush.
- Wash your hands before using cosmetics.
- Keep makeup containers tightly closed when not in use.
- Use Q-Tips—regular or new cosmetic-sized—to apply eye shadow.
- If a product needs water, use water, *not* saliva! Never lick an eyeliner brush or spit in any makeup.
- Don't leave cosmetics or a purse containing cosmetics in the sun. Intense heat may make the preservatives less effective.

Another safety tip that may apply to all cosmetic products is this: Read directions carefully and use the product exactly as instructed! If the manufacturer suggests a patch test, do it. Don't use a hair-coloring product on your eyelashes. Don't put cosmetics on already irritated skin.

The more common sense you use and the more you know about what cosmetics can and can't do for you, the less likely you will be disappointed.

SPECIAL PROBLEMS

Ear and Body Piercing

I haven't read anything about this, but I wonder: Can you get AIDS from having your ears pierced? I know that people who share needles when taking drugs can get AIDS, but what about ear piercing? How can I make sure it will be safe?

Erin K.

Ear piercing has been a popular trend among teens, both male and female, for some years now. Done properly, under antiseptic conditions, piercing of the earlobes can be quite safe. Piercing of the upper part of the ear, getting into slower-to-heal cartilage, may be more problematic, making you more vulnerable to infection. If you *do* decide to get your upper ear pierced, be sure to do the follow-up self-care on a daily basis in order to avoid infection.

How can I convince my parents that it's safe to get my tongue pierced? I REALLY, REALLY want to do it, but they are being totally stupid and say it's unhealthy. What should I do to convince them I know what I'm doing?

Austin S.

If you have a tendency to bleed heavily, have allergies to metals, are unusually susceptible to infections, or tend to form keloid scars, you may want to approach ear piercing with caution. Consult your physician first. In cases like this, it is especially important to have ear piercing done by a physician.

Some people try to go the do-it-yourself route and pierce their own ears—or have a friend do it. We don't advise this. Most of those we have seen with adverse side effects—such as infections—have been do-it-yourselfers. Infections like this may cause swelling around the ear puncture and, if unchecked, may lead to more serious health problems as well as scarring of the earlobes.

And while there have yet to be any reports of someone contracting AIDS through blood-contaminated ear-piercing apparatus, this could be a risk, especially if you try to do it yourself or with a friend and share a common needle or an unsterilized one.

The best way to avoid such risks and complications is to have your ears pierced by a physician with sterile equipment. The doctor will use a sterile stainless-steel needle or an instrument much like a stapler, which will insert a spring-loaded earring into your earlobe. Although the procedure is generally painless, the physician may use a topical local anesthetic on the earlobe to numb it.

Many department and jewelry stores have special technicians trained to pierce ears. Here, the ear is often pierced with the sterilized post of the earring itself. As long as your ear is sterilized with alcohol before and after the piercing and as long as the earring has been sterilized and has never been used by another person, such ear piercing is generally safe. But the training of technicians varies widely—as does the level of sterile precautions used.

After piercing, surgical-steel or 14-carat-gold studs are immediately inserted into the earlobe holes and must be worn continuously for about six weeks until the ears heal. Wearing post earrings for about six months before trying wires may also help your ears to continue to heal and may ensure that the holes in your earlobes will remain instead of shrinking down into mere slits.

Other after-care hints:

- As the ears heal, dab the lobes regularly with alcohol or mild soap to keep bacteria away.
- Always dip your earrings in alcohol before inserting them.
- Be patient! Allow your ears to heal before removing or changing your earrings, or you may find that your earlobe holes will close up, making it painful (or impossible) to put the earrings back in.

In terms of piercing other body parts—such as the tongue, navel, lips, nipples, nose, and eyebrow—we don't advise it, no matter how fashionable it may be right now. This body piercing carries considerable risk of infection and can be quite painful. The risk of infection is especially great when it is done in the tongue, the lips, and the inside of the mouth. In addition, metal in the mouth can damage teeth; swelling of the pierced tongue can make breathing, speaking, eating—all those things we hold dear—much more difficult.

Given the risks involved, if you are still determined to do this, have the piercing done by a physician. It is much more likely that proper technique,

sterile conditions, and good follow-up care will be part of your treatment package.

Even better, *don't do it!* There are less painful, less dangerous ways to look cool.

We would say the same thing for tattoos. Again, there can be danger of infection if a tattoo is applied under less than sterile conditions. And tattoos have a way of going from cool to burdensome very fast. Maybe you break up with "Amy" and no longer want her name immortalized on your arm (or your new girlfriend is less than excited about this part of your body art). Maybe you're trying to get a job and that serpent curling around your ankle isn't helping you make the impression you'd like. Or maybe you just get sick of a tattoo and decide you want a new look. It isn't as if you could just wash it off.

A better idea: Try temporary tattoos, especially the herbal variety that are applied with a brush or plastic cone and last two to four weeks. Press-on tattoos and body painting kits can be fun, too. You can have all the fun of looking different—or like your friends—or shocking your parents or other adults without the painful removal part.

Excess Hair

Help! I'm a 15-year-old girl who is HAIRY! I have hair on my chin and a few hairs around the nipples of my breasts. The hair on my chin really looks awful. What can I do about it? My mom says it runs in the family. Help!

Maria G.

Excess hair growth, particularly on the face, can be an embarrassing problem. For many, the cause may be genetic. If your ethnic origin is Mediterranean (Italian, Spanish, Semitic, Greek, and so forth), you may have a greater-than-average tendency to have more body and facial hair than, say, someone of Scandinavian or Asian origin.

I have excess hair on my upper lip and break out from using chemical hair removers. I've seen ads for do-it-yourself electrolysis devices. Would this be safe to try?

Eileen S.

For a minority of young people, excess hair may signal a hormone imbalance or gland problem. If you are well into adolescence—in your late teens—and suddenly develop excess hair, you might want to consult your physician. For most, however, the cause is genetic rather than glandular.

What can you do about excess hair? Many women, of course, choose to shave leg and underarm hair (which is perfectly normal—and superfluous only because of fashion and grooming trends) or remove it with chemical removers called *depilatories.*

Depilatories dissolve hair on the skin surface, but do not remove hair permanently. They may also be somewhat irritating to the skin, so try them with caution (on a small area) first. If you have facial hair, use a depilatory designed for use on the face or a general one that is safe for facial use.

When a few hairs are involved on the chin or breasts, some women prefer to pluck the hair. This may be a bit painful and, again, does not remove the hair permanently.

Another effective, albeit temporary, treatment is the hot wax method. This can be done at home (following instructions from the hot wax hair removal kit *exactly*), but especially when a large area is involved, it is best done by a professional in a beauty salon or a special waxing salon. Here, hot wax is applied to the skin and then, after cooling, is pulled off, taking excess hair with it. One treatment does not remove hair permanently, but treatments over a period of time *may* retard hair growth. Waxing is not entirely painless and may cause an inflammatory reaction. Also, individual results vary widely.

I have a lot of hair on my back. It looks weird. I'd like to have it removed. Obviously, I can't shave it myself. Should I try something like electrolysis or waxing? I heard these are good ways to get rid of hair like this. I'm a 21-year-old male college student.

Mark M.

Someone like Mark, who has extensive hair on his back and limited funds, might try this method

instead of the more expensive *electrolysis.* Electrolysis is a method of permanent hair removal. Here, a tiny electrode placed, via a needle, into the hair follicle discharges a high-speed electric current, destroying the hair root.

This method of hair removal usually works well, but there are some drawbacks. It is expensive and time-consuming, may be painful, and can produce scars, especially if it is done by an inexperienced technician. For this reason, we don't recommend homestyle electrolysis. You may not be able to locate each hair follicle exactly and, in addition, the do-it-yourself units usually don't have automatic shutoff devices that stop the electric current after a few seconds to help prevent scarring.

Shop carefully for a qualified electrologist. Your search might begin with recommendations from your physician or your county medical association.

For women whose excess hair is the result of hormone imbalance and who have large amounts of such hair, there may be some hope via treatment with one of several prescription drugs. One of these drugs, cimetidine (Tagamet), has been used to treat ulcers in the past and was recently discovered to block the effects of male hormones on hair growth. The other drug, aldactone, is a blood pressure medication that also lowers male hormone levels. Since these drugs are not without risks and side effects, they should be taken only in instances of extreme *hirsutism* (excess hair) and then only under the close supervision of a physician.

Perspiration

I sweat a lot under my arms. By a lot, I mean my shirts get armpit stains and big wet marks. I usually wear big, baggy sweatshirts so it won't leave a wet mark. Once in a while, I'll sneak on a short sleeve shirt. If I'm lucky, it'll last me about ten minutes before the wet marks appear. This has been going on for about a year and I use deodorant and stuff. My mom says I'll outgrow this, but I'm afraid I won't. Do you think I'll grow out of it soon?

J. C.

My armpits sweat and smell even though I wear deodorant. It usually happens when I'm around this guy I like. Never when I'm around my mom. It's very embarrassing to walk around like this. Help—and thank you verrrry much!

Christina P.

My hands used to sweat so bad that when I was doing my school work my paper would be soaked when I got done. My mom took me to the doctor and I got this wonderful stuff (my mom read about it and took the clipping to my doctor who hadn't heard of it but gave me a prescription to try). It's called Drysol. You put it on your hands before going to bed and put rubber or plastic gloves on over it. You might have to do it one or two nights in a row at first but then all you do it is once every one or two weeks as needed. I've been using this for two years now and my sweaty hands are gone!

Amanda S.

As these letters show, excessive perspiration can be a huge embarrassment in the teen years. When your body is growing and changing in so many ways, the sweat glands are also developing fully and, at times, they may seem to be working overtime.

What can help?

- *Check with your physician if perspiration is persistent* despite use of antiperspirants, or if you have really sweaty hands. As Amanda's letter shows, there are special preparations he or she can suggest or prescribe.
- *Use antiperspirants* exactly *as instructed on the label.* Some product labels advise you that, for maximum effectiveness, you should use the product at bedtime rather than first thing in the morning. Others may suggest, too, not to apply an antiperspirant right after emerging from a steaming shower; your perspiration from the shower may simply wash the antiperspirant away. Dry yourself thoroughly and let your body cool down a bit. Then apply the antiperspirant.

- *Keep learning to manage stress and overcome social fears.* As Christina's letter shows, being close to someone you like or feeling stressed out can work you into a sweat when you *least* want it. When you work on stress management (see Chapter 4), you may find, as an added bonus, that you're able to stay dry, too.

It's true, too, that time can help. We've seen a number of young adults who were plagued with perspiration problems as teenagers dry out remarkably when they hit their twenties. This may simply be an adjustment of the body to adult functioning, more expertise at dealing with stress, or perhaps a combination of the two.

Questionable Beauty Aids

I saw an ad for some device that would make me lose a lot of weight in an hour with no pills, no diet, and no exercise. Is this possible, do you think?

Sheila B.

Tell me the truth: Do those bust developers that you see advertised in all the magazines REALLY work? Do they increase your bust like they say? If not, how do they get away with such ads?

Mary Q.

Some beauty devices promise more than they could possibly give you: instant (and seemingly effortless) weight loss or a quickly blossoming bosom! Many people—especially the young— would like to believe such promises. Being a smart consumer, however, means using common sense and recognizing some basic facts:

1. True weight loss is never instant, nor does it happen without some sensible, moderate eating and regular exercise. Some "instant weight loss" devices come with diet recommendations and, in most cases, if you simply followed the diet itself, you would probably lose weight even-

tually. Keep in mind that there are no miracles or shortcuts to weight loss. It takes time and effort!

2. Creams cannot really increase your bust size. Such creams usually contain hormones and may cause an inflammation of your breasts (which may be harmful), but will not bring about a true increase in the size of your breasts.

3. Bust developers do not increase the size of your breasts. These devices, if used over a period of time, may increase your bust size overall by exercising your pectoral (chest) and back muscles. This will perhaps lead to an increase in your all-around bust measurement (as it is measured around the torso), but it will not increase your actual breast (cup) size.

A study by the Good Housekeeping Institute's Beauty Clinic confirmed that cup size was not increased at all by the use of several bust-developer devices. Their conclusion: Eternal hope rather than effectiveness accounts for the sales success of such products.

Don't let money-back guarantees cloud your skepticism. In some cases, the money-back guarantee time limit expires before the product has a chance to show whether it will be effective. In many cases, the manufacturer is betting that you will be too embarrassed, too lazy, or too eternally hopeful to return an ineffective device and demand your money back.

One fact to keep in mind as you scan the ads: If it sounds too good to be true, it probably *is* too good to be true!

It may be helpful, too, to keep all legitimate beauty aids—from cosmetics to plastic surgery—in perspective. These aids might help you to look more physically attractive—but that's all. Looking more attractive may help to improve the quality of your life, but it will not change your life or the person you are. The growth and development of the person you would like to be and the lifestyle you would like to have are very much up to *you*!

CREATING A BEAUTIFUL, HEALTHY FUTURE

When I look at my mom and some of her friends, who are all in their early forties, I see a big difference between those who look old and those who don't. It may seem strange to be worried about looking old when I'm only 17, but what can I do to make sure that I look good as long as possible?

Beverly B.

We all would like to look good well into older age and to live long, healthy lives. Whether we can actually do this is, in part, out of our control. Our genes play a part in determining how we age, how healthy we are, and how long we live. However, lifestyle is also a major factor. And here you have choices. You *can* be in control!

Preventive medicine is an important aspect of medicine today. The purpose of this is to try as much as possible to prevent common killers such as heart disease, cancer, strokes, high blood pressure, and diabetes. Although the possibility of developing such disorders may seem remote to you right now, what you do or don't do now in your teen years may have a great impact on your health in later life. And the beginning of some of these common killers may even be seen among teenagers! So what can you do right now to look and feel good now *and* later in life?

1. *Eat a healthy diet.* Do we sound like an endless recording on this? The reasons: It's so important to your health and it's so within your control. Eat more vegetables and fruit. Cut way down on fatty meats that contribute to high cholesterol.

If you think you have to wait years to see the impact of too many cheeseburgers, think again. A survey sponsored by the American Health Foundation and *Current Science* magazine examined the health habits and food preferences of almost 22,000 young teenagers in 46 states. Researchers concluded that many of those in their early teens are already in trouble.

The survey revealed that *as many as 30 percent of the 11- to 14-year-olds surveyed already have high cholesterol levels.* High cholesterol, which can stem from a diet high in animal fats and cholesterol, is related to atherosclerosis, or hardening of the arteries, and may lead to heart disease and strokes later in life.

The survey also revealed an alarmingly high salt intake among American teens. So what? Too much salt in your diet (translate that to mean salt on your food and salty snacks) can lead to hypertension (high blood pressure), a widespread health problem among Americans that may lead to life-threatening crises such as heart attacks, strokes, and kidney failure, as well as serious vision problems.

2. *Don't smoke.* Nearly 10 percent of the younger teens surveyed smoke cigarettes; it is estimated that up to 40 percent of them (more girls than boys) will be smokers by high school graduation.

Don't smoke! Smoking not only exposes you to health risks, but also makes you wrinkle sooner and more severely than you might otherwise. Cigarette smoking, it is estimated, caused about 75 percent of the nation's 89,000 lung cancer deaths in 1998. Smoking may also be a factor in cancer of the lips, mouth, and esophagus, and in emphysema. Chewing tobacco, popular among some teens, has been known to cause cancer of the mouth.

3. *Don't drink—especially when you drive.* Alcohol, which high numbers of teens (11- to 13-year-olds included) drink in some form, can have a number of tragic consequences if abused. Shattered lives, fatal liver damage, and possible cancer are longer-term future possibilities for young alcoholics.

Tragedy, however, can happen much faster than that. The most common cause of death in teenagers is accidents—usually car or motorcycle accidents—and about 42 percent of these are alcohol related. Don't drink and drive. Don't ride with a driver who has been drinking or taking drugs. Alcohol has also been implicated in skateboard, cycling, and boating acci-

dents, among others. Not abusing alcohol or hanging out with others who do will do more to protect your health and your life right now than *any other single lifestyle choice or change.*

4. *Exercise.* Lack of exercise can be a killer—eventually. American teens, especially girls, do not get enough exercise. Only 58 percent of the girls surveyed were getting *any* form of strenuous exercise!

Get regular exercise. This can help your heart to become more efficient, your bones to grow stronger, and your weight to stay at its best. Especially for girls, getting lots of exercise and eating calcium-rich food is important in the teen years—when the bones are still adding mass—in order to prevent osteoporosis, a crippling disorder linked with loss of bone mass in middle and old age.

Lack of exercise can lead to obesity, which carries with it a greater risk of developing diabetes, high blood pressure, strokes, atherosclerosis, and heart attacks later on. Even if you *don't* become obese via a sedentary existence, you are at a greater risk of having a heart attack or stroke if you continue to avoid regular exercise.

Right now, exercise can make you feel good and look great! You just need to take that first step.

5. *Keep your weight down close to what you and your doctor determine is your ideal weight.* Don't be a yo-yo dieter. It's too hard on the body. And obesity ages you inside—as well as making you look old before your time!

6. *Safeguard your skin.* Use sunscreen whenever you are outdoors (even in cloudy or hazy weather).

7. *Don't use and abuse drugs—legal or illegal.* This goes for prescription as well as street drugs. All can take a toll—as we will see in the next chapter.

8. *Don't take chances with sex.* These days, sad but true, sex can be hazardous to your health and your future fertility—and may even ultimately endanger your life. If this sounds impossibly melodramatic, turn quickly to Chapter 12 to

read about how sexually transmitted diseases can threaten your health and fertility. Abstinence is the only way to be completely safe from these diseases. The next best choice is to be in a monogamous (faithful) relationship with someone who has never had another sex partner. Beyond this, safe-sex practices may decrease your risks.

9. *Learn healthy stress management.* Learn to deal with stress in constructive, healthy ways. Talk with people you trust. Write in your diary or journal. Take a walk. Listen to some of your favorite music. See a counselor or therapist if there are things in your life that you can't handle. Use relaxation techniques or exercise when you're feeling tense and stressed out. Act in ways that make you proud of yourself. Building good self-esteem is a major part of lifelong health and well-being!

10. *See your doctor and dentist for regular checkups.* Seeing your doctor and dentist at least once a year for checkups can help with early detection of problems before they become major, as well as helping you take advantage of preventive medical and dental care. These visits also give you a chance to ask questions and get information that will help you take better care of yourself for now and for a lifetime.

These are the basic health maintenance rules. And they're important to remember and follow *now*! It's important that you work to maintain your good health while you're young and healthy and while whatever damage there may be is reversible and/or not extensive. While it's impossible to predict how long you will live or to say, "If you do this and this, you will never have a major health problem," it *is* possible for you to be healthy—and happy—for many years to come. But whether or not you will be is very much up to *you*.

GOOD HEALTH AND GOOD LOOKS

✔ If you have acne, even a mild case that doesn't respond to over-the-counter treatments, see your doctor. There are prescription medications that *will* help.

✔ Brush, floss, and see your dentist twice a year. Good dental health is vital to your overall health.

✔ Plastic surgery can change a feature—such as your nose—but not necessarily your life. It is real surgery—with discomfort, some scars, and necessary healing time.

✔ Piercing your earlobes can be safe if done under sterile conditions, but piercing other parts of your body, especially in the mouth, can be hazardous to your health.

✔ If a beauty aid seems too good to be true, it probably *is* too good to be true!

CHAPTER EIGHT

Drugs, Drinking, and Smoking

WHY SAYING NO IS VITAL TO YOUR HEALTH

Me and my friends are really sick of all the stuff we get from our parents and at school about not drinking or smoking or doing drugs. It isn't like we're addicts. We like to party. It's our choice, right? All the bad things happen when you're old anyway and we can always quit before then. So what's the big deal now?

Adam N.

W e're all for parties and fun. But there are many different ways to enjoy yourself—and some of them, unfortunately, are quite hazardous to your health and your future. It's true that how you have fun and what you put into your body is *your* choice. But it's important to know what you're choosing.

Why are adults so concerned about teen substance use and abuse? Adults worry a lot about the numbers of young people risking their health and lives at a time when most age groups are becoming more health conscious. They are concerned that teens aren't looking at the facts about substance use and abuse when making choices that can change their lives.

Is there reason for them—and for you—to worry? A number of recent studies and many public health experts say yes. For example:

- In addition to alcohol and tobacco, teen illegal drug use has risen more than 78 percent since 1992. Nearly 11 percent of U.S. teens say they use illegal drugs each month. By far, marijuana is the drug of choice, cited by 8.2 percent of teens surveyed. In another study, 51 percent of high school seniors and 45 percent of sophomores admitted some drug use.
- Heroin (usually in capsule form) has killed numerous teens nationwide, including eleven in Plano, Texas, between 1996 and 1998. Emergency-room visits related to teen heroin overdoses have risen 58 percent since 1992.
- Use of LSD and other hallucinogens has risen 54 percent since 1992. Crystal meth and Ecstasy are new drug favorites as well among teens.
- Alcohol and tobacco are the substances teens use and abuse most often. In a recent survey, more than 40 percent of 12- to 17-year-olds admitted drinking, 35 percent smoke cigarettes, and 12 percent had used marijuana recently. In another survey, 50 percent of all eighth-graders said that they have used alcohol. Why do these statistics matter? Because some experts believe that teens who begin drinking or smoking at an early age are setting the stage for lifelong use or abuse. One study found that 43 percent of teens who began

drinking before age 14 developed alcoholism. And most lifelong smokers report having started the habit by age 14.

■ According to an American Academy of Pediatrics study, one million teenagers take up smoking each year. An early start of the nicotine habit (before age 15) has been found to increase the risk of lung cancer by close to *20 times more than that of nonsmokers.*

■ Experts estimate that 3,000 children and adolescents begin smoking every day. While smoking has decreased among adults, it is on the rise among teens—and this is true of all ethnic groups (though African Americans have the lowest rate of smoking among adolescents, the number of smokers in this ethnic group is increasing as well). According to the Centers for Disease Control in Atlanta, teen tobacco use increased by nearly one-third in the years between 1992 and 1998. About 36 percent of teens are habitual smokers and six million teens report that they smoke cigars. Ethnically, 39.7 percent of white teens smoke while 34 percent of Latino teens and 22.7 percent of African American teens smoke regularly. When cigars and smokeless tobacco are included, the numbers of teen users are 46.8 percent of white teens, 36.8 percent of Latino teens, and 29.4 percent of African American teens.

■ Teen smokers don't have to wait years to suffer health consequences. A recent study found that cigarette smoking damages lung development in teens, most dramatically in girls. Researchers at the Harvard School of Public Health found that even as few as five cigarettes a day can reduce lung function and growth.

■ The Alcohol, Drug Abuse, and Mental Health Administration has reported that addiction to alcohol or drugs can happen more quickly in teens than in adults because young people tend to consume greater quantities. According to this special report, alcohol addiction could happen in six months or less.

In some young people, there seems to be a genetic vulnerability to addiction. Studies of adoptees have revealed that alcoholism can be hereditary, at least in part. Further studies of alcoholics and drug abusers have also revealed a higher incidence of such addiction problems when one of the biological parents was an alcoholic (even if the child was raised in a nonalcoholic adoptive home).

■ Funneling and binge drinking are increasingly popular among high school and college students—and are responsible for a number of deaths.

■ Alcohol-related car accidents are a leading cause of death for teens and young adults. Alcohol is also a factor in other accidental deaths, including drownings and suicide.

■ Anabolic steroids are being used by a small but growing number of teens. Use among teen girls has doubled since 1991. This is of great concern because anabolic steroids can have serious, permanent side effects and long-term life-threatening consequences.

The choice to say no to harmful substances is a health-affirming one in many ways. Today's illicit drugs are more dangerous than ever—with marijuana, for example, generally stronger and quite different from the typical joint of the sixties or seventies. The substances most often abused—the ones we too often don't take seriously—can be the most hazardous to your health. Alcohol, a factor in a rising number of fatal accidents that take young lives each year, kills more teens than any other drug. And although the harmful effects of smoking tend to be more long-term, more and more is being discovered each year about this habit's awesome potential for harm, not only to the smoker, but also to those around him or her and even to that person's future children.

To begin to make your own healthy choices, you may need to begin to think in a whole new way about your life and the role substance abuse may play in it. If you do use or abuse substances—or are tempted to do so—this does not make you a bad person. Most people begin ultimately harmful habits because they want to feel better. They want to feel less shy, less awkward, less lonely, less depressed. They want to belong and be part of a group of accepting and caring friends. Wanting and needing to belong is something that we all feel. All of us have coped—with varying degrees of distress and eventual success—with shyness and social awkwardness. Doing this is part of growing up and part of simply being human. This fact of life can't be changed or alleviated in the long run by any chemical substance.

You also need to know and accept the fact that the dangers of drugs, alcohol, and nicotine are real. Bad things *can* happen to you if you take drugs, drink (especially if you drink and drive or ride with a drinking driver), or smoke. These dangers aren't scare tactics dreamed up by fun-shunning 40-year-olds. These are facts. You need to get past the "It can't happen to me!" mindset and look at the facts in a new way. Developing a realistic attitude about the risks and the possibilities you face will help you make choices that are best for you. This may be the beginning of a new balance of healthy habits *and* all the fun that is part of being young.

What Does All This Mean for You?

If you're like a lot of people, you've seen all the facts, scary statistics, horror stories, and maybe even a few real-life examples of the impact substance abuse can have on young lives—such as people you know in your school or community who have been killed in grad-night or prom-night car crashes or a classmate who disappeared into rehab or, worse yet, dropped out of school and into a questionable future. And yet it may all seem pretty irrelevant to your own life:

Maybe you smoke a little—but feel you can stop whenever you want.
Maybe you drink more than a little—but it doesn't feel like a real problem to you.

Maybe you've used drugs now and again or even pretty regularly—and nothing horrible has happened. In fact, you like the way you feel.

Before you can begin to sort out your healthy choices from the less healthy ones, you need to ask yourself some direct questions about how what you're choosing right now is affecting your life. You don't have to write to us with the answers. You don't have to tell your parents or even your best friend. You just need to be honest with yourself as you consider the following questions:

1. Have you lost time from school or work due to drinking or drug use?
2. Has drinking or drug use made it difficult for you to get along with your family?
3. Do you drink because you're usually shy—and can only relax and open up when you've got a buzz on? Do you use drugs or smoke when you're feeling tense? Are you finding that you really *need* substances in order not to feel shy or tense or depressed?
4. Has drinking, drug use, or smoking affected your reputation? Have you lost longtime friends because of this? Has your circle of friends changed to a faster-moving crowd (and sometimes it's a little scary or exhausting or just a pain to keep up with them)?
5. Have you ever felt unhappy after drinking or drug use? (This can be unhappy with how you acted when under the influence or just depressed in general.)
6. Do you crave a cigarette, a drink, or your drug of choice at a certain time every day or in specific situations?
7. Do you ever want a drink the morning after (even if you're feeling fairly hung over)?
8. Is your drinking or drug use making it difficult to do well in school? Have your grades (not to mention your motivation) dropped since you began using?
9. Have you ever had a loss of memory after drinking or drug use?

10. Do you ever drink or use alone?

11. Do you ever drink, use drugs, or even smoke to build up your self-confidence? Do you find it difficult, if not impossible, to get through school or a social event without this confidence crutch?

12. If you smoke, have you been having more colds lately? Has anyone told you that you have bad breath and/or refused to kiss you? Have you been burning holes in clothes due to dropped cigarettes or ashes? Do you find yourself on the outside looking in—hanging outside of food places while friends or family enjoy themselves inside—because you have to have a cigarette? Has your smoking caused conflicts between you and people who really matter to you?

13. Has your habit—drinking, drug use, or smoking—caused you to break a law?

14. Have you ever been sent to a hospital or jail as a result of drinking?

15. Have you ever stopped caring about how you look?

16. Do you eat irregularly while drinking or using drugs? Or do you smoke a cigarette instead of eating a meal?

17. Do you stay drunk or stoned for long periods (such as several days)?

18. Are you noticing any physical symptoms that you didn't have before, such as fatigue, frequent colds or other illnesses, or feeling hung over in the morning? Or do you just not feel quite as well as you used to feel physically (except when you're using)?

19. If you're an athlete, have you noticed your performance slipping or becoming harder to maintain?

20. If you're taking anabolic steroids, have you noticed any physical symptoms such as an increase in acne or, if you're a girl, a deeper voice, increased body and facial hair, or thinning hair on your head? Have you noticed that you're getting into fights or flying off the handle

at other people over stuff that didn't bother you as much before?

If you could honestly answer yes to any of these questions, your substance use is a problem. Even if you answered no to all and are still using, your choices could bring problems in the future.

THE REAL DANGERS OF THESE PROBLEM SUBSTANCES

People use drugs, alcohol, and cigarettes for a variety of reasons: to cope with shyness, nervousness, loneliness, anger, or social awkwardness, among many other problem feelings; to appear sophisticated and with it, to be part of the group—and share the group's experiences. The problem is that these substances are artificial means of coping. They don't really make you courageous or socially adept. If you take substances instead of learning to cope with the pressures and important lessons you face during these growing years, your social and emotional skills will lag behind your physical development well into adulthood—and maybe even forever. Letting substances mask your feelings and substitute for vital learning experiences will only perpetuate shyness, discomfort, loneliness, alienation, and depression.

In short, substances will only add to your problems instead of solving them. Why make adolescence any tougher than it already is?

THESE SUBSTANCES ARE HAZARDOUS TO YOUR HEALTH—AND YOUR LIFE!

Smoking

What Is It?

Teens who smoke may smoke cigarettes, cigars, pipes, or a combination of all of these.

So What's the Problem?

- *Smoking can shorten your life significantly.* A habitual smoker may be giving up six to nine years of life! You're at higher risk for several kinds of cancer (lung cancer as well as cancers of the lips, mouth, pancreas, esophagus, bladder, and uterus). Smokers have a two or three times greater chance of dying from a heart attack than nonsmokers. They also have many more strokes than nonsmokers and are nineteen times more likely to become victims of emphysema, a crippling respiratory disorder that destroys the lungs' elasticity and leaves the victim gasping for breath.

- *Smoking can make you a lot less attractive.* As well as bad breath, smelly clothes, and stained fingers now, smokers get wrinkles sooner than their nonsmoking friends. Medical studies have found that the level of wrinkling in women who smoked heavily was equivalent to that of women *20 years older!* This wrinkling pattern may be due to the fact that smoking causes constriction of blood vessels and may make the skin more susceptible to wrinkles.

- *Your secondhand smoke can hurt those you love.* Recent studies have found that women who smoke during pregnancy are almost *twice* as likely to miscarry or spontaneously abort. They are more likely to have a stillborn baby or to give birth to a smaller-than-normal child. Studies indicate that children of smokers are also more vulnerable to SIDS (Sudden Infant Death Syndrome) and respiratory problems. Also, children of mothers who smoke more than ten cigarettes a day have a 50 percent higher risk of developing childhood cancers. They may also have lower IQ scores, have difficulty reading and adjusting socially, and be significantly shorter than children of nonsmokers.

- *If you smoke, you have a greater risk of dying in a smoking-related accident.* More than 25 percent of all fires are caused by smokers, and so many car accidents are smoking-related (caused by a smoker taking his or her eyes off the road or hands off the wheel to light up or to retrieve a dropped cigarette) that some auto insurance companies offer discount rates to nonsmokers.

- *All smoking injures you to some extent.* If you're lucky, you may simply experience more than your share of illnesses every year, missing more work or school than a nonsmoker.

Smokeless Tobacco

What Is It?

Called *dip* or *snuff*, this is tobacco that is placed between the lip and the gum. A number of teens, especially those involved in team sports such as baseball and who feel that smoking is unhealthy but that smokeless tobacco is a less harmful substitute, are taking up this habit.

So What's the Problem?

Unfortunately, this habit is terribly unhealthy in its own way, putting users at considerable risk of developing oral cancer. Teens as young as 15 have suffered—and died—from this disfiguring cancer.

Alcohol

What Is It?

Alcohol is a drug that is being abused more and more by teenagers and young adults—and this fact is causing widespread concern. Nearly half of male high school seniors and one-fourth of female seniors who drink are problem drinkers. (This means that they get drunk six or more times a year or have problems in three or more areas of their lives because of drinking.) Of particular concern are drinking behaviors such as funneling (putting a funnel in the mouth and pouring beer or another alcoholic substance down the throat, enabling a teen to drink much more at a faster rate) and binge drinking, which is defined as having five drinks or more at one sitting.

So What's the Problem?

- *Funneling and binge drinking can kill.* As a number of well-publicized college campus tragedies have shown, alcohol ingested in this manner can kill in a number of hours. (Teens who die may do so because of alcohol poisoning or by choking on their own vomit.)
- *Alcohol-related auto accidents (as well as drownings, suicides, and homicides) kill a shocking number of teens each year.* Drinking and driving—whether it is a car, motorcycle, bicycle, boat, Jet-Ski, or other recreational vehicle—can be deadly, even if you don't feel drunk.
- *Regular use of alcohol in the teens can put one at risk for alcoholism.* As we saw in the statistics at the beginning of this chapter, teen drinkers are at high risk for becoming problem drinkers or alcoholics later on. Those from families with a history of alcoholism or other substance abuse are at highest risk.
- *Alcohol is hazardous to your health—especially if you're a female.* Alcohol can affect women faster, more seriously, and in a shorter time because they have more body fat and less body water than men, and this causes the alcohol to enter their bloodstream in a less diluted form. Women tend to develop health-threatening complications from alcohol in less time than men and by drinking less alcohol.

Overall, teens who drink are likely to have poor eating habits, more respiratory problems, general fatigue, and sleep disorders. Long-term health risks of alcohol abuse are much more serious, including severe liver damage that, in some instances, can kill while a person is still in young adulthood.

- *Alcohol can have a devastating impact on the life and health of a female drinker's unborn baby.* Fetal alcohol syndrome (FAS) in newborn babies is a tragic disorder that has been linked to drinking during pregnancy. These babies may be mentally retarded and have heart, facial, and body defects. A study at Boston City Hospital found that 74 percent of infants born to women who had ten to fifteen drinks a day suffered one or more symptoms of FAS. Scientists in Seattle discovered something even more alarming: In a group of 164 women who drank two ounces of whiskey a day during pregnancy, 9 had infants with FAS.

Subsequent studies have found that even a can of beer, a glass of wine, or a cocktail twice a week is enough to increase by 30 percent a woman's chance of either miscarrying or having a brain-damaged baby. And recent research from the University of Washington and the University of Michigan has revealed that heavy drinking (two drinks daily or at least five in one sitting) on the part of a baby's *father* during the month before conception can significantly lower the birth weight of the baby. (Low-birth-weight infants are more likely to die during their first year and are more likely to have birth defects or respiratory problems.)

The National Council on Alcoholism recommends that pregnant women stay away from liquor altogether during pregnancy. Men who have the potential to—or are trying to—father children would also do well to abstain from alcohol.

■ ■ ■

Marijuana

What Is It?

The substance most commonly used by teens (after alcohol and tobacco), marijuana is made from the hemp plant and is usually smoked in a *joint* or with a pipe or *bong* (though it can be ingested as an ingredient in cookies or brownies). It causes a sense of euphoria and relaxation as well as increased appetite. On a positive note, it has been used by cancer patients to help decrease pain and nausea after chemotherapy.

So What's the Problem?

- *Marijuana can have some undesirable short-term side effects.* These include lethargy, lack of motivation, bloodshot eyes, and dry mouth. Some report paranoia and impaired memory or reflexes.
- *Marijuana can come laced with other drugs—and give you a nasty surprise.* Some teens have the misfortune to smoke a joint laced with PCP ("angel dust") and suffer violent hallucinations, impaired judgment and muscle coordination, and at times aggressive, even violent behavior.
- *Smoking marijuana may be even more damaging to your lungs than smoking cigarettes.* An increasing number of medical studies are finding links between smoking marijuana and conditions such as chronic bronchitis, coughing, wheezing, frequent respiratory infections, and a greater risk of lung cancer, especially in people who also smoke tobacco. Researchers estimate that smoking three or four joints a day does as much damage to the lungs as smoking a pack of cigarettes! Joints are unfiltered and thus deposit four times more tar on the lungs than cigarettes. Also, people smoke marijuana differently: It tends to be more deeply inhaled and held in the lungs and airways longer.
- *Marijuana can impair the immune system.* Researchers at the University of Illinois at Chicago have found that THC, the active ingredient in marijuana, may disrupt the complex chemistry of the immune system, diminishing the body's ability to fight off disease-causing viruses and bacteria.
- *Marijuana can cause your brain to age faster.* A study at Wake Forest University's Bowman Gray School of Medicine reports that laboratory animals exposed to THC five times a week for a period of eight months showed a significant decrease in nerve cells in the vital part of the brain that plays a role in emotional behavior. This decrease in nerve cells seems to mimic the aging process. Thus, someone who smokes marijuana regularly and loses 30 percent of brain nerve-cell density at a young age may not notice the effects immediately. However, the normal aging process may account for another 30 percent loss over time. Reaching old age with a 60 percent loss of brain density could seriously affect one's quality of life.
- *Marijuana may affect your future fertility.* Heavy use of marijuana can disrupt hormone production in both males and females, cutting down the level of testosterone and sperm cells in men and interfering with menstrual cycles and ovulation in women. There is no proof, as yet, for pot-induced infertility (thus marijuana should never be considered as a contraceptive!). However, in pregnant women, THC can cross the placenta and cause damage to the developing fetus.
- *Marijuana can linger in your body and impair performance in a number of ways.* Unlike other drugs, which are fairly quickly processed out of the body, THC lingers in the body for four or five days. If a teen smokes marijuana even once or twice a week, this means that he or she may

have a constant level of the drug in the body. THC tends to accumulate in the reproductive organs and in the brain. The results may be difficulty concentrating; impaired reflexes, depth perception, and sense of time; sleep disorders; and personality changes. The habitual marijuana smoker may be just as unsafe a driver as a teen with a drinking problem.

- *Marijuana in cookies, brownies, and other foods can give you intestinal problems.* Those who ingest marijuana in cookies, brownies, or tea are at risk for *salmonellosis,* a common intestinal disease linked with ingesting marijuana contaminated with untreated animal manure.

- *Secondhand marijuana smoke can pack a punch.* This is important to know if you are tested for drugs at school or work or for a sports team. Hanging out with marijuana-smoking friends and inhaling secondhand smoke from their joints can affect you more than you realize. According to a recent study at the National Institute of Drug Abuse's Addiction Research Center, being exposed to the equivalent of only four joints in an hour can make *you* come out positive on a drug test!

Inhalants

What Is It?

Inhalant abuse—often called *huffing*—is a growing practice among young preteens and teenagers who inhale solvents, typewriter correction fluid, Scotchgard, and other household products. (One manufacturer—3M—has been so concerned about this that they have sponsored a rock video warning teens of the dangers of huffing.)

So What's the Problem?

These toxic fumes affect the nervous system and can cause paralysis and also sudden death by cardiac arrthymia. These health- and life-threatening

events could happen the first time you try huffing or the 100th time you try it—or maybe nothing terrible will happen. But why take the chance?

Stimulants

What Is It?

Stimulants include such popular teen drugs as crystal methamphetamine (crystal meth) and Ecstasy, as well as herbal Ecstasy. Cocaine and crack also fall into this category. Crystal meth, crack, and cocaine are usually snorted or smoked. Ecstasy and herbal Ecstasy are taken orally. These drugs can give a quick and intense high. While crack and cocaine highs are short, the high from crystal meth lingers for hours (but can be followed by a depression that lasts for days!). Ecstasy-induced euphoria and energy can also last for several hours.

So What's the Problem?

- *Some stimulants are highly addictive.* Among these are crystal meth, crack, and cocaine. This addiction can change your life in devastating ways.

- *Stimulants are unpredictable.* You may get a pleasurable high—or you may get a medical emergency. Crystal meth, for example, in addition to the previously mentioned depression, can cause increased blood pressure, rapid heartbeat, high fever, and nausea. Some users have suffered strokes, lapsed into comas, and died. Crack and cocaine can cause fatal seizures or heart attacks. Ecstasy and its herbal cousin can also cause high blood pressure, seizures, high fever (even heat stroke), heart attacks, and sudden death.

  If you think heart attack and stroke can happen only to some aging baby boomer tottering around snorting cocaine, think again. In studies of cocaine-related heart attacks, researchers have found that in most cases, these were healthy young people who had taken relatively small doses of cocaine. Many were not chronic users.

- *Abuse of some stimulants can damage your central nervous system.* Studies have shown that habitual use of stimulants, especially cocaine, can also cause a younger person to develop Parkinson's disease, a disabling, progressive disorder of the central nervous system. This apparently happens when cocaine upsets the balance of essential brain chemicals and at the same time destroys vital brain cells connected with motor skills. While Parkinson's disease—characterized by tremors, rigidity of muscles, and progressive crippling—occurs most commonly in the elderly, some cocaine users may develop this disorder some 20 years sooner than susceptible individuals in the general population.

- *There are uncomfortable side effects between amphetamine highs.* Snorted amphetamines can cause ulcers inside the nose; all amphetamine use can result in insomnia, anxiety, and paranoia.

LSD

What Is It?

LSD is a hallucinogenic drug. It can be licked off a postage stamp; ingested in sugar cubes, pills, or liquid; or eaten off one's clothing. Under the best of circumstances, it can cause a euphoric "trip" that can bring pleasant hallucinations and go on for hours.

So What's the Problem?

LSD is highly unpredictable. LSD trips tend to be highly individual—some are reported to be pleasant, some nightmares—and it's impossible to tell when a bad trip or "bummer" will happen. Dilation of pupils, flushing, occasional chilliness,

and increased pulse and respiration rates are some of the minor side effects. Paranoia and hallucinations are common major side effects, often lasting for the twelve to eighteen hours that LSD usually remains active in the body. For some, however, these effects can linger—or come back—for weeks, months, and even years. Long after taking the drug, a user may be confused and paranoid and have flashbacks of the LSD experience.

Heroin

What Is It?

Heroin is a highly addictive narcotic drug. It can be smoked, snorted, or injected. Most teen users these days tend to buy heroin in antihistamine capsules that are broken open and snorted. Heroin causes a euphoric high that can last for several hours.

So What's the Problem?

It's easy for teens to overdose on heroin—and the consequences can be deadly. This drug can cause the lungs to fill with liquid. It can also cause convulsions, coma, and death. Users who inject heroin into their veins with needles face another risk—AIDS—if they use or share needles contaminated with blood that has the AIDS virus present.

Anabolic-Androgenic Steroids

What Is It?

These synthetic derivatives of testosterone, the male sex hormone, are used by many athletes to build muscle mass and strength in a relatively short time. Unfortunately, use is not uncommon among high school athletes and enthusiastic teen weight lifters and body builders. As noted earlier, an increasing number of teen girls are using steroids, often in an attempt to build leaner bodies.

So What's the Problem?

Using this drug can be a shortcut to a lot of trouble. As well as triggering aggressive, violent behavior, anabolic steroids can lead to the following:

- *In males*: a decreased level of male reproductive hormones, permanent short stature, breast enlargement, high blood pressure, liver damage, and perhaps, some forms of cancer.
- *In females*: an increased level of male hormones, resulting in shrinking breasts, male-style hair growth (on the face and body), male-pattern baldness on the head, a deepening of the voice, enlargement of the clitoris, and menstrual problems. Some of these side effects are permanent. Long-term problems include cardiovascular disease, liver damage, and reproductive illnesses.

It's possible to excel in sports and to build a lean, strong body the healthy way: with good nutrition, responsible training, and the patience to let the body grow and develop in its own way.

MAKING A DECISION ABOUT DRUGS, DRINKING, AND SMOKING

Everyone in the world keeps saying "Just say no," but I don't think adults realize how hard it is. If I said no all the time, I wouldn't have any friends and everyone would make fun of me. Do you know what it would be like to be going through high school with everyone hating you?

Talia C.

Saying no to alcohol, drugs, and/or smoking is much easier said than done. And we never said that stopping a habit like smoking was easy. But it's possible to do both—and live a happy, healthy life.

I've been smoking since I was 13—so it has been three years. Sometimes I think about quitting, but it's SO hard! I can't begin to explain it to someone who has never smoked. They think it's so easy, just a matter of stopping one day. But it's not like that. I get really nervous and jittery and feel awful when I go without cigarettes. And, also, I'm scared of gaining a lot of weight if I stop smoking. I'd rather take my chances on some health risks later on than be fat now (and besides, being fat is a health risk, too, isn't it?). If I'm going to risk my health, I'd rather risk it looking good!

Marti Y.

Saying No from the Beginning

While it's easier to never start smoking or drinking or taking drugs than to stop a substance use or abuse habit, it isn't always easy to say no. Some of the most common obstacles to saying no include the following:

- *"I'm afraid of losing my friends. They'll think I'm a prude or a baby."* Some of the people you know may think that. But having your own point of view and your own strong feelings about what's right for you is a sign of *maturity*. Also, a friend worth having and keeping will respect your choices, even when these differ from his or hers. A real friend respects you as a distinct individual and wants the best for you. A friend who doesn't feel that way would probably be simply a temporary friend anyway. So when you lose a friendship like that, you're not losing as much as you're gaining: good health, self-esteem, and the respect of people who really care about you.
- *"I'm going through a tough time right now and I need something to make me feel better."* Feeling hurt by a special problem such as a romantic breakup, the death of someone dear to you, a parental divorce, an alcoholic or abusive parent, or a major disappointment can make you want to grasp onto anything that will ease your pain, if only for a little while. Feeling frustrated by school problems or lonely due to a

family move, a change of schools, or feeling intrinsically different from your classmates can also make you want to escape your problems.

Using alcohol or drugs to escape or smoking to mask your social shyness and awkwardness are only temporary measures. They don't do anything to solve your very real and painful problems. There *are* other, more constructive ways to cope; if you think about it, you can probably come up with some that sound possible to you.

✔ Talk with someone: a special friend or relative, an empathetic teacher, a school counselor, a hotline listener, or even a professional therapist or clergyperson.

✔ Listen to music that makes you feel better. (Studies show that this is what a *lot* of teens do when they're feeling depressed and down.)

✔ Exercise your anger, anxiety, or depression away. Regular exercise can release natural body substances called *endorphins*, which can make you feel better emotionally as well as physically.

✔ If you're facing a difficult situation at school or at home, consider your alternatives, by yourself or with the help of someone else. What can you do to change this problem situation to minimize or eliminate what is causing you pain? If nothing can be done right now, or the loss has happened and is final, take a deep breath and *feel* your pain, crying if you need to. Crying and grieving over a major loss are important steps toward healing and resolving your pain.

All of these alternatives can help you to grow, to cope more readily and constructively next time. All are far superior to postponing your resolving and healing with artificial substances.

■ *"I don't want to be considered 'out of it.'"* You will not be out of it if you pass up drugs, alco-

hol, or smoking. When you look at the statistics, *most* people, including teens, don't use these substances. It is becoming more and more acceptable and is considered quite sophisticated among adults and older teens *not* to smoke, drink, or use drugs.

Saying "No Thanks" Without Transforming into a Dork

■ *Say no and move on—without making a scene.* You don't have to rant, rave, and give long, impassioned explanations. A simple "No, thanks" or a short reason will do.

The following are some reasons we've heard from teens who have said these in a number of situations without any major problems from friends or acquaintances:

"I'd rather not."

"I tried it and didn't care for it."

"I get sick when I drink."

"One of us has to be sober to drive, and I've decided to be the driver."

"I'm allergic to it."

"I have a physical condition that makes it dangerous to do that."

"I feel better when I *don't* (drink, do drugs, smoke) and I want to make the most of this time with you."

■ *Seek help and ideas from others you respect.* Talk with older teens and adults who have said no successfully. They can help you feel good about your own choices and give you some ideas that have worked for them.

Stopping a Harmful Habit

Stopping a habit, especially one you've had for a while, isn't easy. It takes effort. It takes time. It takes patience with yourself. If you try and fail today to give up smoking or drinking or a drug, don't give up. Just try again. And don't be embarrassed to ask for help. If you have a serious drinking or drug problem, you may well need outside help to get you through, at least at the beginning.

Where can you get help?

■ *Check with your physician.* If you want to stop smoking, your physician may be able to help you or to refer you to a stop-smoking program. Some of these treatment plans include not only support during the difficult time when you're trying to stop, but also medical help such as a prescription-only nicotine patch (doctors report that teens tend to prefer the patch over nicotine gum). This can help ease the difficulty of withdrawal from nicotine, which is one of the most addictive substances known and a major reason why people find it so hard to quit smoking. Such programs will also help you develop other behaviors to replace the calming, soothing, mellowing impact smoking has had in your life.

Your physician will also be able to refer you to appropriate inpatient (in the hospital) or outpatient (you go to the hospital at certain times for treatment but don't stay overnight) treatment for drug or alcohol abuse treatment.

■ *Make use of self-help support groups.* This can include so-called 12-step groups founded on the model of Alcoholics Anonymous. There are 12-step programs for many different additions, including drug abuse (Narcotics Anonymous). You can find listings for these organizations in the white pages of your phone book. Members get together—on a first-name-only basis—and work through the steps of the program. Quite often, participation in a 12-step or similar group support program is a mandatory part of drug or alcohol rehab. But even if you aren't in a formal program or don't

feel your addiction is *quite* so bad, participation in one of these programs can help you to sort out your choices and priorities. Some offer groups for young people so that you will have the support of peers as you go about the difficult task of overcoming your addiction and building a new life for yourself.

Many people have a lot of resistance to joining a group or getting professional help to overcome a habit or addiction. "I can do it on my own anytime I want!" you may be saying. Really? Think about it. If you could have done it on your own, you would have done it already. While it's true that some people *can* stop smoking or drinking on their own, it's best to have medical supervision when stopping a serious drug or alcohol habit. And many people find that they need extra support in stopping smoking, too.

Remember: knowing and accepting the fact that you can't conquer a harmful habit alone is a sign of strength—and the first step toward recovery.

You can help yourself in many ways—whether you're going it alone or in a treatment program. Here are some suggestions.

■ *Stop your habit "just for today."* Don't tell yourself that you will never, ever have another cigarette (or drink, or joint, and so on). Tell yourself, instead, "*Just for today*, I will not smoke (or drink, or use drugs)." Stopping a habit forever is too formidable a task. Just do it day by day. You will feel your strength, your resolve, and your self-esteem grow over time as one daily success follows another.

■ *Take responsibility for your choices.* No one forced you to smoke, use drugs, or drink—really. You chose to do this. So you can choose to change the habit. Knowing that you have power over your life—and your habits—can help a lot!

■ *Don't put yourself in situations where the pres-*

sure is greatest. If there is a particular crowd whose major activity seems to be drinking or taking drugs, stay away from that crowd, even if you like certain individuals in it. (It's easier to say no to one or two people you see individually than to a crowd.) Avoid unsupervised parties. When someone whose parents are gone for the weekend is throwing a party, you know going in that there is likely to be more pressure of all kinds: to drink, to use drugs, to engage in sexual activity. If you have doubts, don't go. It's better to miss a party than to get talked into doing things you don't really want to do. Don't get into a car with people who are stoned, drinking, or drunk—even if it means calling your parents to pick you up.

- *Learn from the pressure.* Remember that peer pressure and taunts can be a learning experience. It's all part of learning to think for yourself. If you can withstand the pressure and make your own decisions, you'll have a good head start toward healthy adulthood.

- *Announce your new intentions to family and friends who care.* Those who love you most are most likely to help and cheer you on. They also have great memories for this kind of thing, and, if your resolve is wavering, will be quick to remind you of your good intentions.

- *Seek the best way of stopping—for you.* Some people do better in a group—for example, a stop-smoking clinic sponsored by the American Cancer Society, or similar services for others with substance abuse problems. Others can do it on their own. Those with certain drug problems—such as addiction to prescription drugs—may need to cut down gradually, under medical supervision, to minimize the danger of serious withdrawal symptoms. Others, particularly smokers, may do best if they simply stop "cold turkey." (Some medical studies have found that smokers who cut down to a few cigarettes a day were inhaling so deeply that they were really

minimizing the benefits of cutting down.) If you're stopping smoking or another substance habit, keep in mind that the first day is the hardest and that the urge to indulge will usually go away after a few minutes. Tough it out. You can do it.

- *Seek healthy alternatives.* If you're dying for a cigarette, a drink, or a drug, ask yourself what else you can do to ease whatever feelings or situation is contributing to your longing for this substance.

  ✔ Find new ways to feel less awkward socially—such as easing your expectations for yourself (you don't have to be witty and brilliant or the life of the party to have a good time and be liked by others) or learning social skills in stages (for example, focus on saying hello to and talking with one person at a party, in the school lunchroom, or wherever you feel awkward before you contemplate mixing in a crowd.)

  ✔ Explore alternatives for dealing with loneliness, depression, or tension. Talk to a friend or relative. Take a walk. Listen to music. Read a book. Answer a letter. Plan for the future. Make a list of things you like about yourself—or of five people you can really count on. There are many alternatives you can pursue—if you choose.

- *Be patient with yourself.* If you slip and have a cigarette, a drink, or a drug, don't consider the battle lost or label yourself as a hopeless addict. You're just human. You had a slip. Admit it and limit it to that one instance rather than using it as an excuse for a binge of substance use. Decide what you can learn from it—such as how to overcome the temptation better next time, what feelings or situations or people were connected with your slip, and how you can cope better in the future.

You *can* do it! In saying no to drugs, alcohol, and smoking, you're making a positive choice: You're saying yes to personal growth, self-discovery, and a healthier, happier life!

DRUGS, DRINKING, AND SMOKING

✔ The substances teens most often use and abuse are alcohol and tobacco. Studies show that the earlier you start drinking or smoking, the more likely you are to develop an addictive problem. Those who start drinking before age 15 are at higher risk for becoming alcoholics, and most lifelong smokers report having started their habit by age 14.

✔ Marijuana, the illegal drug most often used by teens, is not as harmless as it seems. In fact, studies are showing that smoking marijuana can be even more harmful to the lungs than smoking tobacco.

✔ Girls pay a particular price for bad habits. Smoking cuts down much more dramatically on teen girls' lung capacity; anabolic steroids can have a devastating and permanent physical impact—balding, deepening of voice, growth of body hair, shrinkage of breasts, and clitoris enlargement.

✔ If you hang out with friends who are smoking marijuana, their secondhand smoke may cause *you* to show positive on a drug test!

✔ You can say no to drinking, drugs, and smoking without being a friendless dork. Say "No thanks" without making a scene or lecturing others about it. Find other ways to ease tension, stress, and social discomfort in your life. You can have friends, fun, and all the advantages of being young without harming your health.

✔ If you want to stop a harmful habit, your doctor is a good person to see. If you have a serious drug or alcohol problem or have been taking too many prescription medications, it's important to have medical supervision and support as you begin to withdraw from your substance of choice on the road to sobriety. Even if you're a smoker looking to quit, medical help may make a difference. Many teens have found the nicotine patch (prescription only) helpful whether they're trying to stop smoking on their own or in a special program.

CHAPTER NINE

Mind over Body

My younger sister (she's 14 and I'm 15) is dieting herself down until she looks like a skeleton. My parents took her to a doctor and they think she has anorexia and she's supposed to eat or else she'll have to go into the hospital. But no matter how my parents or older brother or I talk to her, she won't eat enough to gain any weight. That really makes me mad. It also scares me. Could you tell me more about anorexia and whether people really could die from it?

Sarah J.

Mind and body are inseparable. What affects one will affect the other. So some physical diseases, such as mononucleosis, can bring about depression. And stress and depression can give you headaches, stomachaches, and a variety of other ills. Although the mind-body connection is one of the hot medical topics of the millennium, and more people are understanding the mind-body connection both in terms of diseases and in terms of healing, disorders with a psychological component are all too often misunderstood:

"It's all in your head."

"It's just nerves."

"Forget it. It'll go away."

Have you ever heard of people getting the runs because they're nervous about an exam? I do that during finals every semester and it's really bad. Once I had to leave the room DURING a final. I get stomachaches a lot, too, when I have to give a report in class. My folks put a lot of pressure on me to make good grades, but that's something I want, too. It isn't just them. What can I do about my stomach problems?

Jeremy L.

How many times have you heard this and gritted your teeth as your headache pounded unmercifully or your stomach churned? How many times have you wondered whether symptoms like these might mean that you have a serious health problem? How many times have you thought, "If this *is* just all in my mind, does that mean I'm crazy?"

I get bad, bad headaches about once or twice a month. My mom says they're migraines because she has them. She's getting help for these with something called biofeedback and if that doesn't help her she's going to get acupuncture (with NEEDLES!). I don't want anything to do with any of that. Isn't there a pill I could take? And how do you know if a headache is a migraine or just a plain headache? Can feeling stressed out give you a headache?

Gillian B.

Too often, people dismiss disorders that we call *psychosomatic* (caused, at least in part, by emotional factors) as imaginary and unimportant. Contrary to popular notions, the pains and other symptoms of psychosomatic disorders are connected with the mind and the emotions, but are not imaginary.

THE STRESS CONNECTION

How does the mind enter into these problems? Feelings, especially emotional responses to stress, may help trigger or aggravate certain physical conditions. It's virtually impossible to separate your body and your mind.

What are some of the feelings that can give us physical symptoms? Anxiety, tension, and depression—to name only three—are some of these and may all be related to stress. And no one is immune to stress. It's an inescapable fact of all our lives. We can see—and even expect—stress as we cope with exams, the breakup of an important relationship, the death of someone close, or an increase in fights and tensions at home.

But stress can come from positive events, too. Winning an award, graduating from high school, going away to college for the first time, getting married and/or moving into an apartment of your own, getting your first full-time job, having a baby—all of these positive life changes bring stress along with the challenge and the joy.

Dr. Thomas H. Holmes III, professor of psychiatry at the University of Washington, studied the relationship between illness and the stresses that change may bring. His 43-item stress-rating scale covers everything from the death of a spouse (100 points) or a close family member (63 points) to marriage (50 points), pregnancy (40), outstanding

personal achievement (28), starting or leaving school (26), change in schools (20), a vacation (13), and minor violations of the law (11). Dr. Holmes found that if a person scores 300 change points in a year, he or she has an 80 percent chance of experiencing a change of health as well.

Your body may react to stress by becoming more prone to illness (such as colds), or you may develop one of the more common health problems that may be rooted, at least in part, in stress—and in how you handle this stress. Migraine and tension headaches, gastrointestinal problems such as irritable bowel syndrome and ulcerative colitis, bulimia, compulsive overeating, and anorexia nervosa (compulsive starvation) can bring you very real pain, both mentally and physically.

HEADACHES

There are many types of headaches; not all of them are tied in with emotions. Some, for example, may result from illness: colds, flu, a sinus infection, a dental problem. Others may come from allergies, eye strain, or high blood pressure. Still others may result from something you do—such as eating big bites of ice cream too fast, skipping a meal, drinking or smoking too much, or becoming fatigued. Only in rare instances does a headache signal a brain tumor, although this is a possibility that occurs to anyone who gets headaches regularly.

If you are plagued with regular headaches, however, it's important to see a physician. He or she may help you identify the type of headache you're having and its possible causes. If you're like most chronic headache sufferers, your physician's examination and tests are likely to reveal that there is nothing organically wrong with you.

What can cause chronic headaches? A variety of physical and psychological factors can combine to bring pain and suffering via tension headaches (caused by muscular contraction), psychogenic (depression) headaches, or migraine headaches. Tension and depression headaches are, of course, rooted in the emotions and in muscular responses to these feelings.

Tension Headaches

Tension headaches are most often felt at the front and/or the sides of your head or at the base of your skull. These headaches are often caused by stress-induced anxiety, which also causes muscular tension and tightness in your shoulders and neck. Aspirin or other analgesics and rest are the best way to deal with tension headaches.

Depression Headaches

Depression headaches, stemming from depression and anxiety, may involve tense muscles in the face, head, and neck, and/or a pattern of pain that may feel like a band circling the head. These headaches are more likely to strike early in the morning or in the evening and on weekends. They are the result of longstanding depression. Other signs of depression may be present.

Sleep patterns, researchers have found, can help one tell the difference between tension and depression headaches. A person with tension may have trouble getting to sleep at night. A depressed person, on the other hand, may fall asleep readily, but his or her sleep pattern may be fitful—with awakening during the night or early in the morning.

Pain relievers are only part of the answer in combating a depression headache. It's also important to deal with the feelings behind the physical pain. You may do this with the help of a professional or maybe combine professional help with support from family and friends.

With tension and depression headaches, it's vital to attack the source of your pain, not just the symptoms.

Migraine Headaches

Migraine headaches are something else again. They can be extremely painful, with severe, sometimes throbbing pain, usually on one side of the head. There may be nausea, blurring of vision, sensitivity to light and noise, and dizziness.

There are several different types of migraine headaches, but all are classified as *vascular* headaches. That is, they are triggered not by muscular tension, but by changes in blood vessels. Contrary to widespread opinion, the blood vessels that change are not *in* the brain, but *around* the brain.

What happens when a migraine strikes? For reasons as yet unknown, there is a change in the concentration of a substance called *serotonin*. This causes the blood vessels in and around the brain to experience changes, too. In some people who suffer from migraines, these blood vessels will *constrict* first, causing a phenomenon known as an *aura*. This is characteristic of the *classic migraine*. The person may see flashing lights or colors, spots before the eyes, or blind spots, or may experience extreme sensitivity to light and visual distortions—with people or objects growing smaller or larger. (It is said that Lewis Carroll wrote much of *Alice in Wonderland* while under the influence of migraine headaches.) Mood changes may accompany the aura, or may occur even without an aura. The migraine victim may feel giddy and euphoric. Then the pain hits. The pain of the migraine headache, which comes when the blood vessels dilate (swell), can be intense.

What causes migraine headaches? Heredity can be a factor in migraines. If both of your parents suffer from migraines, you have about a 70 percent chance of doing so. If one parent had these headaches, your chance of having them is about 45 to 50 percent. Of all migraine sufferers, 65 to 80 percent have a family history of these headaches. Some researchers theorize that there may be a migraine-prone gene at work here, giving you a physical, genetic predisposition. Others contend that migraines may be learned or acquired from your environment. You may imitate your parents or experience migraines as a reaction to an atmosphere of tension and high expectations. Whatever the reasons behind this phenomenon, migraines can, indeed, run in families.

Stress can also figure prominently in migraine attacks. The headaches may come in times of stress or in the letdown period after a stressful time (the weekend after final exams, for example, or on the first day of a long-awaited vacation).

Hormones may also influence your headaches. Some women experience increased migraines just before or during menstruation or in response to the synthetic hormones in birth control pills. For this reason, women who begin to suffer migraine-type headaches while taking birth control pills should consult their physician and, possibly, switch to another brand of pill or another form of birth control.

Certain emotions—such as anger and frustration (particularly if these feelings are repressed)—may be a factor in migraines.

What you eat may also bring on a headache. The chemical *tyramine*, which is found in most cheeses, many citrus fruits, freshly baked bread, lima and navy beans, pork, vinegar (except wine vinegar), onions, and nuts, has been pinpointed as a possible migraine trigger. Chinese food containing the food additive MSG, chocolate, and, in some instances, the artificial sweetener aspartame (NutraSweet) can also cause problems. Some feel that alcohol may also stimulate the blood vessels and should be avoided if you suffer from chronic migraines.

What treatments are available? Some prescription drugs can prevent or interrupt a developing migraine. Some of the newest of these include Amerge and Zomig, medications in pill form that alleviate migraine symptoms. Also quite promising are the nasal sprays: Imitrex (it gives relief in a matter of minutes, but can leave a temporary, unpleasant taste in the mouth) and Migranal (which can offer relief in 30 to 60 minutes along with a temporarily stuffy nose). Maxalt, a quick-dissolving wafer, is currently being tested and has been found to ease migraine pain within half an hour.

Some people find that nonprescription drugs such as aspirin and ibuprofen may help during the painful part of the migraine. There is a fairly new product called Excedrin Migraine (which contains caffeine as well as aspirin) that a number of people have found helpful.

There are also some alternative-medicine migraine prevention measures, which we will discuss in more detail in the "Alternative Medicine" section of this chapter. These include the herb *feverfew*, as well as biofeedback and acupuncture.

STRESS AND YOUR STOMACH

The gastrointestinal tract—most notably the stomach and intestines—may also be affected by stress. Some of us, in fact, are so good at burying our feelings that it may take a stomachache, diarrhea, or more alarming symptoms to tell us just how tense, frightened, or angry we feel. Often only a physician can tell the serious from the minor, so if you do experience frequent gastrointestinal problems, it's a good idea to consult your physician.

The following descriptions are included not so that you can diagnose and self-medicate your condition, but simply to give you an idea how stress can affect your stomach—and how important it is to seek help and treatment early.

Many young people suffer from stomach pains. A recent study at the University of Connecticut evaluated 507 junior high and high school students and found that 75 percent of them reported abdominal pain from time to time. About 15 percent reported stomach pain on a weekly basis. And 8 percent of the junior high school students and 17 percent of the high school students reported symptoms of irritable bowel syndrome.

Irritable Bowel Syndrome

Irritable bowel syndrome (IBS) is one of the most common gastrointestinal problems in teens. Symptoms include abdominal pain with bloating, alternating bouts of diarrhea and constipation (or just diarrhea), nausea, and a feeling of faintness. Many teens with this condition also report feelings of anxiety and depression.

With IBS, it is important to avoid spicy foods, as well as alcohol, coffee, or tea and foods high in fiber (also called *roughage*).

Learning to manage stress and your feelings in general—whether these are fear (before exams, a special date, or any other event in your life), anger, or general anxiety—is probably one of the most effective ways to combat this stress-related intestinal ill.

Some young people suffering from irritable bowel syndrome may need professional help to deal with the troubled feelings that can be linked to this problem. A study at the University of North Carolina found that more than half of 206 young women patients with irritable bowel syndrome had a history of physical and/or sexual abuse. If that describes your situation, you may need some psychotherapy or other counseling that may be comfortable for you before your physical condition begins to improve.

STRESS AND EATING DISORDERS

Stress and pressure to meet our society's unrealistic standards of model-thinness puts many adolescent girls at risk of developing eating disorders. A relatively small number of males develop eating disorders, too, usually because they are engaged in sports such as gymnastics or wrestling that tend to have strict weight requirements.

What are the most common eating disorders and who is at risk? Fear-of-obesity syndrome, anorexia nervosa, bulimia, and compulsive overeating are the eating disorders most likely to afflict teens—and we'll be describing these in detail in a moment. But since the risk factors for developing an eating disorder are quite similar, let's take a look at those first.

Who is most at risk of developing an eating disorder?

- *An adolescent girl.* This may be due to the fact that women in our society are more likely to be judged by how they look, and female standards of beauty are more geared to the media ideal of model thinness than are male standards of attractiveness.

- A *person with a perfectionistic personality.* These are often excellent students, well-behaved and intent on doing everything just right—including pursuing the elusive ideal of svelte perfection.

- A *person from a family where weight is an issue.* Parents may put a great value on slimness; the teen may either try to please parents by becoming perfectly slim or rebel by overeating and becoming obese.

- A *person who has had early sexual trauma.* Studies show that those who have had sexual trauma (abuse or molestation) may unconsciously try to protect themselves by making their bodies sexually unattractive and by focusing their attention on something safe—such as food—rather than dangerous—such as human contact and sexual relationships.

- A *girl who reaches physical maturity earlier than her peers.* Early-maturing girls, who experience the normal puberty weight gain while their classmates still have the slim, straight shapes of preadolescence, may be incorrectly identified as overweight by peers, parents, and themselves. Studies show that these girls are particularly likely to have poor body image.

- *Girls with authoritarian parents.* Those raised by strict, authoritative parents or who feel compelled to please their parents may see control of their weight and body shape as their only means of independent choice and expression.

- *Teens growing up with a substance-abusing parent or in an otherwise dysfunctional family.* Having an alcohol- or drug-abusing parent can create a lot of stress. So can being in a family where expressing feelings, especially angry feelings, is taboo. Some teens may eat compulsively when they have these unexpressed feelings or when they're feeling depressed or lonely. Others may react to this stress by compulsively dieting or binging and purging.

- *Teens who are depressed and/or have low self-esteem.* These young people may be especially sensitive to critical remarks and suggestions that they may be overweight—whether or not this is really the case.

Fear-of-Obesity Syndrome

What It Is

Fear-of-obesity syndrome is characterized by self-induced malnutrition due to an exaggerated fear of becoming fat. It differs from anorexia nervosa in its intensity and the fact that teens with this syndrome do not exhibit some of the emotional problems common in those with anorexia nervosa. However, some of the behavior patterns are the same.

Symptoms

Food avoidance, stringent dieting, and body image distortion (thinking you're fat when you're really not).

Special Characteristics

These teens have an exaggerated concern with obesity, regardless of actual body weight.

Dangers

Fear-of-obesity syndrome can evolve into an eating disorder such as anorexia nervosa or bulimia. In the meantime, it can also interfere with a girl's growth and development, since this self-induced malnutrition comes at a time when the body needs nutrients and a certain level of body fat to complete the growth and maturation process. It can be hazardous to self-esteem as well, since model-thinness is often an elusive goal.

Treatment

Fear-of-obesity syndrome can be treated with nutritional and behavioral counseling. Check with your physician for help.

Anorexia Nervosa

What It Is

This disorder is a serious psychosomatic disorder. Characterized by compulsive dieting and self-starvation, anorexia may have some contributing physical as well as emotional factors. A recent study at the National Institute of Mental Health found that a group of women with anorexia had unusual brain secretions of a hormone called *vasopressin*, which regulates the body's water balance. The effects of this hormone on behavior are not yet known, but researchers theorize that this unusual hormonal response could be a factor in tipping the balance between an ordinary diet and compulsive starvation.

Symptoms

Food avoidance, compulsive exercise, intense fear of fat, distorted body image (feeling fat even when emaciated), refusal to maintain a body weight at or over the minimum normal weight for age and height, amenorrhea (cessation of menstrual periods), obsession with food and cooking (while not eating), heavy use of laxatives, and occasional binges punctuated by self-induced vomiting.

Dangers

The dangers of anorexia nervosa are well documented medically. Even when not fatal—as it is in 5 to 15 percent of cases—anorexia can cause severe malnutrition, very low blood pressure, cardiac arrthymia (irregular heartbeat), bone weakness, and general poor health.

Treatment

Prompt medical help—preferably early, before a dangerous amount of weight has been lost—is vital. Treatment is often multifaceted, with medical treatment—sometimes inpatient hospitalization— used in conjunction with individual and family therapy. In this era of managed care, it can be difficult for a family to get either sufficient coverage or sufficient inpatient treatment in some instances. This phase of treatment, however, can be crucial; it's important to work with your physician and your insurance company to get as comprehensive a program as possible. In addition to medical care, family therapy is especially effective since anorexia nervosa can be a symptom of family and parent-child relationship problems.

There is increasing interest these days in drug treatment for anorexia, with research being done with a class of drugs called *opioid inhibitors*. These drugs block the action of pleasure-causing brain opioids and help to break an anorectic person's addiction to dieting. The results of treatment with the drug in several studies have been promising, with 75 percent of patients treated with the drug Naltrexone gaining a healthy amount of weight.

Bulimia

What Is It?

Bulimia is a common eating disorder affecting 4 out of every 100 women between the ages of 17 and 25 (while anorexia affects about 1 in every 100 girls). The major characteristics of this disorder are binge eating followed by purging via self-induced vomiting and laxative use.

Both psychosocial and physical factors can be involved in developing bulimia. Some studies show that as many as 75 percent of bulimics experience major depression; other studies link bulimia with both major and manic depression, anxiety disorders, and substance abuse. Other medical experts believe that bulimia and some forms of depression

may be caused by the same underlying chemical imbalance involving lower than normal levels of the neurotransmitters that facilitate commands between nerve cells in the brain.

Symptoms

A person with bulimia alternately binges on food, sometimes consuming thousands of calories an hour, and then purges via self-induced vomiting, enemas, and laxative abuse. Unlike people with anorexia, those with bulimia tend to be within their normal weight range, so the disorder can remain undetected for years. However, some signs that may appear over time include severe tooth decay (from stomach acids eating away tooth enamel during purging), swollen salivary glands, and irritated mouth tissues.

Dangers

Like anorexia, bulimia can be fatal, with most deaths occurring as the result of rupture of the esophagus from vomiting or from ipecac poisoning or cardiac arrest, the latter most common in women who abuse laxatives or diuretics or who are also alcoholics. A person with bulimia may also suffer from ulcers, hernia, and dangerous body chemistry imbalances that can lead to kidney and heart failure.

Treatment

Bulimia is usually treated with a combination of medical care and psychotherapy. A number of antidepressant drugs relieve symptoms of bulimia. In recent years, Prozac has become, perhaps, the most frequently prescribed medication for bulimia. Like other serotonin reuptake inhibitors, Prozac's side effects are few and patients may actually lose some weight on this medication.

Many experts feel that though drug therapy can be helpful for some people with bulimia, there is no substitute for psychotherapy in helping a patient overcome this disorder.

Compulsive Overeating

What Is It?

This eating disorder is characterized by a large intake of food, more often than not as a result of emotional factors rather than physical hunger. Since this binge behavior takes place without purging, the compulsive overeater's weight may range from slightly to significantly overweight or obese.

Symptoms

Eating large quantities of food, often in secret, without the purging behavior characteristic of anorexia and bulimia. Compulsive overeaters may eat normally at mealtimes, but eat large quantities of food secretly between meals. They often eat in response to emotional rather than physical cues, binging when angry, sad, nervous, or depressed or even when excited or happy about something. Food is often used as a stress reliever or a way to silence angry, hostile feelings the person feels he or she can't express.

Dangers

An obese teenager's greatest dangers are social: He or she tends to be ridiculed and excluded, facing discrimination not only from peers but also from employers and, in some instances, from college admission officials. There are some long-term physical dangers, however, since an estimated 80 percent of obese teenagers become obese adults at risk for life-threatening cardiovascular disease, adult-onset diabetes, and some forms of cancer.

Treatment

A well-balanced eating plan that can be maintained long-term (rather than relying on stringent diets, liquid meals, or prepackaged-food diet programs), combined with regular physical exercise, is the best way to overcome the physical results of compulsive overeating. A doctor- or nutritionist-supervised regimen of participation in programs such as Shapedown or Weight Watchers, which also feature behavior modification help, are commonsense alternatives.

However, as well as treating the symptoms, the underlying pain of this eating disorder needs to be addressed in individual or family therapy for best long-term results.

HYPERTENSION (HIGH BLOOD PRESSURE)

Hypertension, or high blood pressure, can strike at any age, including childhood, adolescence, and young adulthood. High blood pressure means increased stress on the walls of the blood vessels. This can be serious if the pressure becomes so great that it actually causes a break in the vessel wall and bleeding into surrounding tissues. If this occurs in the brain, it is called a *stroke* and can be most serious. Bleeding into the delicate tissues of the brain can result in paralysis and even death. The higher one's blood pressure, the higher the risk of stroke.

Some people are more likely to develop hypertension than others. For reasons not fully understood, African Americans suffer a much higher incidence of high blood pressure. So do people who are obese and those with serious ailments such as kidney disease. High blood pressure may occur for a number of physical reasons; stress and anxiety may also be major factors influencing your blood pressure.

The blood vessels are regulated by the nervous system. Given the body's "fight or flight" response to severe stress, tension, and anxiety, these blood vessels may constrict and high blood pressure results, especially in someone who may already have a pre-existing tendency toward hypertension.

How do you know if you have high blood pressure?
You won't know unless you have your blood pressure checked. Many victims of hypertension have no

symptoms. Others experience dizziness, headaches, and nervousness, symptoms often associated with high blood pressure. But it is possible to have one or all of these and not have high blood pressure.

Two readings—*systolic* and *diastolic*—are taken in a blood pressure examination. In a blood pressure reading of 120/80 (considered normal for young adults), 120 is the systolic. This means the higher pressure achieved each time the heart pumps. This may be affected by tension and anxiety. (If you had a bad day, for example, your systolic might be 150.) The diastolic reading is the low pressure as the heart is filling up once again with blood. This is usually considered the more significant reading, as it reflects the true estimate of the dynamics of the body regarding blood pressure.

Although the blood pressure reading for those in their mid-twenties or younger should not—as a rule—be higher than 120/80, there are significant variations of normal. Athletes, for example, have *wide pulse pressure* with a strong cardiac output. *Wide pulse* means that the person has an efficient cardiac output, requiring fewer heartbeats to circulate the blood. Consequently, an athlete's blood pressure might be 110/50. Children and very young teenagers whose vessels have not aged may have a 90/60 reading.

When does a reading cause concern? Generally, a flag goes up if you have a diastolic of 90 or greater as well as a systolic of 140 or above. If you have high blood pressure, your physician will investigate possible causes. If you show no evidence of a disease that might be a factor, your doctor may advise you to cut your salt intake, avoid taking birth control pills (which may elevate blood pressure), and, possibly, take diuretics. A diuretic will cause you to urinate more frequently and thus help to remove salt and fluid from your body. If you're overweight, this, too, may be contributing to your hypertension. Losing weight may also mean a drop in your blood pressure.

A *point to remember*: If you do have high blood pressure, you *must* be under the care of a physician. But you can care for yourself in important ways, too,

since hypertension can be tied to stress. Taking time out from your hectic daily schedule just for you—to listen to music, just stare at the ceiling, write in your diary, or take a walk—can help alleviate some of the stress you may be feeling every day. Learning to say no when you want to and taking care not to overload your already busy schedule are important preventive measures. You need time to just *be*.

ALTERNATIVE MEDICINE: NEW/OLD WAYS OF HEALING

Yoga Lotus

Especially when it comes to mind-body concerns, alternative medicine offers relief and new hope to many. Even though some people see these techniques as quite new, many are rooted in folk medicine—from Asian, Native American, and African healing methods. Some techniques, too, are products of modern technology, but enable you to use the power of your mind to help ease your physical symptoms.

Chiropractors, who treat pain and injuries via manipulation of the spine, are probably the most common and familiar "alternative medicine" practitioners now being recognized by traditional medicine—with many more insurance companies and HMOs covering expenses for such treatments. Other somewhat less familiar forms of alternative medicine include the following:

■ *Biofeedback.* Biofeedback is one of the most common nondrug treatments used for treatment of migraine headaches. Here the patient, hooked up to the electrodes of a biofeedback machine, learns to relax by listening to the sounds emitted by tensing and relaxing muscles, and learning to control other functions at will. Many migraine victims learn, via biofeedback, to concentrate on raising the temperature in their hands. Some feel that warm hands mean relaxation, while cold hands mean you're tense. Concentrating on warming your hands, then, may also cause you to relax. It may also mean sending more blood to your hands—and away from your head. When the patient learns how to control body responses like this, he or she can do it anywhere, any time, without having to be hooked up to a feedback machine.

■ *Herbal remedies.* Some folk remedies have become positively mainstream as people become dissatisfied with traditional medicine. Ginger is being rediscovered as a remedy for upset stomachs—from stress to motion sickness to morning sickness. Feverfew can help to prevent migraine headaches. And some neurologists now recommend riboflavin (400 mg/day) for those who suffer from migraines. St. John's wort is newly popular as a mild antidepressant. Chamomile (most often ingested as tea) can help gastrointestinal ills and menstrual cramps. Echinacea can help prevent a cold or flu from developing into a full array of symptoms.

Caution:

✔ Don't overdo it with herbs. Take only the dosage recommended by your physician or other licensed medical practitioner. Don't mix a lot of different herbs.

✔ If you have a pre-existing condition, such as diabetes or epilepsy, it's important to check with your physician before taking any herbal medicines. One teen patient we saw recently had a seizure while taking St. John's wort. It appeared that this teen, who had a seizure disorder that had been well-controlled by medication, had her seizure threshold lowered by the addition of the St. John's wort. If you have a similar condition or are taking regular medication of any kind, check with your doctor first before even trying an herbal medicine.

✔ If your physician or pharmacist isn't knowledgeable about herbs, check with a licensed naturopath. (To find one, call the American Association of Naturopathic Physicians at (206) 323-7610.) Or you might look for a doctor of Oriental medicine (or a licensed acupuncturist who has received special training in Oriental medicine) if you're interested specifically in Chinese herbs.

■ *Guided imagery and music therapy.* This has become newly popular with tapes and CDs on the impact of the Mozart Effect—a technique of relaxation and imagery while listening to specific classical music by Mozart. However, guided imagery and music therapy have been around for years. You can find many different relaxation tapes using this technique. Also, many psychotherapists use this tool to help clients deal with stress and anxiety. A combined technique, using soothing music while a patient imagines a tranquil scene, has been found useful in the treatment and prevention of migraine headaches.

■ *Hypnosis.* Far from being the strange stage trick where a hypnotist gets people to cluck like chickens and otherwise make total fools of themselves, seemingly against their wills, hypnosis, when it is used by a licensed medical or mental health professional, can be very therapeutic. It is often used to help patients deal with stress and anxiety or a specific phobia—such as fear of dentists or of a specific medical procedure. Many reputable professionals these days are trained in hypnosis. All of them would tell you that it is impossible to make you do anything against your will. Hypnosis may be quite useful in getting past a feeling or fear that has been an obstacle for you. Hypnosis can also be useful in stress management, anxiety, and phobias and is sometimes used as an adjunct treatment for compulsive overeaters.

Caution: We highly recommend that, if you are interested in hypnosis for a specific problem, you go to a licensed physician or a psychotherapist who is trained in hypnosis rather than someone who is listed as a certified hypnotherapist (CHT). Although there are undoubtedly some capable, highly professional CHTs, many, unfortunately, are very poorly trained, with only a weekend course in hypnosis and little if any knowledge of medicine or psychology or any legal obligation to observe specific professional ethics. Since hypnosis is most often used as an addition to medical or psychotherapeutic treatment, it is better to see a licensed professional in either field who can offer you a full array of treatment.

- *Acupuncture.* This ancient Chinese healing remedy uses fine needles at very specific points in the body (depending on the ailment). It has received increasing acceptance by Western medicine in recent years and has been found useful for treating many different kinds of pain, perhaps by triggering pain-blocking endorphins. Although there are licensed acupuncturists (in some states that require it) and many others who are certified by the National Commission for the Certification of Acupuncturists (call (202) 232-1404 for a referral to one in your area), it's also important to know that many traditional physicians are trained in acupuncture. If your doctor doesn't have this training, you can find one who does by calling the American Academy of Medical Acupuncture at (800) 521-2262.

- *Meditation.* There are a number of ways to meditate. Some people do it on their own by finding a quiet place, relaxing, and imagining a peaceful scene. Others practice religious meditation. Still others find healing in a more formal program of meditation such as Transcendental Meditation, a highly effective technique for gaining deep relaxation, managing stress, promoting inner peace, and alleviating the symptoms of a variety of medical problems. Studies have shown, for example, that Transcendental Meditation was more effective in alleviating anxiety than other forms of meditation. It has been shown scientifically to relieve high blood pressure, insomnia, and other physical manifestations of stress. To find training for this in your area, call the toll-free number (888) LEARN-TM.

If you're simply interested in trying meditation gradually, tapes or classes at your local community college or adult school may offer some useful techniques.

- *Diet, nutrition, and lifestyle changes.* As we noted in Chapters 5, 6, and 7, choices you make about what you eat, how you exercise, and how you take care of your body can have a huge impact on your continuing wellness. Medical science is recognizing that exercise can help you manage stress; this, in turn, can help prevent some stress-related physical illnesses. In the same way, watching what you eat can alleviate the symptoms of conditions such as irritable bowel syndrome, migraine headaches, and high blood pressure. In a growing number of medical centers, nutritionists and exercise physiologists are becoming valued members of preventive-medicine teams.

This approach also gives you more power in your own health maintenance. Instead of expecting a doctor or a pill to fix a condition, you can prevent it or control it by wise and healthful lifestyle choices.

MAKING SENSE OF THE MIND-BODY CONNECTION

It's important to see your health in a holistic sense with emotional health, stress management, and good self-care (in all ways) just as important as good nutrition, regular exercise, good health habits (such as brushing and flossing your teeth), and regular checkups are to your overall good health. With all the stresses in your life—because you're a busy teen who is juggling school, work, friends, and family as well as dealing with a body that is constantly changing—it's not surprising that stress-related physical ailments happen. It's important to understand your psychological needs as well as your physical needs and ask for help when you need it. It may be easier when you see counseling as necessary for healthy, strong people who want to grow.

Growing may mean accepting responsibility for your health: asking for help when you need it and helping yourself when you can. It may help a great deal to realize that feelings must be expressed in some way. If you can't express your feelings in a way of your choosing—talking or writing, for example—these feelings will choose their own way to come out. If you let anger build up, for example, it may burst out in a temper tantrum, a throbbing headache, or stomach cramps—or even trip you up in an accident! In the long run, then, it may be much less painful to say "I feel angry" than to find yourself yelling "Ouch!" or moaning "Oh, my aching head!"

It's important, too, not to put yourself down for feelings or characteristics that you consider negative. We *all* get angry. We *all* have flaws and failings. Having compassion for your faults and accepting feelings such as anger as normal may reduce stress in your life considerably.

A certain amount of stress, however, is inevitable. So it's important that your body be ready for it. Regular exercise, for example, will not only help you work off some of your tension and frustration, but it will also increase your body's capacity to handle stress when it does come. A physically fit body and the knowledge that a rich assortment of professional help—from traditional medicine to alternative medicine—is available when you need it can be reassuring as you face the rigors of daily life. Even more important, however, is the conviction that *you* have the power—if you use it—to keep a healthy balance in your life and to prevent many feelings from hurting you physically. If you know where to turn for help and how to manage stress, you will be well equipped to handle those stresses that are simply part of being alive and a part of the world of the 21st century.

MIND OVER BODY

✔ *Mind and body are inseparable.* Many disorders that affect your body can also cause emotional symptoms. And some emotional states—such as depression—can bring physical symptoms such as psychogenic headaches.

✔ *Some of the most common teen physical disorders can have an emotional component.* These include tension and depression headaches, migraine headaches, stomachaches, irritable bowel syndrome, eating disorders, and hypertension.

✔ *There are traditional and alternative ways to treat mind-body ills.* Traditional medicine has a number of remedies, but alternative medicine can help, too. Biofeedback, acupuncture, meditation, guided imagery, and herbal remedies, to name a few, can be helpful.

✔ *You have the power to keep balance in your life, by taking responsibility for your own health and well-being.* This is accomplished primarily by living a healthy lifestyle and learning to manage the stress that is inevitable in all our lives.

CHAPTER TEN

Your Special Medical Needs

I have diabetes and I'm really sick of it. Everything in my life is so complicated. I hate the insulin shots and having to test my blood all the time. And it's so hard sometimes to do things with my friends when I have to be so careful about when I eat and stuff like that. Sometimes I feel on the verge of giving up. Will it always be this way for me?

Tonia P.

Special medical needs can have a considerable impact on your life. *Any* kind of illness or physical problem can be especially hard on you during the teen years. You're so conscious of and concerned about your body. When something goes wrong, it's easy to get scared—and to feel very much alone. If you're like most people, you want to be active and may resent any illness that you feel keeps you from doing what you want to do, either temporarily or permanently. You may also feel that a special medical need is keeping you more dependent than you would like to be on your parents, and your parents may— even with the best intentions— tend to foster such dependence.

You may hate feeling different, yet when you have special medical needs, you may be intrinsically different. You may have to take medications and be on a special diet. There may be certain procedures you have to follow that make it necessary to

have detailed plans for simple things that other teens take for granted, such as slumber parties and field trips, which point up the fact of your difference even more.

Maybe you don't have a special medical need yourself, but you know someone who does: a college roommate with mono, a cousin who has asthma, the girl next door who has scoliosis (curvature of the spine), or a boyfriend with diabetes. If someone you know and love has a special medical problem, it's natural to be concerned. We have received a number of letters from teens asking questions such as the following:

"My boyfriend is diabetic. Is it true that he'll die young?"

"My sister has asthma really bad. Can she ever get better?"

"A friend of mine at school has epilepsy. If she would have a seizure at school, how could we help her?"

So this chapter is for everybody—for those who may have either temporary or chronic medical problems and for those who know and love someone who does. We hope we can help you to better understand some of the common medical problems that adolescents can have and, most important, to learn how to *live* with these special medical needs.

We are focusing on medical problems that are most likely to be part of your life, either directly or indirectly. Some are temporary. Others may be chronic. Some of the problems may be relatively minor. Others can have serious consequences. All may cause pain, upset, or a feeling of being different, and may impinge on your life in a number of ways.

What problems are we talking about? All kinds, including mononucleosis, urinary tract infections, bed wetting (nocturnal enuresis), allergies, asthma, anemia (iron-deficiency and sickle cell), diabetes, scoliosis, Osgood-Schlatter disease, and epilepsy.

We hope that this information will give you new insights into special medical needs, whether they are your own or those of someone close to you.

ALLERGIES

Since coming to college in the Midwest this fall (I'm from California) I feel like I've got a cold all the time! I'm beginning to think I might have an allergy. But I've never had any problems with allergies before. What could be causing this?

Puzzled

Allergies afflict people of all ages, causing a variety of uncomfortable symptoms including nasal congestion, sneezing, nasal dripping with throat discomfort, redness and watering of the eyes, itching, hives or skin rashes, nausea, diarrhea, and, in some serious types of allergies such as asthma (which we'll discuss in detail a little later on), respiratory disorders and difficulty in breathing.

What exactly is an allergy? It is a reaction by the body against a substance that it recognizes as foreign. Such a substance is called an *allergen*. In response to an allergen, the body forms antibodies and releases certain chemicals that, in turn, cause the allergy symptoms. While many people are able to adapt to allergens, many remain sensitive to common substances that may be completely harmless to those without allergies.

Allergies may run in families. If both parents have allergies, you have an 80 percent chance of being allergic, too. Even if only one parent is allergic, you still have a 50 percent chance of developing allergies.

There are many different kinds of allergies:

- *Environmental allergies* mean that you're allergic to certain pollens, plants, flowers, weeds, grasses, molds, dusts, or tobacco smoke.
- *Food allergies* are quite common. The allergens may be common foods such as chocolate or eggs, or unusual foods such as macadamia nuts or shrimp. Reactions may include bronchial congestion, trouble breathing, skin rashes, and diarrhea.
- *Drug allergies* happen when people are extremely sensitive to certain drugs—often aspirin, sulfa drugs, or penicillin. Reactions range from mild itching to severe hives and shock.
- *Cosmetic allergies* are triggered by substances ranging from eye makeup to shampoo. People are often allergic to the oils in some of these products and may suffer reactions such as rashes after using the product.
- *Animal allergies* are also fairly common. Here people may be unusually sensitive to the dander (skin and hair) of dogs, cats, or horses. While a clean, brushed animal may trigger fewer allergic reactions, some people cannot be around animals at all.
- *Contact allergies* are an unusual sensitivity to certain metals such as gold or silver. You may experience redness or itching of the skin when you make contact with the metal in a piece of jewelry.
- *Hives*, incidentally, may be classified as a sign of an allergy, but, especially in teens and young adults, may be a sign of extreme stress and nervousness as well.

How do you know if you have an allergy and what the allergen might be in your case? The answer is not clear-cut. Like "Puzzled," you may suffer what you think of initially as prolonged cold symptoms after moving to another area of the country. It may be helpful to know that certain geographic areas have different allergens. So if you grew up in the East and go off to college on the West Coast, you may find yourself with a long-lasting "cold" that may prove to be an allergy. Some people find that a stressful situation, illness, or injury may lower the body's resistance to allergies. Other people have very mild or seasonal allergies that are often mistaken for colds.

However, if you have more than an occasional problem—if your symptoms are chronic and stressful—you are probably fairly sure *already* that you have allergies. You might not know what may be triggering these reactions, however.

By going to a physician who specializes in allergies or to an allergy clinic, you can get skin tests to help determine your specific allergy or allergies. Here, prepared solutions of common allergens are injected under the skin at different sites to see if any reactions occur. In this way, your specific allergy may be determined.

However, if you have only an occasional problem or already know what your specific allergen is, it may not be necessary to go to the expense and time of having such tests. Some allergies disappear as you grow up; others may be with you for a lifetime.

How are allergies treated? There is some debate about this. Some physicians feel strongly that patients should have desensitization shots. This series of injections, which may go on for years, usually on a weekly basis, helps build up protection against an allergen and makes allergy symptoms less severe. This traditional approach is becoming less practiced as these shots not only require a regular, longstanding time commitment, but they may also be very expensive. Often, avoiding a particular allergen whenever possible may be quite effective in the long run and much less costly than desensitization shots.

Many physicians advocate treating allergy symptoms with drugs such as antihistamines. This treatment may be especially helpful for the patient with occasional allergies. Also, there are now more new drugs for allergies that do not have the undesired side effects of drowsiness and can be taken just once daily. Ask your doctor about these.

You can help yourself in specific ways, too. Probably the most important part of managing an allergy is avoiding your specific allergens as much as possible. This may mean working with your family to keep your home as dust-free as possible, parting with (or keeping your distance from) the family pet, avoiding offending foods, and, especially, staying away from friends who smoke or smoky rooms, which often can trigger allergies.

ANEMIA

I've been sort of tired lately and was wondering if I might be anemic. Can anemia be caused by heavy menstrual periods? How can I find out if I'm anemic and what can I do about it?

Barbara F.

Thanks to certain television commercials, the word *anemia* is often used to describe everything from depression to legendary "tired blood" malady. We obviously do not support such television diagnoses. Anemia is a very specific problem that must be diagnosed by a physician (via a blood test) rather than by symptoms alone, since some victims have no unusual symptoms. There are many types of anemia, and while it is beyond the scope of this book to cover every type, we will discuss two forms that are commonly seen in teens and young adults: iron-deficiency anemia and sickle cell anemia.

I've been hearing a lot about sickle cell anemia the past couple months. What is it? Can anyone get it? What are the symptoms?

Tom W.

Iron-Deficiency Anemia

This type of anemia is often mislabeled as "tired blood." When you have this condition, your blood is not tired, but is lacking sufficient iron supplies to manufacture a constant supply of red blood cells. When the body lacks sufficient iron, the number of red blood cells may decrease, causing so-called iron-deficiency anemia.

What causes it? Many factors can cause the body to lack iron. Among these may be a heavy menstrual flow. While actual blood lost during menstruation does not have to be replaced, lost iron may need to be.

One of the best sources of iron is a good, well-balanced diet. However, many young adults favor junk foods, which do little, if anything, to help replenish the body's nutrients and iron supplies.

It is quite common, then, to see an active teen with regular menstrual cycles (and often a heavy menstrual flow) who favors a predominantly junk food diet develop iron-deficiency anemia.

How do you know if you have it? You may feel fatigued. But it is also possible that you will have no symptoms at all. A simple blood test is the only reliable way to tell whether you have this form of anemia.

What can you do about it? For some, if it is only a mild anemia, diet may correct the anemia. Others may require additional iron supplements. You and your physician together need to work out the best treatment method for you.

Sickle Cell Anemia

Sickle cell anemia is an inherited disease, most often seen in African Americans, in which there is a genetic defect in the structure of the red blood cells and, as a result, a decrease of healthy red blood cells in the body. An estimated 80,000 African Americans suffer from this disorder.

Due to this structural defect, the red blood cells are shaped like sickles or half moons, instead of being round, and cannot carry on the functions of normal cells—specifically, that of oxygen–carbon dioxide exchange in the lung tissues. Because these red blood cells have an unusual shape, they cannot pass through the rounded blood vessels easily and may become lodged in them, causing congestion in the part of the body where it occurs. This congestion can become very uncomfortable, with leg, abdominal, or chest pain; impaired circulation; and possibly skin ulcers.

This serious disorder may become even more critical in instances where the oxygen level of the blood is affected—for example, during anesthesia or when an infection occurs in the body. For this reason, it is vital to know whether you have sickle cell anemia or may be a carrier. It is estimated that one in every twelve African Americans may be a carrier of the sickle cell trait.

If you are African American, we strongly urge you to be tested for this trait. In many cities, there are testing centers for sickle cell anemia and even vans that enable medical personnel to do free testing in certain neighborhoods. Today, many states require that all newborn infants be tested for sickle cell disease. The test for sickle cell anemia is a simple but important blood test.

You may not have the disease yourself, but you may be a carrier. If you conceive a child with a person who is also a carrier, it is possible that the child will have sickle cell anemia. It is important to know the possibilities—and the risks—in advance. It is also important to know whether you have the disease, since it does require the ongoing care of a physician.

There have been some promising breakthroughs in the treatment of this disease. Although bone marrow transplants have given some severely ill children healthy new lives, relatively few get this treatment because it can be dangerous and requires a sibling who is a good tissue match as a bone marrow donor. Only about 7 percent of sickle cell patients qualify for this procedure. However, the most promising research is in the area of gene therapy. Here physicians remove some of the patient's bone marrow (via a needle and usually from the hip). This bone marrow is then treated with DNA/RNA fragments, dissolved in fat globules to enable them to get into the cells, which then correct the genetic defect. The marrow is then infused back into the patient. As of this writing, this new therapy is still being tested, but shows great promise for the future.

ASTHMA

I first got asthma at the age of 2. I'm now 15. I've heard things about its causes, but nobody has really talked to me about it. Is asthma an allergy or tied to the emotions or inherited?

Sue A.

Asthma may mean an occasional wheeze or, in its most severe form, it can kill. In fact, over the past ten years, there has been a worldwide increase in deaths from asthma. This is causing medical science to take a closer look at the causes and complications of asthma and to begin to treat this disorder in entirely new ways.

Anyone with asthma should have a regular physician and work with him or her in a team effort to monitor and control the asthma—not just to manage crises. In the past few years, there has been a significant change in asthma treatment. The focus used to be on bronchial dilation, opening up the airways. Today, it is on reducing the underlying inflammation of the airways with new drugs, preventing inflammation with new drugs, and closely monitoring air flow. Inflammation and swelling are predominant features of asthma; reducing these in addition to treating bronchial constriction can lead to better management of the disorder.

Close monitoring of air flow is vital. More physicians are monitoring asthma patients—not just during or after an acute attack, but also regularly to see whether medication is helping. Air flow is measured in the physician's office (and can also be monitored at home) with the use of a *peak flow meter*. These readings—which, ideally, are kept in *peak flow diary cards* by the patient on a daily basis at home—are important in two ways: First, they can tell your doctor if your medication is working; second, they can serve as an early-warning system to help you get treatment early on and, quite possibly, avoid a major health crisis. (Studies of young people who died during a severe asthma attack have found that these young people and their families often didn't pick up early-warning symptoms or realize the severity of the problem until it had become a life-threatening crisis.)

New guidelines for self-monitoring from the National Institutes of Health were stated in its National Asthma Education and Prevention Program in 1997. This system involves using a peak flow meter at home and recording the readings on a daily basis, using a traffic-light concept of rating how you're doing and what action, if any, may be required. For example, if your readings are 80 to 100 percent of expected flow, you are under a "green light." This means that things are going well and that no special actions, beyond your usual self-care and regular medications, need to be taken. If, on the other hand, you have a reading between 50 percent and 80 percent of predicted flow, you're in the "yellow light" category and should increase medications as previously directed by your physician. Your "red light" alert is triggered by any reading below 50 percent. That means you or your parents should call your doctor *immediately*.

While asthma is usually considered a severe form of allergy, recent research reveals that viral infections may play a major role in triggering asthma attacks in young children. According to researchers, a genetic predisposition to a defect involving the airways in the lungs or the bronchial tubes may underlie the reaction to the virus. However, when asthma develops after early childhood and before middle age, it may indeed be caused by an allergy. As an allergy, asthma can run in families.

What happens during an asthma attack? The lung tissue begins to secrete a substance that causes the air passages of the lungs to become blocked. The tiny bronchial tubes squeeze shut, making the victim fight desperately to breathe. The victim may experience a sensation of tightness in the chest, shortness of breath, wheezing, rapid breathing, or all of these symptoms at once; it can be very frightening.

The picture at left shows a normal bronchial tube. The picture on the right shows a bronchial tube that has been blocked by a substance secreted by lung tissue and is squeezing shut during an asthma attack.

Asthma/Bronchial Tubes

The attack may be brought on by a specific allergen, such as being in a room with people smoking, or by the flu or an upper respiratory infection, or even by a stressful situation. Stress may involve a specific situation in the young person's life or may be the result of ongoing family problems. Because of this, some physicians may treat asthma patients with a combination of drugs, psychotherapy, and family counseling. In severe cases, the asthma patient may be removed from the home for a time. Asthma can be an extremely serious lifelong problem for some, while others find that symptoms ease or disappear as they get older.

If after removing specific allergens such as a pet, smoke, or dust or mold in the house, you still have asthma attacks, then specific drugs may help prevent or alleviate your symptoms. Today, we know that a combination of drugs may work better for many patients. Physicians often combine drugs such as inhalers, which prevent asthma attacks, with specific drugs that work during an asthma attack.

Today much new treatment is aimed at using inhalers rather than oral medicine, since these drugs work directly *in* the lungs, rather than on the lungs through the bloodstream and thus via the whole body, where the drug is not needed. Many drugs such as albuterol (Ventolin, Proventil) are *bronchodilators*; that is, they are inhaled by the patient and open up the air passages of the lung directly in an acute attack. Other inhaled drugs are *anti-inflammatory*, such as cromolyn sodium, and inhaled steroids, which act by preventing the chance of having an asthma attack. For example, cromolyn sodium or Azmacort, an inhaled steroid, are inhaled though a dispenser called a *metered-dose inhaler*. These drugs work to prevent asthma attacks in most cases. Also, attachments known as *spacers* hook onto the inhaler and provide better penetration into the lungs.

No matter how mild or severe your asthma may be, teamwork is essential. It's important to understand your disease and how to make self-monitoring a regular part of your life. Your physician, your family, and your environment are all important in the unified effort to make treatment effective. But *your* efforts, most of all, are crucial in controlling this disorder.

BED WETTING (NOCTURNAL ENURESIS)

I'm almost 16 and wet the bed sometimes. I'm so ashamed I could die! I've thought about asking my doctor about this, but I'm too embarrassed.

J. B.

It's easy to feel embarrassed or like a baby if you have a problem with bed wetting (medically termed *nocturnal enuresis*). It may be some consolation, however, that you are far from alone. This condition is not uncommon in teens and young adults. In fact, a recent survey found that 3 percent of all 12-year-olds have this condition. Another note of optimism: Nocturnal enuresis is *not* a sign of emotional immaturity and it *can be treated*.

What causes this condition? Some research has found that nocturnal enuresis is related to a specific stage of sleep. The fourth stage (deep sleep) may be so deep for some people that muscle control of the bladder may be lost, causing urination during sleep. Other studies are conflicting and do not relate bed wetting to sleep stage.

What can you do if you have this problem? First, don't let embarrassment keep you from asking your doctor for help. Remember: This is not uncommon and it can be treated.

There are two medical therapies now used. One of the most common medical approaches to nocturnal enuresis is a drug that, when taken before bedtime, causes the sleep level to be more active, preventing the sleeper from going into such a deep fourth stage. It has been clinically proven that these drugs, by elevating the sleep level, decrease the incidence of bed wetting.

Another more recent medical treatment for bed wetting is a nasal spray called *desmopressin acetate* (DDAVP or Stimate), which is an antidiuretic hormone effective in treating adolescents. One spray in each nostril at bedtime has reduced bed wetting in as many as 75 percent of adolescents with this affliction.

There are some commonsense ways you can help yourself, too. Don't drink fluids, or at least cut down on fluid intake, in the evening. And don't forget to urinate just before you go to bed. Also, if someone in your home goes to bed later than you do, you might ask them to wake you just before they go to bed so that you can urinate at that time, too.

■ ■ ■

DIABETES

I have diabetes and I hate it. It's too hard to do things with my friends. I'll have eaten dinner and then some friends come by and say, "Let's go have pizza." I feel embarrassed not being able to have any. I have to wait until later in the evening for a snack, but I feel silly telling them that. What can I do?

Casey K.

Even though the young people who wrote these letters are feeling very much alone and very different, they have lots of company. It is estimated that 1 in every 1,000 people age 17 and younger has diabetes. They're also far from alone in their unhappy, in some cases, desperate feelings.

I just found out that I have diabetes. I wish I was dead. My friends and parents treat me like a cripple. I've also read stuff about all kinds of complications connected to diabetes, and, frankly, I don't see any reason to go on living.

Lisa M.

What are the real facts about diabetes—and the realities of living as a teenager with diabetes? *Diabetes mellitus* is a chronic metabolic disorder that occurs when special cells in the pancreas are inactivated or severely impaired and are thus unable to manufacture *insulin*, a hormone necessary to convert food into glucose, the body's major energy source.

There are two major types of diabetes. Type I, or insulin-dependent, diabetes, can occur at any age, but most of those with this form of diabetes are first diagnosed in childhood or adolescence. Since those with type I diabetes typically have little or no natural insulin production, they must take insulin shots.

Those with type II diabetes, on the other hand, tend to be older adolescents and adults who are overweight, often middle-aged, and may still produce some natural insulin; because of this, they can control the disorder simply with oral medications and diet.

The symptoms of diabetes include sudden excessive hunger and thirst, unexplained weight loss, frequent urination, fatigue, irritability, confusion, genital itching, skin infections, and/or sudden vision changes.

If you have such symptoms, your doctor will test your blood and urine to discover whether there is excess sugar in your urine and bloodstream and to determine how well your body absorbs and utilizes sugar. By the way, have you ever wondered why so many school, camp, and sports physicals require a urine test? Now you know: It's to detect diabetes. Many cases go undiagnosed for quite some time. But the earlier you're diagnosed, the sooner you can begin to safeguard your health.

What causes diabetes in a young person? Many researchers now believe that type I diabetes may occur in those with a genetic predisposition as the result of a viral infection. A number of researchers, too, are beginning to regard type I diabetes as a possible autoimmune system disorder; that is, for reasons not yet fully understood, the body's own immune system produces antibodies that attack the insulin-producing cells of the pancreas as foreign invaders. Much more research needs to be done, however, before the exact causes of diabetes are known.

What medical experts do know is this: Diabetes is *not* a contagious disease or one that occurs as the result of eating too much candy. It also does not mean that you can't live a full and active life—doing what you love to do, having a satisfying career, and, someday, marrying and having children.

When diabetes is the diagnosis, however, your life does change in some ways. There is the challenge of keeping the amount of glucose in the body—measured in the blood—as close to a normal level as possible. Insulin injections, replacing the body's normal insulin production, are part of this. But since injections can never quite replace the body's fine-tuned accuracy in calculating how much insulin is needed, people with diabetes must

monitor the level of glucose in the blood several times a day. This can be done very easily, at home or at school, with a special portable blood-testing device called a *glucometer*. A drop of blood from the finger applied to a special monitoring strip can tell you whether the glucose level is too high (more insulin may be needed) or too low (you need to eat more food to increase the amount of glucose in the blood). This home blood-monitoring device can help you to control your diabetes better and possibly avoid some of its medical complications.

There are also other considerations. You need to eat well-balanced meals on schedule. You must learn how to adjust the amount of insulin you'll need depending on how much exercise you'll be getting on a certain day or what foods you may be eating. Also, a cold or attack of the flu may increase your insulin needs. While this may all sound complicated at the beginning, it doesn't have to be. With time and guidance from your physician and/or nurse practitioner, you may find that these special needs quickly fit into your normal daily routine.

You will find, too, that controlling your diabetes and having a decent social life are possible and manageable. For example, if your friends want to go for pizza and you've already eaten, go along and have a diet drink. Many people who are watching their weight would do the same thing. Your friends may be so busy enjoying the pizza and your company that they won't notice that you're not eating. Taking good care of your diabetes does not mean that you can't have fun with your friends.

Think about it this way: Caring for yourself—with insulin shots, blood testing, and meal planning—doesn't have to take more than 20 minutes a day. The rest of the time is yours to do just about anything you want. You can enjoy sports, eating out with your friends, and going to parties. Some of the things you *can't* do and stay healthy—such as drinking a lot of alcohol or eating a lot of junk food—aren't healthy for *anyone.*

It's important, in taking responsibility for your health, to be aware of the symptoms of an *insulin reaction* (too little sugar in the body), which could lead to a *hypoglycemic seizure*, as well as the symptoms of too high a sugar level (which, if ignored for days, could lead to serious consequences such as *diabetic coma*). While diabetic coma is quite an unlikely event in someone with a well-controlled diet and insulin intake, an insulin reaction or insulin shock leading to loss of consciousness or a seizure can happen on occasion. So it's important to be prepared with a snack—for example, carry a small box of raisins around with you—that will boost your blood sugar level rapidly.

In the past, many people thought that this meant carrying extra sugar cubes or candy around all the time, but many experts insist that this is not the best measure. A sugar cube will quickly raise the blood glucose, but the glucose can fall again quickly unless you also eat some form of protein. Milk is good for these reactions, as are raisins, other fruits, and cheese.

It's important, also, to wear an ID bracelet giving your condition, name, doctor, and instructions for emergency treatment. This could safeguard your health or maybe even save your life if you were found unconscious, as in insulin shock or diabetic coma, or if you were injured in an accident, since there are certain drugs diabetics should not take.

This may seem like a long list of requirements. Some diabetic teens feel helpless and overwhelmed at first. Some try to ignore the reality of their special medical needs. Many teens rebel. It's tough to be different and have to remember so many things. It may be difficult, too, to assert your independence when you are dependent on a drug for your life and when your parents may be concerned and even overly protective. However, making the decision yourself to know and regulate your disease can be a real life-enhancer.

What is in the future for diabetic teens? Many wonder if they can have normal lives and fear suffering from serious complications.

The possible complications are not to be minimized. Diabetes is the third leading cause of death in the United States, after heart disease and cancer. It can lead to kidney disease, nerve damage, heart disease, gangrene, and stroke. It is also the leading cause of blindness in adults. Damage to the blood vessels in the retina is common among the majority of those who have had diabetes for 20 years or longer.

But it's important to remember that excellent control of diabetes is possible with the more accurate monitoring of home blood tests. And this better control will diminish or delay the more serious consequences of this disease.

A lot of ongoing medical research may also help you in the future. For example, insulin pumps, which deliver measured doses of insulin throughout the day without the need for insulin injections, are being improved. These pumps were once worn only on the outside of the body, but a newer version of this pump has recently been designed. This device, a computerized titanium disc that can be programmed—and reprogrammed—to deliver correct doses of insulin, is implanted under the skin of the abdomen. Its supply of insulin would be refilled by a doctor every three months via an external needle. There has also been experimental surgery with transplanted insulin-producing pancreatic cells to help restore, partially or fully, the body's ability to make its own insulin.

One of the most exciting new possibilities is an inhaled form of insulin. Here, the person inhales a fine powder form of insulin as an aerosol cloud. Reaching deep into lung tissue, the insulin passes into the bloodstream, where it controls blood sugar levels. In clinical trials, researchers have found no difference in the blood sugar levels of those who used injected insulin and those who used inhaled insulin. There were no problems with lung function associated with inhaling the substance twice a day before meals. (The study participants still had to take one injection of slow-acting insulin at bedtime in order to regulate insulin and blood sugar overnight.) At this writing, trials were going into a third phase, with hopes that this new treatment could be available to the general public within the next two to three years.

Even today, your chances of living a full life are much greater than the prospects faced by young people with diabetes a generation ago. And along with the responsibilities your special medical needs require can also come some positive changes. Taking responsibility for yourself can give you a new feeling of independence. You may find that careful planning of your day allows you not only to regulate your diabetes but also to organize your work and leisure time better. You may find, too, that little things like taking your own supply of sugarless diet drinks to a party will not set you apart in a major way. Some of your weight-conscious friends may be doing the same thing. You may find, too, that by keeping your diabetes under good control, you'll really start to feel better—and able to do more things you enjoy. Being in control will give you the freedom and the opportunity to live an active, normal life.

In fact, by keeping your weight down, your body trim and well-exercised, and your diet balanced and nutritious, you may even be in better shape and live longer than people without diabetes who eat junk foods, get overweight, don't exercise, and otherwise abuse their bodies.

EPILEPSY

> I'm 14 years old and have epilepsy. I'm afraid to ask my doctor some of these questions, so I'm asking you. What is epilepsy? (I know what it is, kind of, but want to know more.) Is it hereditary? Will I have to take pills all my life? Is it true that it's harder to get a job if you're an epileptic? If so, why?
>
> Want to Know

Epilepsy, a general term used to describe a variety of seizure disorders, is an often misunderstood disorder of the central nervous system that, due to uncontrolled electrical discharges in the brain, will cause seizures. Seizures may not be the major problem, however. Lack of public understanding—and a number of myths—may be the greatest prob-

lem that those with epilepsy face. It's important to know that epilepsy is not a mental illness or a sign of mental retardation (although some developmentally disabled young people do have seizures). It is not contagious, nor is it, strictly speaking, hereditary, although a certain tendency or genetic predisposition may be found in certain types of epilepsy.

> I'm 15 and my boyfriend is 16. I found out that he has something called "temporal lobe epilepsy" and gets stomach pains because of this. I don't understand and he doesn't want to tell me about it. Could you please tell me what it is? (In English, if you know what I mean!)
>
> Anne A.

There are a number of possible causes of this disorder. It can be caused by head injuries from accidents, birth injuries, infectious illnesses, brain tumors, or other disease. Some causes may remain a mystery. Research into more causes and treatments of epilepsy is being done.

There are also a number of different types of epilepsy. The most common fall into three general categories:

- *Grand mal seizures* cause the victim to experience a blackout and convulsions of the entire body for a minute or longer. Then, feeling tired and confused, he or she may fall asleep. This can be frightening, not only to the patient having the seizure, but also to those around the patient who do not know what to do or how to help.
- *Petit mal seizures* may be mistaken for a period of staring or daydreaming. The patient, usually age 6 to 14, will stare, blink the eyes rapidly, or have minor twitching movements before resuming normal activities. Prior to diagnosis, some young people raise the ire of teachers for "daydreaming" in class.
- *Psychomotor* or *temporal lobe seizures* may involve staring, abdominal pains and headaches, chewing and lip-smacking move-

ments, picking at clothing, pacing, buzzing and ringing sounds in the ears, dizziness, and, in some cases, sudden feelings of fear or anger followed by a desire to sleep and, later, amnesia about the whole attack.

In many cases, seizures can be controlled. While there is no cure for epilepsy, it is estimated that 50 percent of those with some form of this disorder achieve complete control of seizures with anticonvulsants and lead essentially normal lives. Another 30 percent gain partial control of seizures through medication. In fact, some people with epilepsy have not had a seizure for ten years or more, and according to a study at Washington University in St. Louis, some (though not all) of these patients may even be able to stop taking medication after a certain number of seizure-free years.

However, most people with epilepsy face a lifetime of medication, and some will continue to have seizures. The need for continual medication, the fear of having a seizure, and a feeling of being different plague many people with epilepsy, but this can be especially painful in adolescence.

You may rebel at having to take medications. You may feel smothered and angry when your parents remind you about your medications or show unusual concern. You may feel ashamed about having epilepsy and may feel afraid to tell anyone. You may be terrified of having a seizure at school and may be mortified if you do. Some kids, it's true, can be pretty cruel and callous about other people's pain. Often, however, such a reaction may be due to fright, ignorance, and embarrassment.

You may feel embarrassed about feeling different in rather obvious ways. It can be particularly tough when everyone else is getting a driver's license and you're stuck trying to make excuses about why you don't have one yet. While those with epilepsy may get driver's licenses in most states, you must submit written proof from your physician that you have been free of seizures for a certain period of time (two to three years in many states). If you have to wait for this time to pass, it can be difficult.

You may also worry about your future. Many people with epilepsy (and those with other chronic diseases) go to college and do well and go on to excellent jobs. Others, however, are still victims of the old myths about epilepsy.

Discriminatory employment laws and practices regarding epilepsy are now being challenged legally. And victories have already been won in other areas. It is now possible for people with epilepsy to marry and have children. So? Big deal, right? Guess what? In the not-too-distant past, this was forbidden in some states, due to a common misconception that epilepsy is, invariably, hereditary.

More people need to understand that a person with epilepsy can live a full, essentially normal life and has as much to offer society as anyone else. Proper education will also help members of the public to deal properly with a grand mal seizure when they see one happening. In such a case, according to the Epilepsy Foundation of America, make sure that the person is in a safe place and loosen tight clothing. DO NOT force a hard object between the person's teeth or give him or her anything to drink. Just stand by until the person has fully recovered and is able to go about regular activities.

On a final note, a spokesperson for the Los Angeles County Epilepsy Society observes that more and more young people are getting epilepsy as the result of head injuries from auto, motorcycle, or skateboard accidents. So it can happen to anyone. That's why it's important to understand what epilepsy is—and is not.

INFECTIOUS MONONUCLEOSIS

I'm 20 and a college student. I have just been diagnosed as having mono. My doctor was most emphatic about my getting a lot of rest. He said something about complications if I don't take proper care of myself. What complications can happen? Is there something I can do for myself besides just resting?

Doug W.

Infectious mononucleosis is a very common problem among young adults, especially college students. A lot of research has been done on the disease that most young people call "mono"; it has been found to be caused by a virus. How this virus is spread, however, is still subject to debate.

In the past, mononucleosis was often called "the kissing disease," but that has proved to be something of a misnomer. You can have close contact with a victim of mono and not get it. Some evidence suggests that people who are fatigued and exhausted may be predisposed to the disorder because their immune system is weakened, which makes them more susceptible to certain infections. Infectious mononucleosis is caused by the *Epstein-Barr virus*. The exact method of transmission is unknown.

What are the symptoms of mono? They vary a great deal, but the most common tend to be extreme fatigue and the need for a lot of sleep. Of course, if you're exhausted to begin with, it may be difficult to tell whether your problem is simply fatigue or whether it is mono. However, when you're tired, you can usually pull yourself together and function pretty well when you want or need to do so. If you have mono, on the other hand, you may not be able to function even if you want very much to be awake and alert.

Other symptoms of infectious mononucleosis include swelling of the lymph glands (especially those in the neck), headaches, and a very severe sore throat. There may also be a skin rash and, in some cases, enlargement of the liver and/or spleen. Sometime you may have a fever, and with a severe sore throat this may be confused with a strep throat. It is important to have this condition diagnosed by a physician, which he or she will do via a physical exam and a blood test.

How is mono treated? With lots of rest and a good diet. These simple instructions are important. If a patient doesn't get proper rest, avoid contact sports (if so directed by the physician), and eat well, enlargement and possible rupture of the spleen could result.

How serious is that? While rupture of the spleen would mean emergency surgery, one can live a normal life without this organ. But *who needs* complications like that?

Many teens with mononucleosis risk such complications by resuming normal activities too soon. It's sad but true that mono seems to strike at times when you don't really have time to be sick—such as around exam time or graduation. Yet sufficient rest is vital to complete recovery.

How long could mono keep you sidelined? This can vary a great deal. Some are only out of step with their normal activities for a week. Others may take a month to recover. It's a highly individual matter. Your body will usually let you know when it's ready to function at full capacity again.

OSGOOD-SCHLATTER DISEASE

I have been having a lot of swelling and pain in my knee and lower leg. I'm active (co-captain of our varsity basketball team) and hate having this pain. What could it be and what can I do to get rid of it?

Rusty C.

Osgood-Schlatter disease, a disorder of the mineralization of the leg bones, is quite common, especially in active young people between ages 10 and 15.

This condition, which can cause swelling and tenderness around the knees and pain in the lower leg, may be caused by stress on the tendon that attaches the *patella* (knee bone) to the *tibia* (front leg bone). The stress is due to the changes of puberty: increased muscle mass in the legs and active use of the upper leg muscle, the *quadriceps*. The stress of the patellar tendon on the upper prominence of the tibia and irregular calcium deposits in the upper tibia cause the painful swelling and pain in this part of the bone. This is a common condition of early puberty when growth is very rapid. It is also a *temporary condition* that is usually self-healing.

To facilitate healing, a physician will usually recommend that you stay away from vigorous sports and exercises involving bending for a certain amount of time—usually a few weeks or sometimes several months of inactivity. It depends on you. If you find that after a few weeks, you can play sports without pain and without increasing the swelling, then it may be OK for you to resume playing. However, if playing a sport causes the pain and swelling to increase, then you will need to take additional time off. This doesn't mean that you can't still be active. Just limit your activities to those—such as swimming—that don't put stress on the knees.

Those with unusually severe cases of Osgood-Schlatter disease may require casts to help healing, but usually a relatively brief period of rest is enough. While this period of reduced activity may seem to go on forever, it may be some consolation that, once healed, you'll be as good as ever—as the following testimonial from a teen named Beth shows:

I'm 16 and two years ago I had Osgood-Schlatter disease bad enough to have a cast on my knee for two months. But now I'm going strong. I'm a cheerleader, a majorette, and I'm on the girls' basketball team. I just wanted to tell other teens to follow their doctors' instructions and take care. You'll be OK, too!

Beth

SCOLIOSIS

I'm supposed to get a brace at the end of July for my back because I have a curvature of the spine—scoliosis—and I'm scared. I know I'll feel like such a jerk running around with a thing like that on my body!

Scared

Scoliosis is a correctable deformity in which the spine curves to one side instead of growing straight. It is especially common in girls (who are eight times more likely to have it) in the growing years between ages 10 and 16. The usual ages of onset are 9 to 10 for girls and 11 to 12 for boys. There is some evidence that this condition may be inherited, although certain diseases such as rheumatoid arthritis and cerebral palsy as well as spinal injuries may also be factors. Most cases of scoliosis, however, have no easily determined cause. But we do know that this condition afflicts about 10 percent of young adolescents to some degree.

Early symptoms include shoulders that are not level, uneven hips, and prominent shoulder blades. An S curve in your spine may also be observed if you have a friend or family member look at your back as you bend over. A number of school districts across the nation have special screening programs to detect scoliosis in its early stages.

Scoliosis

When there is less than a 20-degree curvature of the spine, no treatment is necessary. However, the physician must watch the curvature over a period of time to make sure that it is not increasing. The possibility of increasing curvature can depend largely on your age at diagnosis and how much growing you have left to do. For those diagnosed with scoliosis before age 12, there is about a 75 percent risk of curve progression, compared with 30 percent for those between ages 12 and 15 and only 10 percent for those over age 15.

If the curve progresses or is more pronounced to begin with and is greater than 20 degrees, you may need to wear a *Milwaukee brace* for a period of time and do special exercises. The brace, while it may look cumbersome, doesn't have to interfere with your normal activities and may help a great deal to move your spine back into a normal position.

In severe cases of scoliosis, if the curve of the spine is greater than 40 degrees, surgery and casting are required. Here, an adjustable *Harrington rod* is surgically implanted to help straighten the spine. However, this procedure is quite rare.

Treatment for scoliosis—whatever the method—will keep the curvature from progressing and causing serious deformities in later life. So if you notice any indications of scoliosis, don't be afraid to tell your parents and your doctor. Treatment now will be of lifelong benefit, and the earlier you seek help, the less help you're likely to need.

URINARY TRACT INFECTIONS

I have pain and burning when I go to the bathroom and a friend of mine told me that this is a urinary infection. How do you get it? I heard it may have something to do with sex, but I don't have sex! How do you get rid of it?

Ally D.

Urinary tract infections are common in young adults, most often in young women. Quite frequently, these may be young women who are having their first sexual experiences. But sex is not the only factor in urinary tract infections. Bubble baths may cause irritation of the urethra and, as a result, a urinary infection. Careless wiping after a bowel movement can be another cause. The rectum is close to the urethra (urinary opening) in the woman and it's easy for bacteria from the rectum to invade the urinary tract. This is especially likely if you have a habit of wiping toward the vagina (forward) after a bowel movement. Wiping *away* from the vagina and urethra (backward) will minimize this risk.

How can sexual activity increase your likelihood of developing a urinary tract infection? During intercourse, the man's penis—while thrusting—may touch areas near both the woman's rectum and urethra and may thus spread bacteria from the rectum to the urethra. For some sexually active women, this may mean almost continuous urinary infections.

How can you avoid such problems?

- *Use good hygiene.* Bathe or shower regularly, taking care to wash the genital and rectal areas thoroughly.
- *Urinate as soon as possible after sex.* This can help to wash out any bacteria that may be present in the urinary tract.
- *Drink water after sex.* Some urologists recommend drinking water after sexual intercourse. This will be flushed rapidly through the kidneys; thus, further urination will help to wash any remaining bacteria out of the urinary tract before the bacteria have a chance to multiply.

How do you know if you might have a urinary tract infection? In some cases, it may be difficult to distinguish a urinary tract infection from a vaginal infection. However, with a vaginal infection, you will usually have a vaginal discharge as well as painful or burning urination.

Symptoms of a urinary tract infection include pain and burning on urination and greater frequency of urinating (not as a result of drinking lots of fluids), blood in the urine (when you are not having your menstrual period), and in some cases a concurrent kidney infection with pain in the lower back.

If you have such symptoms, don't just wait and hope that they will disappear. See a physician. A urinalysis will reveal whether you have such an infection. If you do, your physician will usually treat the condition with antibiotics.

■ ■ ■

LIVING WITH SPECIAL MEDICAL NEEDS

Anyone can have a special medical problem. But it can be especially hard to cope with if you're a teen and if your problem is *chronic* and not likely to change. Besides whatever discomfort your physical condition may bring, there will be trying times emotionally.

There will be times when you'd like to throw your medicine out and pretend that you don't need it. There will be times when your parents seem to nag or overprotect you, or take over your illness instead of giving you the space and the responsibility to care for yourself. There will be times when you feel guilty about the time, expense, and emotional strain that your special needs may be putting on your family and times when you try to reassure your parents.

And there may be times when you find yourself almost enjoying the attention and special privileges or considerations you may get because of your condition, times when you may use your illness as an excuse to get out of doing things for yourself that you know you can do. There will be other times when you may feel enraged at being different. You may feel like screaming, "I hate this! Why me?" And there may be times when you fear the future and what it may bring.

The fact is, though, that not one of us knows what the future will bring. For example, most teens who die this year will do so in accidents. Discovering that you have a chronic disease such as diabetes or epilepsy does not mean that your life is over. Part of living fully with (or despite) a special medical need means accepting your feelings of rage, rebellion, and depression as entirely normal.

If you've ever wondered "Why me?" you're far from alone. It can help a lot if you talk these feelings over with someone who understands—a special friend, a family member, your doctor, a counselor, or a medical center social worker. Once you begin to accept your feelings, it is usually easier to get past the negative ones, to accept your special needs, and to take responsibility for your own care as much as possible. Control of your condition—even in little ways—can give you a new feeling of power in your life. When you have a chronic medical condition, it's easy to start feeling that things are constantly being done to you rather than doing things for yourself. It may help you achieve a real sense of independence if you can assert your right to be involved in your own treatment and to manage your own life as much as possible.

Keeping your condition—whether it's asthma, diabetes, epilepsy, or something else—as well controlled as possible will free you to do other things. You will be able to see past your special needs to your special potential—and the full range of exciting possibilities in your life!

YOUR SPECIAL MEDICAL NEEDS

✔ Doing what you need to do to take care of your special medical need can free you to enjoy the rest of your life.

✔ If you assert your right to be involved in and control your condition, even in little ways, you will have a new feeling of power in your life. For up-to-date information on your special medical need, check the appropriate section of this chapter!

✔ Check with your physician as well as Internet sites for continuing up-to-date information about new findings and treatments.

CHAPTER
ELEVEN
You and Your Sexuality

I'm confused. People talk about sex. And then they talk about sexuality. My friend says that everyone has sexuality even if they don't have sex! I always thought that the two words meant pretty much the same. Is sexuality something everybody has? Even old people and kids?

Wondering

Many people confuse sex with sexuality and many, too, think that sex automatically means intimacy as well.

It's more important than ever—in this era of escalating teenage pregnancy rates and the growing threat of AIDS in the general population (including adolescents)—to know exactly what these differences are in order to make wise, responsible sexual choices.

Sexuality, which includes sexual *feelings* and how you feel about yourself as well as others (as well as sexual activities), is a major part of who you are all your life—from infancy to old age. All too often, however, people see it only in a limited sense. Some see sexuality as a synonym for sexual intercourse. But there is so much more to it than that. Sexual actions are only a *part* of your sexuality. You can be a very normal, happy sexual person without having sex—right now or even for years!

Some people define sexuality in terms of sex roles. They are very concerned about being masculine or feminine according to society's traditional standards and may be afraid of any feelings or actions that might seem to contradict society's images of how a man or a woman should be. A young man may hide tender feelings to protect a macho image. A young woman may feel guilty about having strong sexual desires or may take great pains to hide her intelligence. Yes, despite all the social changes in the past two decades, we still get letters describing these feelings and choices. And when men and women get stuck in these old ways of thinking and acting, they may be sacrificing personal honesty to maintain old stereotypes.

Caught up in roles where "sexuality" may be seen in terms of "sexiness," people may relate to one another as sex objects, forgoing the friendship that gives love and sex new meaning and bypassing the tenderness that makes an intimate friendship so special. Indeed, someone who defines himself or herself in terms of traditional sex roles may have trouble maintaining close relationships with the same or opposite sex, afraid to show tenderness in a same-sex friendship or honest friendship in a dating or sexual relationship.

SEXUALITY AS PART OF YOUR LIFE

Some people see sexuality as a separate entity in their lives. It isn't. Your sexuality goes far beyond labels and stereotypes, far beyond sexual relationships, far beyond whatever sexual actions and options you might choose. The fact is, despite the choices you make regarding sexual activities—even if you choose *never* to have sex with another person—you are an innately sexual being, just like everyone else.

There is nothing strange or mysterious about your sexuality. It just *is*. Like you. How you choose to express yourself sexually, on the other hand, does involve value judgments. Who you are, how you feel, and what you think can't be judged. But you *are* responsible for your choices and activities.

Sexuality is shared equally by males and females. No one sex is more sexual than the other. We're all simply people. And people feel tenderness and passion and love. People feel sexual desires. People have all kinds of sexual fantasies. People of all ages—even infants—feel sexual sensations.

Accepting your sensations, your fantasies, your desires, and your feelings—from tenderness to passion—as normal and natural can help you feel more at ease with others and with yourself. Feeling such comfort with your sexuality can help you make more responsible choices regarding any sexual activities. For example:

- *You can have and enjoy a sexual fantasy without ever needing to act on it and make it reality.* We fantasize about all kinds of things—why not sex? Feelings and fantasies can't be judged. They just happen. However, you *are* responsible for the choices you make and what you *do*. You may have fantasies about things that you wouldn't dream of doing. That's OK. You may find yourself having warm feelings toward someone of the same sex or someone of the opposite sex. These feelings don't necessarily define you one way or the other. Most of us are capable of responding emotionally to people of both sexes with warm feelings, deep friendship and love, and, at times, somewhat erotic feelings. This can happen with people whose primary

sexual orientation is heterosexual as well as with people who are primarily homosexual. Most people, whatever their sexual orientation, age, or marital status have a rich and varied fantasy life.

- *Fantasies can help you act more responsibly by putting sexuality in perspective and balance with the rest of your life.* In a study at Trinity University, for example, people were told either to think about sex or to attempt to keep all thoughts of the subject out of their minds. The mere mention of sex was arousing to all people in the study, but the excitement level gradually diminished among those who were encouraged to think and fantasize about sex. Those who tried *not* to think about sex felt themselves fighting constant, unexpected thoughts about sex and a continuous level of sexual excitement.

- *Real love and intimacy do not need sex in order to grow and thrive in a relationship.* Sexual sharing may be simply a part of some of these relationships when the time is right. If you know the difference between love and sex, you're not as likely to get the two confused and, in search of love, to enter prematurely into sexual relationships.

- *If you feel good about your sexuality, you won't be in a rush to have sex.* You can enjoy all your feelings and sensations. And, when you do have sex eventually, your positive feelings about your choice will lead you to make wise decisions about birth control. (People who don't use birth control because they think that such "planning ahead" is wrong don't feel good about having sex or about their sexuality. So they need to pretend that sex is, invariably, a passionate accident.)

YOUR SEXUAL ORIENTATION

I'm 15 and gay. (It feels funny and yet very normal to write that! It's the first time I've written that on paper yet it's like saying what's been in my heart as long as I can remember.) I knew I was different in some way when I was just five or six, but really started knowing by sixth grade. Just last week, I came out to my parents. They were pretty cool about it overall, but keep saying "Are you SURE? You're so young! How do you know for sure?" I tell them that I'm as sure as anyone else my age who is into dating girls. They have some gay friends who didn't come out until they were in their thirties—one of the guys was actually married and has a son! So I think that's why they're surprised I know so early, but I keep telling them that times are different now and that maybe their friends always sort of knew, but couldn't accept that they were gay because it was so looked down on when they were young. What do you think?

Jason O.

Sexual orientation is a major aspect of our sexuality. Even though, ideally, sexual orientation should be just another part of who we are, some gay people—young and older—still feel the sting of society's disapproval. This is more prevalent in some communities, some schools, and some social circles than others. What it can mean is that some heterosexual teens worry about the fact that they may have warm emotional feelings—and maybe some erotic feelings—about certain people of the same sex: perhaps a much-admired teacher or an especially treasured friend. And some young people who know in their hearts that they are gay may worry about being socially isolated and ostracized by school friends and rejected by their families if they let people know who they are and how they feel.

In both instances, these young people's worries stem from the reality of social prejudice against people whose sexual orientation is gay or lesbian. In both instances, too, these young people are experiencing feelings that are entirely normal for them.

Crushes on teachers or others of the same sex are normal. We admire and love many people, especially in adolescence. Everyone has idols and secret crushes. Admiring someone else may help you discover more about what you would like to grow to become. It can be a positive step in your growth toward maturity.

Close friendships with those of the same sex are vitally important, too. Closeness with a best friend can be great mutual comfort at a time in your life when you face so many changes. In friendships, people express affection in many different ways. Some express their feelings with thoughtful acts or gentle teasing. Some can say how they feel. For others, a touch or hug or kiss says, "You're special. I care." And our sexual orientation—whether heterosexual or homosexual—is a normal part of the people we happen to be.

It may help to know that, although most of us have a definite sexual orientation that is either heterosexual or homosexual, very few people are 100 percent heterosexual or 100 percent homosexual. The Kinsey Institute has devised a scale to rate sexual orientation. An extreme heterosexual, someone who has never responded emotionally or physically to someone of the same sex, would be a "zero," while a "six" would be the other extreme—someone who is and always has been exclusively homosexual. A 1970 Kinsey study revealed that at least 60 percent of American men and 30 percent of American women have had at least one overt, intentional homosexual experience by age 15. Other studies have placed these figures even higher.

So a high percentage of the American population would be neither a zero or a six, but somewhere in between. They would include people who are almost exclusively heterosexual, but who have had a minor homosexual experience; people who have had experiences with both sexes, but who prefer the opposite sex; people who have no special preferences; and people who prefer those of the same sex, but who are not exclusively homosexual.

What about the men and women—"7.2 million Americans under the age of 20 are gay, lesbian, or bisexual" (from Statistical Abstract of the U.S., Washington, D.C., U.S. Bureau of the Census)—whose sexual orientation is primarily homosexual?

How we develop our sexual orientation is still being studied, and so far the findings have been fascinating, if not definitive. We do know that you find your gender identity—seeing yourself as male or female—by age 2. Most of us see ourselves by our anatomically correct gender. (Those who see themselves as the opposite sex are called *transsexuals* and are quite different from transvestites, who are either heterosexual or homosexual and see themselves as the correct gender even though they enjoy dressing in the clothing of the opposite sex.) Homosexuals see themselves as the correct gender. They simply grow up finding that they are physically attracted to those of the same sex.

We know that some people may not come to terms with their true sexual orientation for years. In fact, some people marry and have children before coming to terms with the fact that they are primarily homosexual. This may have much less to do with "turning gay" or choosing to be gay and much more to do with the fact that, in years past and even today, there is so much social disapproval of homosexuality that it may take years for a gay man or lesbian woman to come to terms with his or her sexual orientation and to find the courage to come out of the closet. It's quite possible that this scenario may change for today's teens—some of whom are growing up in a much more supportive social environment than those who came before them.

In fact, the prevailing wisdom used to be that a person couldn't be totally sure of his or her sexual orientation until young adulthood. Now we know that most teens are quite aware of their own sexual orientation at a very young age.

Dr. Gary Remafedi of the Adolescent Health Program at the University of Minnesota headed a team of researchers that surveyed 34,706 teens in grades seven through twelve in that state. His findings: most teens know their sexual orientation by age 17 or 18. At age 12, only 26 percent of young people were unsure of their sexual orientation. By age 17, those who were still unsure had dropped to 5 percent.

Some religious counselors feel that sexual orientation may be learned behavior and, as such, can be changed. Some mental health therapists believe that sexual orientation *may* be changed in instances where the individual is highly motivated and wants very much to change. But mainstream experts are skeptical. There isn't conclusive evidence that such therapy changes a person's actual sexual orientation, but simply his or her sexual behavior. That is, you may learn to behave in a different way, but will your real feelings change? Other unanswered questions: How long can you behave in a way that may be contrary to your true sexual orientation? And what will the psychological cost be?

Many other therapists emphasize the importance of authenticity and self-acceptance. A lot of therapy these days is supportive: helping gay people deal with social pressures and disapproval, to understand and to accept their feelings. Some wonder to begin with, "*Why* am I gay?"

There are many theories. Some controversial studies are focusing on hormonal influences in the womb that may predispose a person to become homosexual. Some experts believe that whether one actually becomes homosexual may depend on these prenatal hormonal influences combined with certain environmental factors. A recent study at a medical center in Boston found that there seems to be a tendency for male homosexuality to run in families. The researchers studied 51 homosexual and 50 heterosexual men as well as their siblings. About 4 percent of the brothers of heterosexual men were gay. Among the brothers of homosexual men, some 22 percent were also homosexual. The researchers have said that, in this particular study, it was not possible to show whether heredity or upbringing was more important in determining sexual preference. Curiously, these differences were not apparent in the sisters studied. The sisters of homosexual men were not any more likely than sisters of heterosexual men to be homosexual.

Obviously, there's a lot more we need to learn about what makes us who we are—whether we're primarily heterosexual or homosexual. What's important to remember in the meantime is:

- Many gay people are at least vaguely aware that they are somehow different in very early childhood.
- While a lot of people worry about gays molesting or "recruiting" young people, the fact is that the vast majority of child molesters are heterosexual.
- There's no reason to fear someone who is gay or lesbian. Generally, they don't want to be rejected socially or physically any more than you do, so they're likely to be attracted to people who share their sexual orientation. If someone does show an interest that makes you feel uncomfortable, all you need to say is "No, thanks."
- Homosexuality is not a disease or a mental illness. In the past few decades, important professional organizations—such as the American Psychological Association—have accepted this fact as policy. There is nothing inherently wrong with someone who is gay or lesbian. Sexual orientation is just another part of who we are as human beings, like having blue eyes or red hair or a family-shared talent for music.
- Reading and learning about gays and lesbians is not going to turn your sexual orientation in that direction unless it was there already. Some people fear that if teens read or hear about homosexuality—for example, in a school sex education class—they will want to become homosexual. Not likely! Given the physical and verbal abuse that gay and lesbian teens still face on some school campuses and the anger and rejection they often face at home when they try to discuss their sexual feelings with their parents, it's unlikely that many teens would be eager to make that choice—if, in fact, being gay were truly a choice.

Think about it. Who could influence a person strongly enough to make such a difficult choice?

Studies show that even parents—who, perhaps, influence us more than we ever know—don't have a definitive influence on their children's sexual preferences—with most homosexuals coming from homes headed by heterosexual parents and gay parents no more likely than heterosexual parents to raise children who grow up to be gay.

If you feel you may be gay or lesbian, accepting this reality can be a painful and confusing process. It may begin when you're very young and realize that you're different in many ways that you can't explain. Or you may only gradually become aware of your feelings, longings, fantasies, and consistent attraction to those of your own sex. You may have times of feeling terribly alone, like you're the only person who feels so different and like if you breathe a word to anyone your whole world as you know it—family relationships, friendships—could fall apart. You may have times of denying your feelings to yourself and to others as a way of being accepted. You may date and even have sex with people of the opposite sex (studies of adult gay men and lesbian women show that most have had heterosexual experiences). You may work very hard to act like everyone else, keeping an important part of who you are hidden even from those close to you for a long time. Then, as your sexual identity seems to be an intrinsic part of you, you may begin to share this part of yourself with others—with widely varying results ranging from loving acceptance to angry rejection. The process of accepting yourself, with such mixed reactions even among those you love most, is not easy. You may need to talk with a counselor or someone else you feel could help you through this time.

As you begin to accept your sexual orientation as part of the complex and fascinating person you are, you may feel less overwhelmed by your feelings. Your sexual preference is only a *part* of your total identity—not the whole thing. You are still the unique individual you have always been—with your own special array of skills, talents, and strengths. Once you realize this—and once your family and friends realize, too, that you're still the same person they've always known and loved—you will begin to move past your pain to new peace. Growing in self-acceptance and in your capacity to relate to others in a non-exploitive way, to give and receive love, is vital—whatever your sexual orientation.

SEX EDUCATION AND YOUR SEXUAL CHOICES

I can't talk to my parents about sex. Their only sex education is "Don't you dare!" Now they're upset about a new sex education class offered next year at my school and I'm afraid they won't sign a permission slip for me to be in the class, which would be so embarrassing, plus I want to know the facts about sex. I don't have any plans to do anything because I do want to be virgin when I get married. I really believe in that. But I feel really stupid around my friends and con-fused, too. I think a sex education class would help. How can I convince my parents to let me take it?

Sarah H.

Our sex education comes from a wide variety of sources—some helpful and some not so helpful. We get impressions about sex by what we see on TV and in the movies. We pick up certain ideas and attitudes from what our parents *don't* say as well as from what they do tell us. We learn many things—some correct, many not—from our friends. And, despite the controversy surrounding school-based sex education programs, we can also learn a great deal from these.

Ideally, a sex education program at school or, less formally, at home from parents, needs to include discussions of all aspects of sexuality, *including* the option of abstinence. There are many good reasons for abstinence from sexual inter-course during the teen years; we'll be discussing these later in this chapter. However, to limit all dis-cussion to this highly suggested option neglects the needs of teens whose values and choices differ. A good sex education course needs to discuss the fol-lowing:

- *Sexual choices*—including abstinence.
- *Respect for yourself and others*, whatever your sexual choices. Teens of both sexes need to be educated about the necessity of respecting another's feelings and values. Both boys and girls need to respect another's right to say no without ridicule. Both sexes need to discuss and learn what responsible sexuality is all about—and what intimacy means, with or without sex as a component of an intimate relationship.
- *Facts about the body and about sexuality.* This includes understanding how males and females differ biologically and socially. Under-standing biological differences—such as the fact that males may become sexually excited faster and more urgently during a kissing or making-out session and, on the other hand, that their health and sanity are not in danger if their sexual urges are not fulfilled on the spot—can help young people of both sexes avoid trouble. Understanding the social pres-sures of being male or female in junior high or high school—the pressures on guys to be macho and "perform" and on girls to have a boyfriend—may lead to more mutual compas-sion and good communication.
- *Practical facts about sexuality*—including information about birth control and sexually transmitted diseases. In many ways, education about birth control underscores one's risk of getting pregnant if one has sex—and may lead to sexual responsibility, not wild abandon. Education about sexually transmitted diseases is also vital—and may deter some teens from having sex at this point in their lives while helping others protect themselves against vari-ous health risks.

It is also vital to know about how one thing can lead to another if you don't realize what's happen-ing. The fact is, some teens engage in activities such as deep kissing, petting, and oral sex without realizing that these are part of sexual foreplay and can lead to unplanned intercourse unless you know specifically how far you're prepared to go and stick to your decision. So knowing explicit details about sex, rather than inciting impulsive action, may actually help you make more responsible choices.

It's important to realize that many parents have difficulty talking about sex because *they* weren't raised to be open about the subject. (Their parents couldn't and didn't talk to them either!) When parents do talk, they may stress abstinence because of their love and concern for you. Most parents are well aware of the bad things that can happen as a result of sex too soon or with the wrong partner: not only the risks of AIDS and other sexually transmitted diseases and pregnancy, but also of the emotional pain that can come when and if the relationship ends. As much as they may want you to become independent, your parents still have a strong inclination to want to protect you from danger and from hurt. So their negative feelings about teen sex may not be coming from lack of caring or from prudery, but from their love for you.

These parents need to understand that correct information—from them and/or from school programs—will help you make more responsible, life-affirming choices. Studies have shown that teens who scored highest on tests of sex knowledge were much less likely to be having sex than their lower-scoring peers. Other studies have found that teenagers who have had complete sex education courses in school that cover all options and areas of information are more likely to use birth control if they do decide to have sex.

- *How to make your own choices and decisions.* Some choices are too important to be left to chance—including choices about sexuality. And these choices aren't always easy. For example, making a decision about whether or not to have sex with someone you truly love, someone who cares about you, respects you, and loves you, too, is quite different from making the decision not to have sex with a casual

date who is coming on strong. Your choice, in both cases, may be *not* to have sex, but saying no to someone who really matters to you is very hard. And saying yes to sexual involvement can be difficult, too, and is not necessarily just a matter of going with the flow and letting your hormones take the lead.

Some people have difficulty accepting the fact that teens have—or should have—choices about their sexuality and feel that parent-mandated rules should be the law. While parental values and wishes *do* need to be respected and considered (because, more often than not, your parents, above all others, have your best interests at heart), your parents can't be with you 24 hours a day or on every date. You will be faced—and probably have been faced—with making choices on your own. That's why it's so important that you know how to think and decide for yourself what's best for you. Many times, this may coincide with what your parents want for you. Sometimes it may not. Either way, you need to feel confident and empowered by your own decision-making ability. You need to be able to stand up for what you want and not let someone else—including a partner—talk you into anything that doesn't feel right for you.

Whatever your choices—right now and in the future—making them with as much information at hand as possible will help ensure that you will make wiser, more responsible decisions.

MAKING SEXUAL CHOICES

I'm 13 and confused. Well, I want to know if you could have any idea when you are ready to have sex? I want to but I'm scared, and all the risks that are involved are holding me back. Can you help me out?

Confused Greatly

You make sexual choices all the time. You don't have to be sexually active to do this. Deciding that you would rather be a virgin until marriage or, at least, for a while longer is a sexual choice—and can be a very positive one!

Deciding how to deal with your sexual feelings is a choice, too. Some people enjoy fantasies. Some masturbate. Some choose to have sex with other people. And some choose all three or varying combinations.

Sexual decision making is an important part of deciding who you are and what your values are. It's vital that your actions match your values. Otherwise, you will feel bad about yourself and guilty about your choice. All sexual choices—from choosing to have sex with someone or choosing, at least for now, to abstain from sexual activity—can and should be joyous ones, made after careful reflection and with a strong sense of what's right for you.

MASTURBATION

Is masturbation normal? Can it harm you? Can you do it too much (and maybe use up all your sperm so that you can't have children when you're grown up and married)?

Just Asking

Masturbation is a natural expression of sexuality for males and females, young and old. It means sexual stimulation of oneself—in some instances, to the point of orgasm. It is estimated that about 97 percent of males and 90 percent of females have masturbated by the age of 21. Contrary to old wives' tales, masturbation will not cause hair to grow on your palms; make you sterile, blind, or insane; give you acne; or take your virginity. It can offer release from sexual tensions, particularly if you are not sexually active in other ways. Of course, many married people and others with satisfying sex lives may masturbate as well.

Masturbation is also the safest form of sexual activity if you're concerned about avoiding the risk of AIDS. (Between two people, the safest sex is in a long-term, mutually monogamous relationship in which both partners were virgins coming into the relationship and who have no other risk factors—for example, IV drug use or a history of blood transfusions before 1985.) Other benefits of masturbation include releasing sexual tensions, growing to learn what you enjoy, and experiencing orgasm.

Orgasm, a normal sexual experience, means reaching a height of sexual excitement. For the male, this usually means ejaculation. Women, of course, don't ejaculate, but have feelings of intense excitement and, sometimes, a throbbing feeling in the genitals followed by the same sense of relaxation and peace that a man may feel after ejaculating. Orgasm may occur when you're fantasizing about sex or masturbating or when you're having some sort of sexual contact—from petting to intercourse—with someone else.

Can masturbation ever be harmful? Only in a few instances. First, if you are extremely religious and/or your values and beliefs are making you feel extremely guilty about masturbation, this may be a problem for you. The self-hatred that may be a by-product of extreme guilt may drive you to masturbate even more. And so you're caught in a cycle of misery.

How can you deal with this? You may want to talk about your feelings with your physician, clergyperson, counselor, or someone else you can trust to listen and who may reassure you that you are, indeed, quite normal. Whether or not you do masturbate is very much a matter of personal choice. If you do, it doesn't make you bad. If you choose not to, due to your personal beliefs, it doesn't make you strange. It's up to you.

Many teens wonder if it's possible to masturbate too often. How often is too often? That's a good question—and one that's difficult to answer. In general, however, masturbation—though healthy and normal—is not meant to take the place of other things in your life. If you find yourself using masturbation as a crutch to avoid problems, facing feelings, challenges, or social encounters with others, you may want to re-evaluate its place in your life and make some changes.

A number of young people feel very guilty about group masturbation, which is quite common especially in early adolescence, especially in boys. This may mean masturbating in the presence of a friend or friends or touching each other in erotic ways. Among boys, some of these group masturbation sessions are almost competitive games to see who can ejaculate fastest and farthest. This can all seem like a good idea at the time, but some teens are plagued with guilt afterward, wondering why they did it and if this means that they're gay.

Especially in the early teens, such group masturbation is quite common and is not considered abnormal. As your own body is developing, you may have an intense curiosity about others, wanting to see if they have the same feelings you do. Finding out that others may look, feel, and respond much like you do may help reinforce your own positive feelings about yourself and your ability to function sexually. Testing this ability around friends of the same sex may be somewhat less threatening if you happen to be quite young and still a bit uncomfortable with the opposite sex. But remember: It's important not to label yourself. Participating or not participating in group masturbation is very much a matter of personal choice. Some do it more than others, and some never try it at all—and that's OK, too.

RELATING TO OTHERS

My boyfriend is trying to talk me into having sex with him, but I'm scared of being used. It isn't that I don't love him, but I don't feel ready to have sex. But I don't want to lose him. What should I do?

Maureen M.

Making decisions about whether to become sexually involved with another person and building non-exploitive relationships with the opposite sex can be extremely difficult when there's so much peer pressure to be sexually active, to "score" and to be popular, and, especially for girls, to have a special boyfriend. In such a pressure-filled atmosphere, it can be difficult to make a few choices about your sexuality, about what you will—or won't—do at this time. Yet free choices are what non-exploitive relationships are all about.

Many young people are choosing to postpone sexual activity these days. A recent government study found the numbers of teens overall who have had sex has dropped noticeably through the 1990s. A Planned Parenthood–Louis Harris poll of American teenagers of both sexes a few years ago came up with similar results. It was discovered that *fewer than half* of the 16-year-old girls *and* boys were sexually active. Only in the 17-and-older age group did the sexually active begin to outnumber the virgins. Of those who were having sex, 73 percent of the girls and 50 percent of the boys cited various forms of peer pressure as the main reason for beginning sexual activity.

It's important to keep in mind that what may be right—or seem right—for some of your friends may not be right for you. There may be some very good reasons for you to say no to sexual activity right now.

12 Reasons to Say No Right Now

1. *You don't feel ready.* This is one of the most important reasons *not* to have sex. Feeling ready—instead of pressured—can make sex a whole different experience, when you freely choose to engage in it.

2. *Premarital sex is against your beliefs and values.* Your values matter—a lot! And if you violate them, the guilt and anxiety you would feel would override any enjoyment. Why put yourself through such an emotionally taxing experience?

3. *You're in love for the first time.* Be cautious. Go slow. You're emotionally vulnerable to pain

when your feelings are so strong and new and when you have so little experience with love and loss. Work on building a strong, stable relationship as well as on your own self-esteem before even *thinking* about having sex.

4. *Your partner is pressuring you.* Beware of the person who ignores your feelings and tries to threaten or bully or cajole you into sex before you feel ready. If he or she really cares, your partner will respect your values, even if they don't agree with his or hers.

5. *You don't know anything about and/or are too embarrassed to use birth control.* This is a splendid reason to wait. Until you can learn which methods of birth control work and which ones don't, you don't know enough to have responsible sex. Furthermore, until you can admit that you are—or will be—sexually active and use a reliable method of birth control, you're not mature enough to cope with the many responsibilities of a sexual relationship.

6. *Pregnancy would be a personal disaster for you.* No birth control method except abstinence is 100 percent effective. If a pregnancy would be a real disaster right now—for reasons of health, education, family, relationship, or other personal matters—abstinence is the best way to avoid this.

7. *You want your first time to be extra-special.* You will probably always remember—for better or for worse—the first time you have sex. Do yourself a favor and wait for the right time, the right person, and the best possible circumstances. Do you really want your first time to be in the back seat of a musty old car? Or a rushed encounter before your parents get home from work? Don't create never-to-be-forgotten memories you'd really rather forget!

8. *Your relationship is in jeopardy.* Relationship problems are not solved by having sex—even if your major problem is the fact that you and your partner differ over sexual choices.

9. *You don't know each other well.* The best sexual sharing comes with someone you know and trust. Sex, under the right circumstances and with the right person, can be very special. Why do it with someone who *isn't* special to you?

10. *You're concerned about sexually transmitted diseases.* You're right—and you're smart—to be concerned. Besides the risk of AIDS, a number of other sexually transmitted diseases can threaten your health and your future fertility in addition to your dignity. If you're sexually active, you are at risk for sexually transmitted diseases. The more sex partners you have, particularly people you don't know well, the greater your risk. It's smart to consider these risks beforehand—and these can be an excellent reason not to have sex right now.

11. *You don't know much about sex.* Read. Take a sex education course. Talk with your parents or other informed adults. Bring a list of questions to your doctor. Become a theoretical expert first. Knowing the real facts about sex can help safeguard your health and your future.

12. *You're tempted to have sex for nonsexual reasons.* Maybe you're not especially popular and think that being sexually active will change all that. Despite what you may think, having sex cannot make you genuinely popular, ensure a lasting, loving relationship, boost your self-esteem, or decrease loneliness. If you have sex to get what you can really only give yourself, you will be disappointed.

Taking the time to learn how to build and nurture friendships can help you grow into a giving and mature person who can fully share with another when the time, person, and circumstances are right.

A Few Words About Dating Violence and Date Rape

As a 19-year-old college student, I am just now finding out there is one area of sex education that I wish my parents had been more explicit about: sexual assault. I believe that most people in my generation have the attitude that women and men can do exactly the same things in the world. In many cases, that is true, but women do need to be especially careful to prevent sexual assault. I received my education concerning this unexpectedly when my roommate was raped. I have since read many books on rape and learned that one in four women is raped at some point in her lifetime. This is not a topic to be taken lightly and more people need to be informed about it.

Laurie T.

Laurie is absolutely right. Unfortunately, one in ten teenagers experience physical violence—often date rape—in their dating relationships.

How can you avoid becoming yet another statistic?

- *Be selective about your dates.* That popular athlete or that incredibly cool frat man can be big trouble. Recent studies show that women most at risk for date rape are those who are high school students or college freshmen, who date athletes or men who belong to college fraternities, and/or who drink on dates. This doesn't mean you should never go out with these guys, but it does mean you should be careful. Don't let yourself get into vulnerable situations when you're with them.
- *Don't mix alcohol and dating.* This is a good idea no matter *who* your date happens to be. To stay in control of your own body and destiny, you need to stay sober.
- *Avoid troublesome situations.* You know what they are—being at a fraternity party where everyone is drinking, being alone with a guy in his dorm room or in his room at home when no one else is around. Don't set yourself up for trouble, especially with a guy you don't know well.
- *Let him know that no means no:* This means being very clear about what you will do and won't do, and that when you say no, you mean it. No one deserves to be raped. It isn't justifiable—ever. But if you waver back and forth between yes and no or tease him sexually, he

may not believe you really mean no. Don't put yourself in that position. Set your boundaries firmly—and mean it!

How to Know When You're Ready for Sex

The decision when and with whom to have sex is, ultimately, entirely yours. How do you make a responsible decision regarding sexual involvement? You might start by asking yourself a number of questions.

- *Am I trying to prove something to others? To myself? How do I really feel about having sex right now? How does my partner feel?* It's important to know why you're thinking of having sex and how you feel about it—and how your partner feels. If you're in a loving, committed relationship and the choice seems right to both of you, it may well be the right decision for you.

    But it's also important to know what sex cannot do for you—in case you may be thinking of sex for nonsexual reasons. Sex cannot fill gaping holes in your self-esteem or make you instantly wise, mature, and adult. Sex also cannot necessarily bind you to another person forever or make love, commitment, and intimacy grow where these qualities never existed before.
- *What feelings do I have for the other person?* If you see your potential sex partner as a challenge, a conquest, or someone who's simply there and available—stop and think before acting. For the best possible sexual experience, wait for someone you like very much or love, someone you know well and with whom you can be comfortably yourself.
- *Do we communicate well?*

    Can you talk openly and honestly?

    Can you share what you're really feeling?

    Can you talk about what sex means to you individually and as a couple?

Can you make a responsible decision together, sharing the responsibilities for being involved and for whatever consequences may occur? Can you talk to one another about birth control, for example?

Can you tell each other if something hurts, is uncomfortable, or is distasteful to you?

Can you talk about your expectations—and your fears?

- *Do I have accurate information about sex?* Sexual/anatomical ignorance can cause a lot of unplanned pregnancies *and* a lot of grief and disappointment when the people involved don't have enough information about their own bodies—and each other's bodies—to fully give and receive sexual pleasure.
- *Are we willing to take full responsibility for our actions?* Responsibility means reviewing all possibilities—and options—in advance. Pregnancy and sexually transmitted diseases are two very real risks of sexual involvement.

What would you do in the event of an unplanned pregnancy? Could you be supportive of one another? What options would you have?

If one of you noticed symptoms of a sexually transmitted disease, could you take the responsibility of telling your partner and suggesting that you both get tested?

Do you know how to prevent an unplanned pregnancy? Have you learned what the most reliable methods of birth control are and how they can be obtained and used?

More to the point: *Will* you take the responsibility of using a reliable method of birth control? Are you mature enough to plan ahead to prevent a pregnancy?

■ ■ ■

"Birth control is like planning for sex and I feel that such planning is wrong. Sex should be romantic and just happen . . . " is a comment we have heard a lot—often from teenage mothers. Some of these teens are victims of the old double standard, which sees the man as the seducer and the woman as the seduced. This old myth seems to say that, unless a woman is quite literally swept off her feet, she's no lady.

A variation on this theme is the romance myth that says that sex is romantic only when it is totally unexpected. Some victims of the "He swept me off my feet!" school of thought feel that they have to get drunk or stoned to make sex OK.

Others feel that just getting carried away with passion justifies the act. This attitude is reinforced by many popular TV shows—especially the daytime and nighttime soaps—where characters lead active sex lives, but only rarely seem to concern themselves with birth control.

The fact is, planned sex can be extremely romantic. In some cases, it may be much more so than the so-called spontaneous variety of sex. Taking birth control precautions to avoid an unwanted pregnancy and to help alleviate the fear of such pregnancy can free you both to enjoy sex.

Birth control should be a mutual decision and discussed well *before* having sex, not during or after. Seeking a reliable method of birth control means admitting to yourself and, possibly, to others that you are—or soon will be—sexually active.

Can you do this?

If you're not ready to face this responsibility, you're not ready to have sex.

- *Are we loving, caring friends?* There's a lot to be said for waiting until you can have sex with a very special friend:

A friend will not make fun of you or criticize you if you're clumsy, uncertain, or scared.

A friend will enjoy sharing all kinds of experiences—some sexual and some not—with you.

A friend is not likely to say, "You got pregnant? That's *your* problem!"

A friend will not brag and tell all.

A friend will ask, "How do you feel?" and value your beliefs, your opinions, and your feelings.

A friend will care about you—as a person.

When we're just learning about our sexual selves and having our first sexual experiences, it really helps to have a partner who is also a caring friend.

Sex vs. Intimacy

Many people think that sex and intimacy are the same. But this is not so. Ideally, of course, emotional intimacy is a vital part of a sexual relationship, but this is not always the case. Some people have sex without emotional intimacy. Many others have intimate relationships that don't include sex. And some people are able to build a lovely blend of the two.

Intimacy means that you feel safe in a relationship—safe enough to be yourself and to be vulnerable with another person—and that this other person feels the same safety and freedom. It means honest communication and nonjudgmental emotional support. Real intimacy isn't instant or easy. It takes time and effort to build.

Being truly intimate with another does not mean constantly baring your soul. It can also mean being comfortable together in silence. It means finding joy in sharing ordinary—as well as extraordinary—moments together.

Sex is not an inevitable part of the ordinary or extraordinary experiences that intimate relationships bring. You can have wonderful feelings of closeness with a variety of people with whom you will never have sex. Intimate friendships—whether these involve friends of the same or the opposite sex or your family members—can be passionate in spirit, feeling, and commitment and can bring a great deal of love, joy, and satisfaction into your life.

With someone who you feel might become a lover or life partner, developing a passionate, intimate friendship is an excellent way to grow into love. In fact, sex—particularly sex too soon in your life or too soon in the relationship—can *interfere* with intimacy if it is used as a shortcut or substitute for all the steps you need to take in order to develop an intimate bond with another person. There are no shortcuts or substitutes for talking, sharing feelings, or taking the time to get to know each other as valuable, distinct individuals and to build solid mutual trust. Substituting sex for any of these vital steps may make true emotional intimacy impossible.

However, intimacy can greatly enhance sexual sharing. While sex with a mysterious, exciting stranger may be a fun fantasy, in real life you may find—when you do feel ready for sex—that sexual sharing in an atmosphere of loving trust and mutual vulnerability is the most rewarding kind of sexual experience you can have.

You may find that each intimate relationship—sexual or not—has a unique and treasured place in your life, in the present or in your loving memories. Developing the capacity to be intimate, comfortable, and caring with others can mean a lifetime of abundance—in love, in friends, and in the very special joy true intimacy can bring.

Growing to be your own person, making your own informed choices, being sensitive to the rights of others to be themselves, and learning to take responsibility for your own actions can greatly enhance your life in many ways—including your sexuality and your relationships on all levels.

With time and personal growth, so much of the pressure, fear, and uncertainty you may be feeling now will fade. In its place may be joy in your uniqueness—your feelings, your fantasies, and your beliefs. There may also be new joy in sharing who you have become with someone else. There will also be the joy of discovering another person in a myriad of ways: talking, touching, laughing, crying, liking, loving, and discovering each other, not only as lovers but also as very special friends!

YOU AND YOUR SEXUALITY

✔ Sexuality is part of who we are; sex is something we do.

✔ Sexual fantasies are normal whether or not you're having sex and can actually reduce sexual tension.

✔ Masturbation is something most people—male or female—do at some point in their lives. It isn't harmful unless it violates your own values and makes you feel terribly guilty or unless it begins to take over your life. But for most people, it is a pleasurable and healthy choice of sexual activity.

✔ Researchers don't know exactly what makes one person homosexual and another person heterosexual. But it's important to know that sexual orientation is part of who we are, like having blue eyes or brown hair or musical talent. It isn't a choice.

✔ What matters most is not whether you are gay or straight but whether you're able to love and have non-exploitive relationships with others.

✔ Don't mix dating and drinking. Alcohol is a major factor in 90 percent of teen date rape cases. To keep control of your body and the situation, stay sober!

✔ If you don't feel ready to have sex or if your partner is pressuring you, DON'T!

✔ Developing an intimate friendship with another person—which may or may not involve sex at this time—is an excellent way to grow in love. Sex too soon can actually interfere with intimacy. Intimacy isn't just closeness and passion; it's feeling safe with another and free to be truly yourself.

CHAPTER TWELVE

The Truth About Sexually Transmitted Diseases

We had this totally disgusting lecture from some sort of expert in our health class today on all kinds of diseases you can get by having sex. I think she was just trying to scare us. I mean, she spent so much time talking about AIDS—which normal people don't get— right? Also, since things like gonorrhea can be easily cured, or so I've heard, what's the big deal if you get something like that? I think that adults are just trying to scare us into not having sex. Am I right?

Michelle P.

Michelle's view of sexually transmitted diseases (STDs)—that they always happen to someone else, that they can be easily cured without any harm done, that they're just too disgusting for a nice person to hear about, let alone have—is fairly common, but quite inaccurate.

The most basic fact about sexually transmitted diseases is this: **If you are having sex, you are running the risk of getting sexually transmitted diseases**.

If you want to avoid getting a sexually transmitted disease, you have several choices:

- You can choose to abstain (not have sex at all).
- You can wait to have sex until you're married and then marry someone who is also a virgin—and be faithful to each other.

- You can take all the precautions you possibly can to cut down the risk of getting a sexually transmitted disease.

Preventing sexually transmitted diseases is especially important these days. Even though new combination treatments have extended HIV-infected persons' lifetimes for years, even decades, young people—both men and women—*are* dying from AIDS. Once you have it, there may be treatments, but there is no vaccine and no 100 percent cure. AIDS is one of the five leading causes of death for adolescents and young adults.

Genital herpes is also incurable, though not fatal. And even diseases that people take more for granted these days—such as gonorrhea—or perhaps have never heard about—such as chlamydia—can threaten a woman's future fertility by causing pelvic inflammatory disease in her Fallopian tubes. Pelvic inflammatory disease (PID) can be very serious, even fatal in some instances.

Particularly in women, a number of sexually transmitted diseases are not easy to detect or to treat. It's important to know, too, that sexually transmitted diseases can happen to anyone—nice people included. You can have only one sex partner, have sex only occasionally, and keep yourself very clean—and still get a sexually transmitted disease. You can have sex only with someone you love and still be infected with a sexually transmitted disease. Love is no protection, unfortunately, against sexually transmitted diseases.

While it may not be pleasant to think about such possibilities, it's vital to know as much as you can about the risks, symptoms, and treatments of the more common sexually transmitted diseases so that you can decrease your risk of infection and know when to check with your physician for diagnosis and treatment. (Early treatment is crucial with several forms of STDs). Since sexually transmitted diseases are at epidemic proportions nationwide, chances are that an STD could happen to you or someone you know. The statistics are shocking:

- It is estimated that up to 25 percent of all new HIV infections occur in adolescents between ages 13 and 20. Most of the young adults in their twenties who are being diagnosed with AIDS were infected with HIV during their teen years.
- Among adolescents, it's much more likely to be infected with HIV as a result of heterosexual (rather than homosexual) sex. According to recent data from the Centers for Disease Control and Prevention, 90 percent of all new adolescent male cases and 95 percent of all new adolescent female cases of HIV infection result from heterosexual sex.
- Sexually transmitted disease infection rates are highest among young adults 15 to 25 years old.
- There are an estimated two million cases of gonorrhea and three million cases of chlamydia infections each year in all age groups. These two diseases, often undetected and untreated until major symptoms develop, are a leading cause of sterility in young people.
- Teenage girls have the highest rate of gonorrhea in the United States. Teen boys run a close second. The rate of gonorrhea infection is *20 times* higher in teen girls than in women over 30, according to statistics from the Centers for Disease Control and Prevention.

- One in four sexually active teens in the United States will become infected with an STD before they turn 20.
- More than five million Americans (and estimates have been much higher) are suffering from genital herpes, with 500,000 new cases each year and, as yet, no cure.

While syphilis and gonorrhea are often the first diseases people think about when sexually transmitted diseases are mentioned, these are much less likely to occur in teens than diseases such as genital herpes or chlamydia, which is the most frequently seen sexually transmitted disease among teenagers.

The following is an overview of some troublesome and common sexually transmitted diseases.

AIDS

Can you get AIDS if you're not gay? How do you get it? I mean, can you get it in ways besides having sex, like from swimming pools or if someone with AIDS sneezes near you or something? Can you get AIDS from donating blood? From kissing? I've heard all kinds of rumors and stuff. What's the truth?

Brad A.

What Is It?

AIDS (acquired immune deficiency syndrome) is a breakdown and failure of the body's immune system and is caused by a virulent strain of a virus called HTLV-III. The virus is usually introduced into the body through intimate sexual contact or by exposure to contaminated blood via a shared hypodermic needle or a blood transfusion. (The AIDS virus is present in the body fluids—primarily blood and semen—of an infected person. And it's possible for someone to have the virus in his or her body fluids without yet having any symptoms.)

According to current research, there is no evidence that you can get AIDS through casual contact with an infected person. This means that being in the same room with a person with AIDS, even if he or she is coughing or sneezing, is not likely to expose you to AIDS. However, if a person with AIDS happens to have tuberculosis (a disease that quite often infects people with AIDS) and was coughing, you could be exposed to tuberculosis—but not to AIDS. You cannot acquire AIDS through hugging, touching, or kissing an infected person on the cheek or closed lips. (It's not yet clear whether the virus can be spread via saliva. So far, no cases have been reported involving the transmission of AIDS via French kissing, but, to be safe, until we have more information, it may be best to avoid such kissing with an infected person or someone in a high-risk category.)

You cannot acquire AIDS by eating a meal or swimming in a pool with someone who has AIDS. (The pool chemicals and water should dilute and kill the virus which, outside the human body, is really quite fragile.) You also cannot get AIDS by donating blood. All needles used on blood donors are sterilized and used only once.

How does AIDS destroy a person's health and take his or her life? Once in the bloodstream, the HTLV-III virus attacks and kills a special kind of white blood cell called a *T-cell*. The T-cells are essential to the effective functioning of the body's immune system. Once these T-cells are damaged and depleted, the body is vulnerable to any number of infections and diseases. Some of these, which would be minor or easily cured in a healthy person, such as a yeast infection, are very serious and long-lasting and can even be fatal to a person with AIDS.

Symptoms

Some people can carry the AIDS virus and have no symptoms at all. A recently developed blood test can detect exposure to the AIDS virus by noting antibodies to the virus in the blood. It is still too early to tell how many people who have antibodies to the virus go on to develop AIDS. It is possible, even if you don't have any signs of the disease, to transmit the virus to others. So anyone who tests positive is advised to either abstain from sex altogether or, at the very least, use strict safe-sex measures.

Please Note: Today there are sophisticated laboratory tests—such as PCR (DNA tests)—to detect the AIDS virus very early. Also, there is current research into AIDS prevention—specifically, treating people who have been exposed to the HIV virus. All of this is important for a number of reasons. For example, if a woman is planning a pregnancy or is already pregnant, knowing her HIV status can be crucial to the health of her baby. Researchers have found that giving the drug AZT to HIV-positive pregnant women and to their babies at birth can lower these babies' infection rate significantly—with fewer than 10 percent of these babies being infected with the HIV virus! In terms of prevention for teens and adults, researchers are currently studying a "morning-after treatment" for AIDS exposure. Who would get this? A person who had unsafe sex the night before (as the result of a condom breaking or impulsive sex without protection, with a partner who is known to be infected with HIV or who is in a group at high risk for HIV infection). This experimental preventive treatment with the drug AZT to see whether a rapid high dose of this medicine can indeed prevent an individual from becoming infected is still in early stages of research and not available to the general public yet.

Treatment

Doctors treat symptoms and infections associated with AIDS and are sometimes successful in temporarily alleviating these. Until the mid-1990s, the best-known drug used in the treatment of AIDS was AZT. Then, in the mid-1990s, a new group of drugs called *protease inhibitors* was developed. These drugs work in a different way on HIV and have actually caused many AIDS patients to improve their health very significantly with weight gain and fewer infections. Some have even been able to return to work. Also, some people infected with HIV are longtime survivors, infected with the virus for over fifteen years, and still have not developed AIDS. Ongoing studies are looking at what keeps full-blown AIDS from developing in these survivors.

Researchers are working intensely on testing trial AIDS prevention vaccines. Unfortunately, at the time of this writing there is no vaccine and still no cure for AIDS. Despite so many new (and expensive) drugs, AIDS often leads to an early death.

Special Risk Groups

Anyone who has sex, particularly with more than one partner and without using safe-sex precautions (to be discussed later in this chapter) is at risk for HIV/AIDS infection. At this time, however, some people are at greater risk than others. These include the following:

- Male homosexuals—with young gay and bisexual men between ages 17 and 25 at special risk. A recent study of young gays by the San Francisco Department of Health's Office of AIDS found that 14 percent of gay and bisexual men between ages 17 and 19 were infected with the AIDS virus and that 30 percent of the survey participants reported engaging in unprotected anal intercourse, the highest-risk sexual activity. Teenage gay men under age 19 were twice as likely to engage in unsafe sex as gay men in their late twenties. These young people told researchers that they didn't feel personally threatened by HIV infection, that they considered it a problem for older gay men.
- Intravenous drug users, who may be exposed by shared needles.
- Hemophiliacs and others who require transfusions of blood or blood products. (However,

this risk has diminished significantly since 1985, when blood supplies began to be tested for the virus and donors screened more carefully.)

- Those who have sex with any of those in major risk groups. This would include women who have sex with bisexual men or IV drug users or men who have sex with women exposed to AIDS by drug use or other sex partners. (That is why, these days, sex with a prostitute is particularly risky. Besides having many sexual partners, many female prostitutes are often also IV drug users.)
- Babies of women infected with the virus. As we discussed earlier, considerable progress has been made in prevention of AIDS infection in infants. The result is that there are fewer HIV-infected babies. However, prevention is the key; to receive prenatal preventive care, a woman has to know that she is infected. So testing all pregnant women for the AIDS virus is vital.
- Sexually active teenagers. There are several reasons for this. Studies show that today's teens are more likely to have sex at an early age, to have multiple sex partners as they go through adolescence, and to neglect safe-sex practices, even when they know better theoretically. The "it can't happen to me" mindset, such a factor in teenage pregnancy in the past, has now, often tragically, become a risk factor for sexually transmitted diseases in teens.

These are just the groups in which AIDS is most often seen right now. But everyone who has sex is at risk. And most victims of AIDS are relatively young—a great many in their twenties. Some experts feel that teenagers are the next major risk group. When you're young, it's very easy to feel immortal and that nothing really bad will happen to you or someone you know. Some health educators sadly observe that teens may not take the risk of AIDS seriously until they see their friends and classmates begin to die before their eyes. But, by that time, it may be too late. Be smart. Take precautions NOW.

BACTERIAL VAGINOSIS

I had this fishy kind of creamy discharge (sorry to be gross, but I want you to know what I'm talking about) and my doctor said it was a sexually transmitted disease! I'm really upset because I've only been having safe sex for two months and only with my boyfriend Kyle, who told me he was a virgin, too, when we made love for the first time. The doctor said it was bacterial vaginosis. What is THAT? I was too shy and embarrassed to ask him.

Shelli K.

What Is It?

Bacterial vaginosis is a very common vaginal infection that is often, though not always, sexually transmitted. If there is a possibility of sexual transmission, the sex partner should be examined and treated, too, since men can carry and transmit this infection without having any symptoms themselves.

But you can get this infection without having sex. You may be at risk when you're under a lot of stress or have been taking antibiotics or because of poor personal hygiene. This infection is annoying, but not serious.

Symptoms

The primary symptom is a heavy, creamy, grayish-white discharge that has a foul, fishy odor. This symptom is most likely to occur in the female partner if the infection has, in fact, been sexually transmitted.

Treatment

This infection can be cured with antibiotics, usually the medication Flagyl (metronidazole) in

pill form and sometimes in one dose at your doctor's office.

CHLAMYDIA

For the past week, I've noticed a clear or kind of milky discharge at the tip of my penis, especially in the morning when I wake up. Also, it sort of burns when I urinate. Could this be gonorrhea? My girlfriend hasn't mentioned having any symptoms and I'm afraid to say anything about it to her. What could be the problem?

Gary D.

What Is It?

Chlamydia is the number-one sexually transmitted disease in the United States. It is much more common than any other STD, affecting about four million new cases each year. It is estimated that one in ten teen girls is infected. Chlamydia is found most often in sexually active adolescents between ages 15 and 19. This disease is caused by the bacterium *Chlamydia trachomatis* and is usually spread during sexual intercourse with an infected person.

Symptoms

There are quite often no symptoms at all, either in men or women. One recent medical study revealed that some 75 percent of those with chlamydia had no symptoms at all. In the Teenage Clinic at Kaiser Permanente Medical Center in San Francisco, we have routinely tested all girls coming in for routine pelvic exams for chlamydia and found that 15 percent of them were infected—often without being aware of any symptoms. More recently, we have been using a special urine test called *LCR* (ligase chain reaction)—a special DNA test that can actually detect DNA strands of the chlamydia organism in the urine. Now being used in research trials, this offers the woman a test for chlamydia without having a pelvic exam. For males, it is a test for chlamydia and even gonorrhea without having a swab inserted in the penis. As technology in this area improves, more and easier methods of diagnosing chlamydia and gonorrhea enable teens to be diagnosed and treated earlier for these diseases.

Males are more likely to have symptoms than females. These may include:

- Mild irritation or burning during urination
- A thin milky or clear discharge which is most often evident in the morning.

Some men mistake these symptoms for gonorrhea, but there are some important differences. The incubation period for chlamydia is longer (two or three weeks after exposure) and the discharge is lighter in color. (It is possible to have both gonorrhea and chlamydia at the same time, so if you notice any discharge from the penis, or irritation or discomfort during urination, check with your physician immediately—and let your female partner know about your symptoms so that she can be tested, too.) Chlamydia can also be transmitted between two males. However, since the disease can have more serious consequences in females, we have focused our discussion on heterosexual couples.

Unfortunately, most women do not have symptoms—sometimes not until damage has already been done to their reproductive organs via a pelvic infection (pelvic inflammatory disease, or PID), which can occur in undetected, untreated chlamydia. You might ask your doctor to do a test for possible chlamydia if you have vague lower-abdominal pain or find yourself in a special risk category for this disease by answering yes to two or more of the following four questions:

- Are you under 24 years of age?
- Have you had intercourse with a new lover within the past two months?
- Do you use a nonbarrier contraceptive? (Barrier contraceptives include the condom and

the diaphragm.) Or do you use no contraceptive at all?
- Have you noticed mild bleeding after a gynecological exam or sexual intercourse?

If you are at increased risk, a test for chlamydia as soon as possible is an excellent safeguard for your health and future fertility. After the initial test, plan to get routine follow-up tests for chlamydia twice a year.

Special Risks

Untreated, chlamydia may spread, causing pelvic or cervical infections in women and inflammation of the major sperm-carrying passage from the testes in men. In both instances, this infection can cause infertility.

In addition, pelvic inflammatory disease (PID) in women—typical symptoms are lower-abdominal tenderness or severe pain, fever, fatigue, a vaginal discharge, and enlargement of the Fallopian tubes—can cause infertility or later tubal pregnancies due to Fallopian tube scarring. It can, in some instances, even be fatal.

Chlamydia has also been linked to conjunctivitis (an eye inflammation) and pneumonia in newborn babies whose mothers have the infection. About one-third of pneumonia cases in infants under six months of age are linked with their mothers' chlamydia. And a University of Washington study associated birth-acquired chlamydial infection with severe eye disease in some older children.

Treatment

Antibiotics in pill form—doxycycline or erythromycin—are usually prescribed. These antibiotics are usually taken for seven to ten days. However, there is a new, one-dose treatment available now: a new antibiotic, azithromycin, that you get in the doctor's office—and that's it!

GENITAL HERPES

How do you know if you have herpes? I really need to know! Does any blister on the penis mean herpes, or does it have to be painful? Is there anything that gets rid of these blisters or do you have them forever? Please hurry and let me know!

Scared

What Is It?

Herpes progenitalis, or genital herpes, afflicts about one in five Americans age 12 or older. The rate of infection in teens nearly quintupled between 1980 and 1994, with about 4.5 percent of all teens now infected.

Herpes is caused by the herpes simplex type 2 virus, which is related to the virus that causes sores in or near the mouth. Researchers are finding that differences between these two types of herpes virus have narrowed in recent years. Some believe that this—and the growing incidence of genital herpes—may be due to an increase in oral sex, which can transmit herpes viruses of both types from mouth to genitals and back again.

Genital herpes has been called "the sexually transmitted disease without a cure" since its victims tend to suffer recurrent attacks, especially in times of stress. The virus, it seems, never leaves the body, but lodges in nerve tissue until conditions are right, when one's resistance is down, for the next attack.

Symptoms

Symptoms, which first appear 2 to 20 days after exposure (sexual contact with an infected person), include the following:

- Tiny clusters of painful, fluid-filled blisters on the labia, around the vagina, or in the vagina in women; on a man's penis; and, possibly, around the anus of both sexes.

- Swollen lymph glands, aching muscles, and fever.

While symptoms usually diminish within a few weeks, the herpes virus lies dormant in the patient's body. Sometimes there is never another active episode of herpes.

Some people who are infected with the genital herpes virus never have any symptoms, but are still capable of transmitting it to others. In a study at the University of Washington, 636 female college students were tested for herpes. Nine percent were infected and 71 percent of these were completely unaware that they had herpes.

This brings up an important point. If, for any reason, you suspect that you have been exposed or may be at risk for herpes, don't rely on your own observation. Consult your doctor.

More commonly, however, the symptoms do recur, especially when the person's resistance is low due to illness or because of emotional stress. It doesn't take another sexual contact to trigger a repeat attack. Some people can feel recurrence coming on for hours or even a few days before the blisters appear. This burning, tingling, itching sensation is called the *prodrome* and appears in the area to be affected.

During this prodrome, as well as when sores are present, the person with herpes is most likely to infect a sex partner. But it's possible to infect another even when symptoms are not present. Some medical experts feel that regular, continual use of the medication acyclovir may reduce infectiousness. Also, those who are most likely to be infectious—those who have eruptions every four to six weeks—may want to protect sex partners during supposedly dormant times by using a condom with spermicidal jelly containing nonoxynol-9. While this doesn't give total protection, it may reduce the risks of transmission.

Special Risks

Genital herpes can cause herpes encephalitis, a virulent, often fatal brain infection in infants born vaginally to mothers who have active cases of genital herpes. This complication can be prevented by Caesarian-section delivery if the disease is in an active stage when the mother is due to deliver. Having a herpes infection when the baby is in the womb or having vaginal delivery when the disease is in an inactive stage will *not* infect the baby.

There may be a link, too, between genital herpes and cervical cancer. While this has not been proven conclusively, some studies have shown that women with a history of genital herpes may have an increased cervical cancer risk.

For this reason, a woman with herpes must get a Pap smear (see Chapter 15) at least once—and preferably twice—a year. According to the American Cancer Society, cervical cancer is easily detected (via a Pap smear) and treated during its early stages, so the possibly increased risk of getting the disease should be a cause for caution, not panic.

Treatment

At this time, for genital herpes, just as with HIV infection, there is no cure. However, the antiviral medication *acyclovir*, taken in pill form, can alleviate symptoms and shorten or prevent recurrences. New research shows that daily use of this drug for three years is safe and effective. In a study of 525 people who had at least six herpes recurrences a year before taking acyclovir, 61 percent were free of symptoms during the third year of acyclovir use. Twenty-five percent of the patients studied were totally symptom-free for the entire three years.

There is also an over-the-counter ointment called ImmuVir that can relieve painful symptoms of herpes in an hour or less. This anti-viral drug, in tests at Oregon Health Sciences University, shortened the duration of the average herpes outbreak by about two to three days, and researchers speculate that it may reduce the chances of infecting another person. This drug is available at pharmacies without a prescription.

Note: Avoid the nonprescription self-treatment BHT, available in many health-food stores. This has a number of unpleasant side effects—severe stomach cramps, vomiting, dizziness, and even loss of consciousness when taken on an empty stomach. There is also no reliable evidence that BHT prevents genital herpes outbreaks.

During an outbreak of herpes, aspirin—if you are able to tolerate it—can relieve pain and fever. Cool baths can also provide some relief.

To help decrease recurrences, avoid hot baths and tight clothing. Also, decrease the chocolate, nuts, and seeds in your diet. These contain phenylalanine, which apparently allows viruses to enter body cells more readily. Learning to control stress, following a healthy diet, and getting enough rest and relaxation can also help to alleviate recurrence—and can make you feel better in general.

Since herpes is painful not only physically, but also emotionally, you might want to get information and support from the Herpes Resource Center at (800) 230-6039.

GENITAL WARTS

I have these funny, skin-colored, cauliflower-like things around my vagina and near my butt and my boyfriend has the same on his penis. What are these things anyway?

Adrienne W.

What Is It?

Genital warts (condylomata acuminata), caused by a variation of the human papilloma virus (HPV), are sexually transmitted. They may occur around the vagina or rectum or on the penis. They may also occur internally on the cervix, in the vagina, or in the urethra in the male. This is the third most common sexually transmitted disease—after chlamydia and gonorrhea—

afflicting about one million people every year. Genital warts are three times more common than genital herpes.

These warts are extremely contagious. It is estimated that about *half* of all sexually active adults are infected, but many of them have never had symptoms and don't know they have genital warts. A growing number of teens are infected, too.

Symptoms

The warts—which appear several months or more after exposure—are skin-colored, cauliflower-shaped eruptions and are sometimes accompanied by itching and irritation. Untreated, these warts can multiply rapidly, so it's essential to seek prompt medical help.

Special Risks

Genital wart infection has been linked to cervical cancer in women. About 10 to 15 percent of women with untreated genital warts develop cervical cancer. Some 28 percent of women with genital warts show *cervical dysplasia*, or precancerous cell changes in the cervix. One study found that 50 percent of women with invasive cervical cancer also have genital warts.

Any woman with external genital warts should also have a careful internal examination to see if there are warts or if the wart virus is present on the cervix. She should also have a Pap smear at the time and twice yearly thereafter.

Treatment

Removal of the warts by a physician is currently the best available method of treatment. This can be done in one of several ways. Your doctor may apply a topical medication called podophyllin on the warts, giving several follow-up treatments as necessary until the warts are gone, or your doctor may burn the warts off with an electric needle. This may be uncomfortable, but it is a highly

effective one-time treatment. Your physician might also use liquid nitrogen to freeze and thus remove the warts. This treatment involves minimal discomfort and is also quick and convenient.

Several recent studies have tested self-administered topical treatment with good results. Here, patients applied the prescription medication *podofilox* to their warts, with promising results. In a study at Sinai Hospital in Detroit of 72 female patients with external genital warts, 75 percent of those given this medication to apply at home found that their warts went away completely. In another study at the University of California at San Francisco, warts cleared completely in 44 percent of those who used self-administered doses of podofilox.

Stubborn or severe cases of genital warts may be treated by laser or with the anti-cancer drug interferon.

GONORRHEA

What causes gonorrhea? Can you get it from anything besides sexual intercourse? I mean, things like kissing? Or sitting on a germy public toilet seat? I really need to know!

Janet

What Is It?

Gonorrhea is a sexually transmitted disease caused by gonococcus bacteria. These bacteria can usually survive only in the warm, moist environment of the human body. Gonorrhea can occur in the cervix, penis, throat, or rectum, and even in the eye in some cases.

Symptoms

When they occur, symptoms (which usually appear in the male) are evident two to nine days after exposure and can include the following:

- Painful urination and an uncomfortable, thick, yellowish discharge.
- vaginal or pelvic discomfort.
- A sore throat, rectal pain and itching, and mucus in bowel movements, if the throat and/or rectum have been infected.
- Eye infections in newborn infants of mothers with gonorrhea.

Unfortunately, about 80 percent of affected women have no early symptoms, and later symptoms (such as pelvic or lower abdominal pain) may signal serious complications such as pelvic inflammatory disease.

This is why it's so important to tell your female partner(s) if you are a male with gonorrhea. If you're a sexually active female with multiple partners, a medical exam and gonorrhea and chlamydia cultures and/or tests every three months is a good idea.

At the time of this writing, there are new, more technologically advanced tests that can actually detect gonorrhea in the urine of males and females.

Special Risks

An undetected, untreated case of gonorrhea in a woman can spread from the cervix into the pelvis, infecting the Fallopian tubes which lead from the ovaries to the uterus. The resulting abscesses and scar tissue in the tubes can cause blockage and, as a result of this, sterility.

In both men and women, gonorrhea, if untreated, may spread throughout the body, affecting joints (especially knee joints) and even heart valves.

Gonorrhea transmitted from a woman's vagina to her infant's eyes during birth can cause blindness in the child. Although most states have laws requiring hospital personnel to put a special protective antibiotic solution into the eyes of all newborn infants to prevent such a possibility, there are an increasing number of home deliveries these days where this may not be done.

Treatment

Because of the prevalence of penicillin-resistant strains of gonorrhea, all gonorrhea is now treated by new drugs such as *ceftriaxone* by injection and even newer drugs that can be administered by mouth in just one dose.

MOLLUSCUM CONTAGIOSUM

I'm really scared because I have some bubble-like bumps on my inner thighs and near my vulva. They don't itch or hurt, but they're sure ugly and noticeable. What could this be?

Samantha O.

What Is It?

Molluscum contagiosum is another sexually transmitted disease caused by a virus.

Symptoms

Smooth, bubble-like, usually non-itchy bumps on the genitals and/or inner thighs are the usual symptoms. This sexually transmitted disease seems to be seen more often in teens than adults.

Treatment

Treatment must be prompt because these bumps multiply rapidly and don't go away on their own. With the patient given a local anesthetic, the physician removes each bump with a surgical curette. To avoid infection, this must be done by a physician only and under sterile conditions.

■　■　■

PUBIC LICE

What causes crabs? Do you get them from having sex? Is there any other way you can get them?

Wondering

What Is It?

Pubic lice are six-legged parasites (also called *crabs*) that live and lay eggs in the pubic hair. These are usually transmitted sexually, but can also be spread via infected bedding, clothing, towels, and toilet seats.

Symptoms

- Intense itching.
- Visible eggs and lice in the pubic hair.
- Tiny spots of blood on the underwear from sites where the lice have burrowed under the skin.

Treatment

A prescription creme rinse—Nix or Elimite (permethrin)—or Kwell shampoo (lindane) is the usual treatment. However, a nonprescription drug called A-200 (pyrinate), a medicated shampoo for the pubic area, may also be effective when used according to instructions. It is also important to wash bedding, towels, and clothing in very hot water to remove any trace of the lice or their eggs.

A follow-up treatment in a week may be needed; in the meantime, it's vital to abstain from sex to avoid possibly transmitting or becoming reinfested with the lice.

SCABIES

Some kids I know went on a camping trip in the mountains and several came back with something called scabies. Is this something you can get from sleeping in the wilds or is it some kind of disease you get from sex? My brother says it's a type of VD.

Cody Y.

What Is It?

Scabies is another parasitic disease caused by a mite. It can be transmitted sexually or acquired through close skin-to-skin contact or via infected bedding, clothing, and blankets.

Symptoms

- Intense itching (especially at night).
- Red spots where the mite has burrowed under the skin.
- Raised red or gray burrow lines in the skin.

Genitals, buttocks, breasts, elbows, and hands may all be affected.

Treatment

The prescription creams Elimite (permethrin) or Kwell (lindane) are the most common. Washing clothes and bedding in very hot water and abstaining from sex for at least a week will help make the treatment more effective.

SYPHILIS

Is it true that syphilis will go away, even without treatment? I heard that somewhere. So why do people go for treatments?

Rance G.

What Is It?

Syphilis is a sexually transmitted disease caused by a tiny corkscrew-shaped spirochete. While it is usually spread by sexual contact, the disease can also be transmitted from an infected sex organ to an open cut in the skin of another person.

Despite rumors that it is a disease of the past, syphilis is still very much with us and afflicts approximately 30,000 people each year. Although cases of syphilis in the United States are leveling off, there is still a dramatic disparity in who has syphilis and where it is occurring. Latino and African American youth have a 5 to 60 times greater risk of becoming infected with syphilis than whites, and the incidence is much higher in the southern part of the United States.

Symptoms

Symptoms appear slowly—10 to 90 days after exposure—and in stages. The first-stage symptom is usually a painless sore on the genitals, rectum, lips, or mouth. This disappears in a week or two. It is followed some weeks or months later by second-stage symptoms, which include a rash spreading all over the body, swollen joints, and a flu-like illness. If you have these symptoms, seek immediate medical help.

Special Risks

Untreated syphilis doesn't just go away. After the second stage, it goes into a latent period that may last for years before the third stage appears. In this stage, the impact on the victim's body becomes tragically apparent, with damage to the nervous system, brain, and/or circulatory systems. This can result in heart and vascular problems, insanity, paralysis, and possibly death.

Syphilis can also be transmitted from a mother to a baby in her womb, causing a number of serious congenital defects including bone deformities, blindness, and facial disfigurement. Women who are pregnant while in the first or second stage of syphilis also have a higher than usual rate of stillbirths.

■ ■ ■

Treatment

Syphilis is detected by a blood test called the VDRL or RPR and is treated with penicillin injections, or, in the case of penicillin allergy, with other antibiotics. If detected and treated in the early stages, syphilis is curable. If you are sexually active with a number of different sex partners, it's a good idea to get regular blood tests for syphilis.

TINEA CRURIS (JOCK ITCH)

I'm on the varsity basketball team and practice every day. For the past few weeks, I've noticed a scaling, itchy rash in my crotch. The coach says it's "jock rot" and told me to get some cream from the trainer, but now my girlfriend has the same kind of rash. What's happening?

Josh

What Is It?

Tinea cruris, or "jock itch," may be caused initially by a fungus that can develop on an unwashed athletic supporter that has been stashed in a closed locker. The fungus may then be transmitted from the supporter to the skin of the man's groin. *Then* the infection may be transmitted via skin-to-skin (usually sexual) contact. In this instance, it would be classified as a sexually transmitted disease.

Symptoms

The usual symptom is a scaly, itchy rash in the genital area.

Treatment

An over-the-counter drug—Tinactin—will destroy the fungus when used as directed over a period of time. However, if the rash does not improve within a week, effective prescription drugs are available from your physician.

There are also some things you can do, in addition to using Tinactin or a prescription drug, to help promote healing: Dry your body thoroughly after showering or bathing, and wear cotton underwear and loose-fitting clothing.

TRICHOMONIASIS

What is trich? My girlfriend went to the youth clinic last night because she had some sort of discharge. The doctor told her she had this disease called trich. Also, he prescribed some pills for me. Why should I take these pills? I don't have any problem! What's the big deal?

Ted

What Is It?

Trichomoniasis is an infection of the vagina in women and of the urethra in men. It is caused by *protozoa*, tiny parasites that thrive in moist environments. Although this infection is usually sexually transmitted, it can also be spread via damp washcloths, towels, and bathing suits shared with an infected person.

Symptoms

Symptoms appear 4 to 28 days after exposure. In women, these include the following:

- A frothy, greenish-yellow, foul-smelling discharge.
- Frequent and painful urination.
- Itching.
- Inflammation of the vulva.
- In some, but not all cases, severe lower abdominal pain.

Symptoms are far less noticeable in men—often little more than mild discomfort in the penis—if any symptoms occur at all.

Treatment

The medication Flagyl—in pill form for men and women—is the most common treatment. It is best for both partners to be treated at the same time with a large number of these pills taken all at once. If both are not treated at the same time, sexual intercourse should not be resumed until the other partner has been treated as well.

THE ABCs OF HEPATITIS

Hepatitis, an infection of the liver, occurs in several serious forms, including *hepatitis* A (infectious hepatitis), *hepatitis* B (serum hepatitis), and *hepatitis* C (previously called non-A non-B hepatitis). Now a hepatitis D and hepatitis E virus have also been described. Most hepatitis viruses are not usually considered sexually transmitted diseases, but some forms, especially hepatitis B, can be spread through contact with an infected person and/or by certain sex practices.

Hepatitis A is most often spread by contaminated food and by food handlers who did not wash their hands properly after a bowel movement. However, it can be transmitted sexually, if there is oral-anal contact.

Hepatitis B, like AIDS, is spread by exposure to contaminated body fluids: transfusion of infected blood, shared needles or accidental needle sticks (the latter, a hazard for health care professionals), and sex with an infected person. Hepatitis B can also be transmitted at birth from mother to newborn infant. In some countries, if the mother is not tested for hepatitis B, her child may be infected and not know it until some years later when he or she tests positive during routine school screening tests or a regular exam.

Those at most risk for acquiring hepatitis B via sexual transmission are male homosexuals and male or female heterosexuals who have multiple sex partners. According to one study, a 20 percent incidence of hepatitis B has been found among college students with five or more recent sex partners.

Hepatitis C has, in the past, usually spread through blood transfusions. But today almost all blood is now screened for hepatitis C before being administered. So now the most common way of becoming infected with hepatitis C is through intravenous drug use and tattoos that are placed without using a sterile needle.

Hepatitis is not a minor problem. It is a serious illness that can be fatal. If you notice symptoms—mild tiredness, exhaustion, loss of appetite, and especially jaundice (yellowing of the skin and the whites of the eyes and dark urine)—call your doctor immediately. If you know someone with hepatitis, avoid close physical relations. If you have had such contact with an infected person, call your doctor. It's important to know what type of hepatitis you have been exposed to, since this will determine your course of treatment.

If You Have Been Exposed to Hepatitis A

Your physician will want to give you an injection of gamma globulin. This may help protect you from acquiring hepatitis A. Today there is a vaccine for hepatitis A. This vaccine is recommended for health-care workers and also for anyone traveling to a country where hepatitis A is very common, usually countries with unclean drinking water.

If You Have Been Exposed to Hepatitis B

Your doctor is likely to give you an antibody shot and then a vaccine to protect you. If you are in danger of being exposed to hepatitis B because of medical work or treatments or because of your lifestyle (if you are very sexually active and/or a male homosexual), you might want to look into a vaccination that could protect you from this disease and maybe

save your life. Recently, several school districts throughout the country are requiring that all students entering middle school complete the hepatitis B vaccine series.

The vaccine series for hepatitis B consists of three separate injections given over six months. Usually the second injection is given one month after the first and the third injection is given five months after the first vaccination. More and more physicians are recommending that all adolescents be immunized against hepatitis B; many colleges are now requiring the complete vaccine series prior to admission.

Avoiding Hepatitis C

The best way to avoid being exposed to hepatitis C or of not getting infected with hepatitis C is not to use intravenous drugs and be very careful if you are having a tattoo that the equipment used is sterile!

WHAT IS "SAFE SEX"?

Is safe sex really safe? As safe as not having sex at all? What romantic things can you do besides making love . . . or is everything risky now?

Caitlin B.

Many teens wonder what "safe sex" really is—and what kinds of choice it involves. Taking responsibility to protect yourself and your partner from infection with a sexually transmitted disease is vital—and has several levels of safety. What is usually termed "safe sex" should probably really be called "safer sex." Why? Because "safe sex" as usually practiced is much safer than unprotected sex, but is still not 100 percent safe.

If you want to be 100 percent safe from sexually transmitted diseases, you have three choices:

1. Total abstinence—no sex with anyone.
2. Masturbation (by yourself).

3. Waiting to have sex until you're married—and marrying a virgin or someone who has practiced safe sex, has not been infected with the AIDS virus, and will be faithful to you (and you to him or her) throughout your marriage.

If these three possibilities don't appeal to you, then you need to take responsibility for protecting yourself—and your partner—in situations that carry risks of infection with sexually transmitted diseases.

TEN SAFE-SEX GUIDELINES

1. *Know what sexual behavior carries risks and what doesn't.* Too many people worry needlessly about catching sexually transmitted diseases from toilet seats, doorknobs, or casual nonsexual contact when they really need to think about— and perhaps change—their sexual choices and practices.

   You need to know, for example, that the more sex partners you have, the greater risk you have of getting a sexually transmitted disease. People in mutually monogamous relationships are at considerably less risk. So are people who are careful about what they do and with whom. It may be more risky to have one or two unprotected sexual experiences than more experiences with protection (for example, condoms).

   It's important to know, among sexual activities, which carry more risks than others. The following lists will give you a general idea.

Very Safe Sexual Activities
✔ Kissing with closed lips (dry kissing).
✔ Rubbing against each other while clothed or partially clothed, avoiding direct genital contact and exchange of body fluids.
✔ Masturbation (by yourself).
✔ Talking about your sexual feelings and fantasies with each other.
✔ Nongenital touching and massage.

Reasonably Safe Sex
✔ Sexual intercourse with the man using a condom and the woman using a spermicidal jelly, cream, or foam containing nonoxynol-9 in her vagina.
✔ Wet ("French") kissing. New evidence that the AIDS virus can directly infect mucus-membrane cells, such as those found in the mouth or vagina, has been presented. However, experts still consider French kissing a rather low-risk activity since an infected person's saliva contains far less HIV than blood, semen, or vaginal fluids. Just the same, you might think twice about deep kissing someone who is (or might be) in a high-risk group for HIV infection.
✔ Oral sex with latex barriers between the mouth of one partner and the sex organ of the other. This means that a man should wear a condom and a woman needs to put a dental dam (a thin, square piece of latex) on her vulva and vaginal opening.
✔ Mutual masturbation (stimulating each other) with a spermicidal jelly or cream and/or latex rubber gloves.

Unsafe Sex
✔ Sexual intercourse where partners are not protected by condom and spermicide.
✔ Oral sex where a barrier is not used and there is direct mouth-genital contact.
✔ Masturbation with or in the presence of another person where sex toys like vibrators and dildos are shared.

2. *Be selective.* It is vital to be selective not only in terms of partners—if he refuses to wear a condom, don't have sex; if she has had a lot of sex partners or doesn't want to practice safe sex, don't have sex—but also in what you do. While safe-sex rules may sound pretty grim on first reading, stepping back and letting your relationship grow in many other ways and gradually increasing your physical intimacy can

make it *better* and more romantic. Think about it. You can have a wonderful time talking, kissing, and caressing each other, gradually building up to sexual involvement with great excitement and anticipation instead of rushing into it because that's the way you've done it before or because you feel it is expected. Taking time to get to know each other first will let you know if you even *like* this person enough to have sex with him or her. With the risks of sexual activity today, it doesn't make sense to have sex with someone who isn't pretty special to you. Also, the better you know and like each other, the easier it will be to talk about safe sex and birth control measures—things that *do* need to be discussed before you ever have sex.

3. *Take the initiative with safe-sex practices.* Don't wait for your partner to get around to purchasing a condom or spermicide. Buy some yourself. That way, at least *one of you* will be prepared for *both of you* to have sex.

Condoms are easier to buy than ever and many women are buying them these days. Many stores carry them on open racks. So you can just buy them and have them handy. It may help to know, if you've never bought condoms before, that they come in one size. If you end up having to ask a pharmacist for some and he or she gives you the old "What size?" line, he or she means the size of the package—for example, a package of 3, 12, or 36.

If a partner is shocked by the fact that you are prepared with safe-sex aids, remind him or her that, these days, it's a smart and loving gesture to be careful and to be prepared in advance for sex. You may explain that you're not implying that he or she strikes you as having a sleazy past or a myriad of unspeakable diseases, but that people—including yourself—can have infections without knowing it, and you want to protect your partner as well as yourself. If your partner says that the safe-sex aids will make sex distinctly non-sexy, you might say that feeling safe will allow you to relax and enjoy each other more—and that people *can* have satisfying safe sex.

4. *Be open-minded about safe-sex aids.* If you feel your libido plummet at the mere mention of a condom (let alone a dental dam or rubber gloves!), don't reject these possibilities until you've tried them. Even though it may seem unbelievable to you right now, some people have actually grown to *like* the soft silky feel of this latex gloved hands or fingers on their genitals. A condom or a dental dam does not have to diminish the pleasures of oral sex. In fact, some young people—particularly males—have told us that they hadn't had the nerve to try oral sex until they used the safe-sex barriers. So these aids may actually expand, rather than limit, your sexual horizons! Also, condoms these days are thinner (and stronger) than they used to be, so sensation isn't dulled nearly as much. So the old line about how wearing a condom is like wearing a raincoat in the shower isn't really true anymore. Sex can be very pleasurable with a condom and spermicide—even more so than unprotected sex because you're at less risk of getting a sexually transmitted disease.

5. *Be aware of the fact that condoms and spermicides can't prevent* all *types of sexually transmitted diseases.* The condom and other barriers cannot prevent pubic lice, scabies, and, in some instances, genital warts or herpes. To avoid these diseases, you need to avoid sex with someone who shows signs of having these. Take a good look at your partner before you have sex. Taking a shower or bath together first can help make this a bit less obvious and more fun. But if that isn't possible, prolong foreplay and look carefully for any signs of lice, herpes blisters, or warts. That may not sound awfully romantic, but getting these diseases isn't at *all* romantic and, in some instances, can be health-threatening.

6. *Practice good hygiene.* This is a way to avoid

getting trichomoniasis and to make yourself less likely to get or have a recurrence of genital warts or herpes. Don't share towels or washcloths with others. Don't swap clothes—especially damp swimsuits—with another person. Don't wear tight, unventilated clothing for long periods, trapping heat and moisture in the genital area. Take regular baths and showers. Wash genital and anal areas before sex. Also, urinating and again washing the genitals after sex may be of some help in preventing some types of sexually transmitted diseases.

7. *If you have suspicious symptoms, seek help* and *tell your partner.* Don't be afraid. County and city health departments, adolescent clinics, free clinics, and youth clinics throughout the nation offer low- or no-cost medical diagnosis and treatment for sexually transmitted diseases. This care is completely confidential and may be given without parental knowledge or consent, in most states, to anyone over age 12. The people who staff these clinics see all kinds of sexually transmitted diseases all the time, know how to treat them, and tend to be quite non-judgmental.

   Notifying your sex partner or partners—particularly if they're female and are less likely to have symptoms for diseases such as gonorrhea or chlamydia—is very important. They may not only continue to spread the disease, but may also develop serious complications if they are not treated. Giving them the bad news is not easy, but it is the decent, considerate, responsible thing to do.

   If you choose, a health worker will call your partner or partners for you. A staff member will take a list of your contacts and their phone numbers from you, then call these people (without mentioning your name), asking them to come in for examination and treatment.

8. *If you have a sexually transmitted disease, don't have sex while you're infectious.* This is a very important way to stop the spread of sexually transmitted diseases. Ask your doctor very specifically how long you should abstain from sexual activities. And then follow his or her guidelines carefully. If you have a chronic condition—such as genital herpes—be especially careful to avoid sex altogether when you're in an active stage and take safe-sex precautions during the times in between.

9. *Get regular checkups.* This is especially important if you're sexually active with several partners. If you have just one partner, a physical and/or gynecological exam once a year will probably be enough. If you have multiple sex partners, plan to have an exam three to four times a year, even if you don't have symptoms of any sexually transmitted diseases. New guidelines suggest that *all* teenage girls who are having sex get tested twice a year for chlamydia. This is an excellent safeguard for your health and fertility and is well worth your time. Regular exams may detect any hidden infections before serious complications arise. You have to request tests for chlamydia, gonorrhea, or syphilis, and even HIV, since they may not be part of every routine gynecological exam.

10. *Learn as much as you can about sexually transmitted diseases.* These days, ignorance can kill—and there is a lot of ignorance around. For example, a survey of some 860 Massachusetts teens between ages 16 and 19 revealed that while 96 percent of them had heard about AIDS, only 15 percent had changed their sexual behavior to lower their risks. And, in San Francisco, a survey of some 1,326 teens found that their feeling of invulnerability to AIDS was growing: 54 percent of those polled said that they weren't worried about getting AIDS, compared to 34 percent in 1985. This lack of worry, unfortunately, is less likely to reflect the security of abstinence and safe-sex practices than it is to point up the fact that too many teens assume that bad things simply happen to other people, never to them.

REMEMBER: IF YOU'RE HAVING SEX, YOU'RE AT RISK FOR SEXUALLY TRANS-MITTED DISEASES.

That's a fact. So the more you know about these diseases—how to recognize them and how to prevent them—the better off you'll be. Read this and other books about sexuality. If you have specific questions about safe sex or sexually transmitted diseases, call the AIDS or other sexuality-related hotlines listed in the appendix of this book. Talk with your doctor. Share your feelings and intentions with your partner. Some of this information may seem distasteful and embarrassing, but it can be health-saving—even lifesaving.

If the current epidemic of sexually transmitted disease is to be halted, prevention must play a major role. At this time, there is no cure and no preventive vaccine for AIDS. There is, as yet, no definitive cure for genital herpes. And more discoveries are being made all the time about the distressing long-range consequences of other sexually transmitted diseases such as chlamydia and genital warts. Medical research is ongoing, but in the meantime, prevention of sexually transmitted diseases in ourselves and our partners is the most valuable defensive weapon we have. Being aware and taking responsibility for safeguarding your own health and that of your partner is a major step toward maturity and growing up to be a healthy, loving, caring person.

THE TRUTH ABOUT SEXUALLY TRANSMITTED DISEASES

✔ If you're having sex, you are at risk for sexually transmitted diseases. It doesn't matter how much you and your partner love each other or, in many instances, how clean you are. Teens are at high risk for sexually transmitted diseases.

✔ The only true "safe sex" is abstinence or sex with a long-term, mutually monogamous partner (and even the latter, if he or she is not a virgin, may be carrying an undiagnosed sexually transmitted disease from a long-ago previous relationship. That's possible with sexually transmitted diseases such as herpes, genital warts, or HIV).

✔ To make sex safer, know safe-sex measures and follow them—avoiding unprotected sex of every kind, every time.

✔ If you notice any suspicious symptoms—unusual discharges, bumps, blisters, warts or other growths, pain in the abdomen, intense genital itching, tiny spots of blood on your underwear—see your doctor or seek help at a public clinic right away. The sooner you get an STD taken care of, the better for your health and future fertility. None of them truly go away on their own. Even if you're really embarrassed, see a doctor *now* rather than later.

✔ You can legally receive confidential medical care for the diagnosis and treatment of a sexually transmitted disease in most states if you are 12 or older.

✔ If you're diagnosed with a sexually transmitted disease, tell your partner(s) so that they can be treated, too. It isn't an easy thing to do, but it's the right and loving thing to do.

CHAPTER THIRTEEN

Birth Control: An Ounce of Prevention

I've heard that it's better to use birth control if you're sexually active, but how active do you have to be to need it? What if you're too nervous to go to a doctor or even talk to your boyfriend about it? Can you get it without your parents finding out? Is it true that you can't get pregnant the first time you have sex? (I really need to know!)

Amber S.

Amber's questions have been echoed by many teens who are confused, scared, and often just plain uninformed about birth control. Too few teens realize the importance of using a reliable method of birth control every time they have sex—*including the first time!* Pregnancy can happen to *anyone* who has sex without using a reliable method of birth control. That's why it's important for you to know as much as possible about contraception, whether or not you're presently sexually active.

A number of studies show that teens are taking big risks by not using reliable methods of birth control consistently or at all. An unplanned pregnancy can mean not only making difficult choices now—an early marriage, being a single parent, having an abortion, giving a baby up for adoption—but living with the consequences of these

choices. The fact is, as hard as it can be to seek and use birth control, doing so is much easier and less embarrassing and distressing than dealing with an unplanned pregnancy.

FIVE LAME EXCUSES FOR NOT USING BIRTH CONTROL

1. *"It isn't romantic."* How romantic is an unplanned pregnancy? How romantic is worrying about pregnancy? Using birth control frees you to enjoy sex more!
2. *"It would be like planning to have sex."* You plan other good things in your life. Why not sex?
3. *"My boyfriend doesn't believe in birth control."* That's fine for him, but *you* need to protect *yourself* against an unplanned pregnancy.
4. *"I'm too embarrassed to talk about it or deal with it."* If you're too embarrassed to admit that you're having sex and that you need to use birth control, maybe you're not ready to have sex.
5. *"Wearing a condom is like taking a shower with a raincoat on. Sex isn't as pleasurable."* Oh, please! Condoms are a vital aid to safer sex as well as birth control and some do not interfere much, if at all, with sexual sensation. And, of

course, there are many other forms of birth control available.

Many teens ask us questions like "Can you get pregnant if . . ." and add any number of situations to the question. Quite often, if intercourse or ejaculation near the vaginal opening is involved, the answer is yes. The following is a quick guide to circumstances under which it's possible to get pregnant.

YOU *CAN* GET PREGNANT IF . . .

- You have sexual intercourse without reliable birth control.
- You have unprotected sex at *any* time of the month (even though pregnancy is most likely during ovulation—about two weeks after your last menstrual period—the exact time of ovulation is hard to pinpoint, especially in teens whose cycles aren't well-established.)
- You have unprotected sex for the first time or the thousandth time.
- He ejaculates close to your vaginal opening and some semen gets into your vagina.
- You don't have an orgasm or even enjoy sex. (He would usually need to have an orgasm— or "come," as many people call it. But you could get pregnant even if he doesn't come *if* he becomes sexually aroused and secretes some lubricating fluid that may have some stray sperm in it.)
- He "pulls out." The problem is, sperm may be in his lubricating fluid before he comes (see the preceding item), or he may not be able to pull out in time to avoid spilling some semen in your vagina.
- You use a makeshift form of improvised birth control, such as plastic wrap, douching, or standing up immediately after sex. Forget these makeshift methods. Use the real stuff. It works.

OUR ALL-TIME FAVORITE
NON-METHOD OF BIRTH CONTROL

(With best wishes to Denise and David)

We've been hearing a lot about this new form for natural birth control and it sounds great! In fact, it's the only method my boyfriend and I would even consider using. All we want to know is how effective it is. The method is that a female drinks ice water right after sexual intercourse to freeze all her organs so she won't get pregnant. Would this work well?

Denise and David

Dear Denise and David and Everyone:

Don't try this at home. Don't try it anywhere! It doesn't work in terms of freezing your organs OR preventing pregnancy. Use a *real* form of birth control!

TEENS *CAN* GET BIRTH CONTROL PRODUCTS

Birth control devices *are* available to teens. These include the following:

Nonprescription Methods

Condoms (male and female) and spermicidal jelly, cream, or foam are generally available over the counter in drugstores, supermarkets, and, in the case of condoms for males, in vending machines in some public restrooms. They are also available at family-planning clinics and at a number of high schools with condom distribution policies.

Prescription Methods

Oral contraceptives (the Pill), Depo-Provera injections, and the diaphragm are available from your physician or from family-planning clinics (such as Planned Parenthood) or your local youth clinic or school-based clinic.

Legal Aspects of Your Access to Birth Control

Contraceptive services are available to minors at clinics in all states. The legal question involved in such services usually does not deal with contraception directly, but with the issue of medical care of a minor without parental consent. Some teens, of course, do have parental consent for contraceptive services. Others don't. Yet these services are, quite often, available to teens without parental consent.

A number of states have *emancipated minor* statutes declaring that legally emancipated minors (for example, those living away from home and/or supporting themselves and making their own decisions or minors who are married) may give their own consent for medical treatment. A variation of this is the "mature minor" rule, recognized by a

---

A NOTE OF CAUTION REGARDING BIRTH CONTROL AND SAFE SEX

I'm confused. My doctor said that if I take the Pill, I won't get pregnant. But a friend of mine said I still would have to use a condom or get my boyfriend to use a condom because of the danger of AIDS. My question is: What's the point of taking the Pill if you have to use a condom anyway?

Cheryl H.

Many teens, like Cheryl, are confused about contraceptive options and the necessary use of condoms to help protect against sexually transmitted diseases. While the condom can offer contraceptive protection and decrease one's risk of getting certain sexually transmitted diseases, including the HIV virus that causes AIDS, some want additional protection against pregnancy. Since the Pill is, statistically speaking, a more effective method of birth control than the condom, those for whom preventing pregnancy is an ultrahigh priority will often choose to take the Pill

continued

BIRTH CONTROL AND SAFE SEX (continued)

as well as using condoms to get the best overall protection against both pregnancy and sexually transmitted diseases.

There are some young people, of course, whose life circumstances may require contraception, but not necessarily the protection against sexually transmitted diseases that their peers require. These would be young people who are married and monogamous and who have not ever had sex with anyone but each other. Unless that describes you, it's vital to use condoms—either as combination protection against pregnancy and STDs, or in conjunction with other contraceptives.

number of states, which states that "a minor can effectively consent to medical treatment for himself if he understands the nature of the treatment and it is for his benefit."

Even in states without such rulings, teens can get help. Although clinic personnel may ask a patient's age and whether that patient is emancipated, they will generally not ask for proof. "Our first concern," says one clinic official, "is for the adolescent who needs help." Many echo this sentiment. In fact, the American Medical Association, the American College of Obstetrics and Gynecology, and the American Academy of Pediatrics have all given public support to the issue of contraception for sexually active teenagers.

So birth control information and help are likely to be available to you—if you take the responsibility for seeking it.

WHICH METHODS WORK?

You have a lot of choices in birth control methods. We recommend that those who are not in a long-term (five years or more) monogamous relationship use a condom and spermicidal jelly or cream as a safeguard against AIDS and other sexually transmitted diseases. Some may want further birth control protection and choose an additional method as well. And, of course, for those in long-term, committed relationships, there are a number of choices.

The right method for you will be one that you will use consistently and that fits your lifestyle. You might want to check out the following chart.

Before making up your mind which method you'll choose, it's a good idea to read about *all* the methods and then to discuss these with your partner and, if applicable, your physician. We can only give you information. The best method for *you* is a very personal decision.

MAKING CHOICES ABOUT BIRTH CONTROL (18)

If You Want . . .	Consider These Methods
Highly effective, continuous protection	• Oral contraceptives (the Pill) • Depo-Provera (3-month shot) • Norplant system
A highly effective method with few, if any, side effects	• Condom with spermicide • Diaphragm with spermicide
Emergency contraception (after unprotected sex or a contraceptive mishap—if, for example, a condom breaks) **Please Note: This option is for true emergencies only and should not be considered a regular method of birth control.**	• Several birth control pills (only certain types are used for this, so see your doctor) taken within 3 days after unprotected sex. This is the preferred "morning after" option.

The Pill (Oral Contraceptives)

Birth Control Pill Packet

What Is It?

There are many different types of birth control pills ("the Pill"), but most are combinations of synthetic preparations of the hormones estrogen and progesterone. There is also a pill containing only progesterone, but the effectiveness of this "mini-pill" has been shown to be somewhat lower than that of the combination pills. *Triphasic* birth control pills most closely approximate the normal hormonal fluctuations of the menstrual cycle.

How Does It Work?

Oral contraceptives prevent pregnancy in several ways:

- The hormones in these pills prevent the ovaries from releasing an egg each month. If there is no egg, there can be no pregnancy.
- The hormones also affect the lining of the uterus so that if, by some chance, ovulation and fertilization should occur, the egg would have difficulty attaching itself to the uterine lining.
- Progesterone may cause cervical mucus to become thick and difficult for sperm to move through.

How Do You Use It?

Birth control pills are available in 21- and 28-day packets. If you have a 21-day packet, you will take a pill every day for three weeks with seven days each, generally starting the new packet of pills on the fifth day after your menstrual period begins. If you have a 28-day pill packet, you will take a pill every day. Seven of these pills, however, are nonfunctional sugar pills. They are included so that you can take a pill every day instead of trying to calculate when you should be starting and stopping your pills.

The newer triphasic pills are taken on a 28-day schedule—with the hormonal content and combinations changing every seven days. Each different type of pill in the packet is a different color—red for the first week, blue for the second week, green for the third week, and yellow for the last week. The yellow pills do not contain hormones at all, but are nonfunctional sugar pills, much like the last seven pills in any other 28-day packet.

Pills should be taken at the same time every day. These should also be taken only as directed by a physician. In other words, do not borrow a friend's pills. You must have your own prescription, tailored to your needs.

Some teen girls run into difficulty in their use of the Pill when trying to decide what to do after a relationship ends. After a breakup, they may stop taking the Pill and then, when they meet someone else or get back together with the boyfriend, either find themselves unprotected for pregnancy or going through a physical readjustment to the Pill. It is best, if your relationship is unstable or has just ended, to keep taking oral contraceptives for several months to ensure continuous contraceptive protection.

How Effective Is It?

Oral contraceptives are very effective, with a failure rate of less than 1 percent. Failures are most likely to happen if you forget to take a pill for one or two (or more) days during your cycle. If that happens, take the forgotten pill as soon as you remember (along with your regular one for that day) and, for the rest of the cycle, use a backup method of birth control—while continuing to take your pills.

Illness can also cause the pill to be less effective. If you're vomiting or having diarrhea, this may affect your absorption of the Pill. Some antibiotics can also decrease the Pill's effectiveness. Check with your physician about this when he or she prescribes antibiotics and, when in doubt, use backup methods as well as the Pill for the rest of your cycle.

Who Can Use This Method?

The ideal candidate for the Pill is a healthy young woman under 30 who does not smoke. (Many of the side effects of the Pill tend to occur in smokers or women over 35.) Generally, a woman who is menstruating regularly and has well-established cycles and no condition that would preclude use of the Pill may use birth control pills.

Who Should Not Use This Method?

- Heavy smokers.
- Those with a history of high blood pressure, abnormal vaginal bleeding, blood clots, liver disease (such as hepatitis), or cancer in the reproductive system.
- Those with migraine headaches or diabetes, who are advised to consider other forms of birth control—or, if the Pill is the method of choice, to take it under the close supervision of the physician treating the pre-existing condition.
- Those who must take certain medications known to interfere with the Pill's effectiveness. If you take anticonvulsants (including phenobarbital), tetracycline, or similar antibiotics; the antibiotic rifampicin; or the antifungal drug griseofulvin, discuss this with your physician. You may need to use another method of birth control.

- If you tend to be forgetful, the Pill may not be for you. To be effective, birth control pills must be taken consistently, on a precise schedule.

What Are the Advantages?

- The Pill is highly effective.
- It is convenient to take and doesn't interfere with sex.
- It may offer some relief from heavy and/or painful menstrual periods.
- Oral contraceptives can significantly reduce your chances of getting ovarian and uterine cancer.
- The Pill can also reduce your risk of developing fibroid tumors of the uterus, which can cause menstrual problems and, in some cases, infertility.

What Are the Disadvantages?

- Side effects such as spotting between periods, headaches, breast tenderness, and nausea may occur. (These may be due to taking a pill with a hormone balance that is not right for you and may be remedied by switching to another brand of pill with a different hormone concentration—for example, if you have nausea, headaches, or breast tenderness, you may be taking a pill that has too much estrogen for you.)
- Birth control pills can contribute to high blood pressure, migraine headaches, and changes in blood sugar.
- Very rare but serious side effects include blood clots, strokes, and liver tumors. If you develop a sudden, severe headache unlike any you've ever had before or have pain in your chest or the calves of your legs while taking the Pill, see your doctor immediately.

Risks can be minimized by not smoking and by getting regular medical examinations to make sure that all is well.

Please Note: When sizing up the risk of the Pill, do consider the fact that the Pill is quite safe when compared to the risks involved in pregnancy and childbirth, especially if you're young.

How Do You Get It?

Birth control pills are available by prescription only from a physician who has taken a complete medical history and performed a physical examination that will include checking your blood pressure, examining your breasts, and doing a gynecological exam, Pap smear, and perhaps a urine test. Annual health checkups are advised.

Depo-Provera

What Is It?

Depo-Provera is the first injectable contraceptive available in the United States. Available only from a physician, it is given as a shot in the arm or buttocks and protects against pregnancy for thirteen weeks. About four of these shots per year will give you continuous contraceptive protection.

How Does It Work?

Depo-Provera works much like the Pill in preventing an egg from being released from the ovary.

How Do You Use It?

Once you get the injection, you don't have to do anything for three months. Every three months, you need to get another shot for continuous protection.

How Effective Is It?

Injectable contraceptives are, like oral contraceptives, about 99 percent effective.

Who Can Use This Method?

Most women can use this method if they so desire. The exceptions are listed here.

Who Should Not Use This Method?

- Those with vaginal bleeding without a known cause.
- Those who have had breast cancer (teens with a family history of breast cancer might want to be cautious as well).
- Those with a history of liver disease, stroke, or blood clots in the legs, or who are allergic to the Depo-Provera injection.
- Those with high blood pressure.

What Are the Advantages?

- Depo-Provera is highly effective in protecting against pregnancy.
- It's a very private method of birth control, with no pills or devices that anyone can discover.
- It's quite convenient, requiring a shot every three months.

What Are the Disadvantages?

- It requires a shot every three months (a problem if you're needle-phobic!).
- It can have side effects such as menstrual changes (heavy periods, no periods, or irregular bleeding or spotting), weight gain, and headaches. (Some side effects diminish with time. Others can be managed with the help of your physician.)

How Do You Get It?

Depo-Provera is available only from a physician and is given as an injection by the doctor or nurse every three months.

■ ■ ■

The Norplant System

What Is It?

The Norplant is a long-term, reversible contraceptive. Six flexible capsules containing the hormone *progestin* are inserted under the skin on the inside of the upper arm. Left in place for five years, they provide consistent contraceptive protection.

How Does It Work?

The hormone action of the Norplant prevents pregnancy by inhibiting ovulation and thickening the cervical mucus to block sperm cells.

How Do You Use It?

Once the implants are inserted, you don't have to do anything. Contraceptive protection is continuous and automatic for the next five years.

How Effective Is It?

The Norplant appears to be highly effective, with typical first-year failure rates of only 1 in 500 women.

Who Can Use This Method?

While, theoretically, any healthy teen could use this method, the best candidates might be teens who have been sexually active with a history of contraceptive failures or problems. This method might work well, too, for a young married couple who want highly effective contraceptive protection while they finish school or get established in their careers.

Who Should Not Use This Method?

- Those with a great need for privacy and secrecy. After the implants are inserted, you will have to wear a noticeable bandage around your upper arm for several days and the implants will be somewhat noticeable, at close inspection, as long as you have them.
- Those who are significantly overweight or have weight fluctuations. Women who weigh 155 pounds or more would need to have the implants replaced after three years (instead of five), and major weight fluctuations can decrease the effectiveness of the contraceptive protection.

What Are the Advantages?

The Norplant, once inserted, needs no action on your part to give you continuous and highly effective contraceptive protection.

What Are the Disadvantages?

- This method isn't as private and discreet as some others. (But usually the implants are not that visible.)
- Some people might be put off by the possible discomfort of the insertion, which is done under local anesthetic by a physician or other specially trained medical professional. (We're not talking major surgery, but a ten- to fifteen-minute office procedure. And the incision is only about one-quarter inch, so there are no big, noticeable scars, either.)

How Do You Get It?

The Norplant must be inserted by a physician or other medical professional who has had special training in the procedure. It is a minor office procedure, usually performed within seven days of the beginning of your menstrual period. After the site is numbed by local anesthetic, the physician makes an incision and inserts six Norplant capsules in a fan-shaped pattern. The incision is so small that it doesn't require stitches. Instead, it is secured with a butterfly bandage covered by a piece of gauze bandage material. The gauze can be removed after a day or so and the butterfly bandage can come off in three days.

The Diaphragm

What Is It?

The diaphragm is a shallow, dome-shaped cup made of soft rubber. It is placed securely over the cervix and is used with spermicidal jelly or cream.

How Does It Work?

The diaphragm is a barrier between the sperm and the uterus. The contraceptive jelly or cream used with it offers added protection by immobilizing and killing the sperm cells.

How Do You Use It?

Contraceptive cream or jelly is applied to the rim and both sides of the diaphragm. Then the rim (which is reinforced by a metal spring) is squeezed and the device is placed high in the vagina, covering the cervix. You can tell whether the diaphragm is properly placed by feeling for the cervix through the dome of the device. It may be inserted some time before intercourse. However, if it has been several hours since insertion, it is a good idea to add some more spermicidal jelly or cream with an applicator before having sex.

If intercourse is repeated within the next few hours, another application of jelly or cream should be inserted. But DO NOT remove the diaphragm! The diaphragm must remain in place for at least

1. To insert a diaphragm, spread contraceptive jelly on both sides and around the rim.

2. Squeeze the rim together.

3. Insert into vagina until it covers cervix.

4. Check proper placement.

5. To remove, hook finger on rim and pull gently.

How to Use a Diaphragm

eight hours after intercourse. After this, it may be removed, washed, dried, and stored in its container.

How Effective Is It?

If fitted correctly and used every time, the diaphragm is a highly effective method of birth control. Recent figures show about a 97 percent effectiveness rate. To minimize the risk of failure, follow directions for use exactly and check the diaphragm before insertion (by filling it with water or holding it up to a bright light) to make sure there are no holes or tears in it.

Who Can Use This Method?

It works best for people who are emotionally mature, responsible, and highly motivated to practice birth control. It is an especially good method for someone who does not have sex regularly, since it is used only when one has sex.

Who Should Not Use This Method?

Anyone who finds it disgusting, distasteful or just too much trouble and who would be tempted to leave it in the drawer instead of using it every time.

What Are the Advantages?

- The diaphragm is completely safe and has no adverse side effects. (The tendency of women using diaphragms to be at higher risk for urinary tract infections has been significantly decreased with the introduction of the wide-seal diaphragm.)
- It is used only when you need it.
- It may provide some protection against several types of sexually transmitted diseases and against cervical dysplasia (abnormal cellular changes of the cervix).
- It can also catch the menstrual flow, making intercourse during menstruation a more acceptable option for some.

What Are the Disadvantages?

- It requires some preparation and planning before sex, and some see it as messy and inconvenient.
- It must be replaced if you lose or gain more than ten pounds. (The wide-seal diaphragm comes in half-sizes and makes an accurate fit more possible.)
- It needs to be replaced about once a year.
- It may become dislodged during intercourse. However, this is less likely with the wide-seal diaphragm.

How Do You Get It?

You must be fitted for a diaphragm by a physician in his or her office or clinic.

The Cervical Cap

What Is It?

The cervical cap is a thimble-shaped, soft rubber device somewhat like the diaphragm, but smaller. It fits snugly over the cervix.

How Does It Work?

The cervical cap works much like the diaphragm, blocking the sperm cells' entrance to the cervix, with extra protection from the spermicidal jelly or cream used with it.

How Effective Is It?

It is somewhat more effective than the diaphragm.

Who Can Use This Method?

The same motivated and mature teens who could use a diaphragm—those who are comfortable with the requirements and routines of barrier contraceptives.

Who Should Not Use This Method?

People who would be tempted *not* to use it "just this once" and who don't feel comfortable with inserting and caring for the device correctly.

What Are the Advantages?

The cervical cap can be more convenient to use than the diaphragm since it requires less spermicide and can be left in place for several days before or after intercourse.

What Are the Disadvantages?

At this time, the cervical cap comes in a limited number of sizes, so not everyone can be fitted. Some have complained that it can be dislodged during intercourse and that, if left in place for more than a few days, can cause an odorous discharge.

How Do You Get It?

You must be fitted for a cervical cap by a physician at his or her office or clinic.

The Condom (Male)

What Is It?

The condom is a thin sheath of rubber or animal tissue that is slipped over the erect penis before intercourse. For best results, it is used in combination with spermicidal cream, jelly, or foam.

How Do You Use It?

Roll the condom carefully over the *erect* penis, taking care to leave space at the end for seminal fluid if the condom doesn't come with a receptacle tip. It's also important to hold on to the condom as you're withdrawing from your partner after sex to guard against spilling the collected semen. Do not

re-use a condom. Use a fresh one each time you have sex.

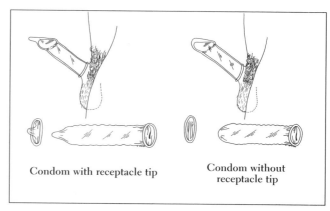

Condom with receptacle tip   Condom without receptacle tip

Male Condoms

How Does It Work?

The condom prevents pregnancy by keeping sperm from entering the vagina. Instead, the semen is deposited in the reservoir tip of the condom or in a space left by the man at the end of the condom. It works best when used in conjunction with spermicides.

Many condoms these days come prelubricated with spermicides. If you're using one that is not and you don't need the extra contraceptive protection because your partner is using the Pill or another effective method of birth control, yet you need extra lubrication, *use only those lubricants that are manufactured for sexual use!* These include products such as K-Y jelly. DO NOT use an oil-based lubricant such as Vaseline with a condom, as it can damage the latex material with amazing speed. One study found, for example, that Vaseline Intensive Care Lotion can destroy a condom in five minutes. Baby oil or mineral oil can destroy one in a minute or less!

How Effective Is It?

Condom-user failure rates range from 10 to 20 percent. This percentage can be cut drastically if the man follows the manufacturer's instructions carefully and uses a spermicide in addition to the condom.

For best protection against sexually transmitted diseases—another *very* important use for condoms—it is essential to use those made of *latex*. DO NOT use "natural" or animal tissue condoms, which do not provide adequate protection against STDs. Use only fresh latex condoms. *Fresh* means that you haven't been carrying it in your wallet for weeks or months.

Who Can Use This Method?

Ideally, just about everyone (except those who have been virgins until now or who have been in a monogamous relationship for five years or more) should use this method to help prevent sexually transmitted diseases—notably AIDS—in addition to pregnancy.

Who Should Not Use This Method?

There isn't anyone who should not use this method. This said, if you are in a long-term, committed relationship, if birth control is very important to you and if you dislike the condom enough to be tempted not to use it "just this once," then you might consider another method. If, however, you're *not* in a long-term, mutually monogamous relationship, *do* use condoms no matter how inconvenient they might seem to you. Condoms can safeguard you against life- and/or fertility-threatening sexually transmitted diseases as well as against an unplanned pregnancy.

What Are the Advantages?

- The condom is safe, with no adverse side effects.
- It is widely available in drugstores, supermarkets, and restrooms. It is also distributed at some schools.
- Particularly when it is used with vaginal spermicides, it can be a very effective method of birth control.
- The condom offers some protection against AIDS and other sexually transmitted diseases.

What Are the Disadvantages?

- Because the condom needs to be put on the *erect* penis, some people feel it interferes with lovemaking. Others, however, make rolling the condom on simply part of foreplay.
- Some complain that condoms may detract from physical sensations. But many condoms today are very thin. Avanti condoms (which are especially thin) and Pleasure Plus condoms (with a special tip designed to be pleasurable for both partners) are made of polyurethane (helpful if you're allergic to latex) and are perhaps the best brands to use if you (or your partner) hate the idea of condoms. (You may be in for a pleasant surprise!)
- The condom can break, spilling semen into the vagina. This is most likely to happen if the man forgets to leave a space at the tip for semen and/or if the condom is old or not of good quality.
- The condom can slip off and spill semen in the vagina. To minimize this possibility, the man should withdraw his penis before he loses his erection and should hold on to the condom as he withdraws.

How Do You Get It?

You can buy condoms anywhere. Drugstore condoms may be fresher and of better quality than those sold in gas stations and restroom vending machines. Condoms are usually displayed on open racks in stores, so you don't have to ask for them. You don't need parental permission to buy them. If you end up having to buy them over a drugstore counter and asking a clerk for them, remember that condoms come in one size. If a clerk asks you "What size?" he or she means the size of the *box*. Condoms typically come in packages of 3, 12, or 36.

■ ■ ■

The Condom (Female)

What Is It?

The female ("Reality") condom is a thin, soft polyurethane pouch with two flexible rings on either end. One ring fits over the cervix while the other covers the outer vaginal area.

How Does It Work?

It covers the cervix, vagina, and outer lips, acting as a barrier contraceptive and also as a protection against sexually transmitted diseases, including AIDS and genital warts.

How Do You Use It?

The woman can insert this device (see illustration) into her vagina up to eight hours before sex. Insertion may seem awkward at first, but with some practice it's not difficult at all. Be sure to insert the condom straight into the vagina. Don't twist it. And use plenty of lubrication (spermicidal jelly, cream, or foam or a simple lubricant such as K-Y jelly).

After intercourse, you remove it and throw it in the trash. You need to use a new female condom for every act of intercourse. Do not try to use a male and a female condom at the same time.

How Effective Is It?

The female condom has about a 20 percent failure rate overall, but its effectiveness in preventing pregnancy rises if you're very careful to use it correctly and every time you have sex.

Who Can Use This Method?

Any woman can, but it may be especially useful for women whose male partners refuse to wear condoms or whose lifestyle involves multiple partners and who are at high risk for exposure to sexually transmitted diseases.

Who Should Not Use This Method?

Ideally, there isn't anyone who shouldn't consider this method for protection from sexually transmitted diseases. But if you would be tempted NOT to use it "just this once," another method might work better for you.

What Are the Advantages?

- The female condom can protect a woman whose male partner will not wear condoms.
- It can also protect a woman more completely than a male condom can, since it also covers the outer vaginal area and labia. This is especially important when protecting against HIV, genital warts, or herpes infections.

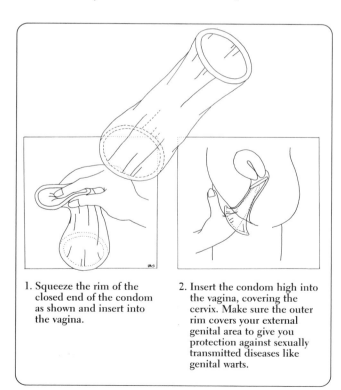

1. Squeeze the rim of the closed end of the condom as shown and insert into the vagina.

2. Insert the condom high into the vagina, covering the cervix. Make sure the outer rim covers your external genital area to give you protection against sexually transmitted diseases like genital warts.

The Female Condom: How to Use It

■ ■ ■

What Are the Disadvantages?

- It can be awkward to insert, at least initially. (Practice helps, so practice before the first time you'll be using it.)
- It isn't quite as effective as methods mentioned earlier in preventing pregnancy—but this effectiveness can be improved by using spermicidal cream or jelly with it.
- You must be very careful when inserting it NOT to tear it with your fingernails.

How Do You Get It?

The Reality female condom is available at most drugstores and some supermarkets and discount stores.

Spermicidal Jelly, Cream, and Foam

What Is It?

Spermicidal jelly, cream, and foam are chemical contraceptives that, when inserted into the vagina via tamponlike applicators, kill sperm. Foam will also block sperm trying to enter the cervix. Foam, which comes in a container under pressure (like shaving cream) is generally considered to be the most effective of these spermicides.

How Do You Use It?

You insert the spermicidal foam, jelly, or cream into the vagina with a special applicator that usually comes with the product (see illustration). If you repeat sex in the same day or night, you need to insert a new supply of spermicide into the vagina.

How Does It Work?

Spermicides immobilize and kill sperm cells as they travel up the vagina.

Foam is inserted into the vagina with an applicator.

Foam in Use

How Effective Is It?

Spermicides vary in effectiveness. Used alone, these birth control methods are considered less effective than the condom or diaphragm. In use without any other device, foam is the most effective spermicide.

Who Can Use This Method?

Anyone not allergic to the chemicals in spermicides can use this method. However, if birth control is especially important to you, it's important to remember that spermicides used alone aren't as effective as previously discussed birth control methods.

What Are the Advantages?

- They're readily available at most drugstores and have few side effects (though they can cause vaginal or skin irritations in some people).
- They need to be used only when you have sex.
- Nonoxynol-9, the active ingredient in most

spermicides, may help to prevent some sexually transmitted diseases.

- These contraceptives, used with a condom or diaphragm, make those methods even more effective.

What Are the Disadvantages?

- Some feel that inserting these into the vagina shortly before intercourse is an inconvenience (but some quite happily incorporate it into foreplay).
- Some feel these are messy, or they are allergic to the chemicals.
- The biggest disadvantage: Spermicides, used alone, just aren't as effective as other methods of birth control discussed earlier.

How Do You Get It?

Spermicides are sold in drugstores, supermarkets, and discount stores.

NOTE: The next two birth control methods aren't recommended for teens, but we're including them because many of you have asked about them.

Natural Family Planning

What Is It?

There are several variations of this method, but all have one goal: helping the woman estimate the days in her monthly cycle when the risk of pregnancy is highest and when sexual intercourse should be avoided.

. . .

How Does It Work?

Natural family planning works by alerting couples to the times of highest fertility so that they can avoid intercourse—and probable pregnancy—during those times.

Those who get the best results tend to monitor a combination of body changes during the month: basal body temperature, changes in cervical mucus, and other signs of ovulation. (This method is *not* simply a matter of counting the days since your last period to determine when you're likely to be ovulating.)

How Effective Is It?

Among mature married couples who carefully monitor body changes and are highly motivated, enough to abstain from sex during the fertile periods, this method may be helpful—especially if their religious beliefs preclude using any other method. For this group, theoretical effectiveness levels may be as high as 80 to 85 percent.

However, teens are less likely to be able to use this method effectively. Why? Because many teen girls do not yet have regular menstrual cycles—and that is a must if this method is to be effective at all. Also, many young people don't have the patience, motivation, restraint, and tolerance for the periods of abstinence that this method requires. The failure rate of this method among teens can be abysmal—and tragic. It is not recommended for teens.

What Are the Advantages?

- Natural family planning has no method-caused side effects.
- It will reduce one's chances of getting pregnant to 20 to 30 percent versus 80 percent probability of pregnancy if no contraceptive measures are taken at all.
- It is also the only birth control method that is officially accepted by the Catholic church.

What Are the Disadvantages?

- It can be risky. No matter how careful one's calculations, ovulation does not always follow a regular pattern. Thus, it can be difficult to determine just when it happens from one month to another.
- This method requires a fair amount of sexual abstinence during "unsafe" days. Patterns of desire do not always coincide with "safe" and "unsafe" days.

Sterilization

What Is It?

Sterilization is a popular method of birth control for married people over 30 who have had all the children they want and for people, married or single, who have decided that they will never have children.

How Does It Work?

When the male is sterilized, the procedure is called a *vasectomy*, which involves cutting and tying of the vas deferens (to effectively block the passage of sperm) via a simple operation that may be performed in a doctor's office. This operation is not the same as castration. The male will be able to function just as well sexually and will ejaculate seminal fluid with no sperm in it. However, it may take ten to fifteen ejaculations after the surgery is performed before the ejaculate will be entirely sperm-free.

Sterilization for women is a bit more complicated, involving a brief hospital stay. In this procedure, called *tubal ligation*, the Fallopian tubes are severed to prevent the passage of the egg from the ovary to the uterus. This operation may be done through a tiny abdominal incision or through the vagina. The tubes may be severed by cutting, by blocking them with special clips, or by sealing them off with electric currents.

■ ■ ■

How Effective Is It?

This permanent form of birth control is practically 100 percent effective. Sterilization operations may be performed on the male or female.

Vasectomy

Tubal ligation

Vasectomy and Tubal Ligation

Who Can Use This Method?

Only people looking for a permanent method of birth control should opt for sterilization. Even though some research is being done on reversible methods of sterilization, at this time it must be considered permanent.

Because of this, sterilization is not a commonly chosen method of birth control among young adults. It is most often chosen by married couples in their thirties or beyond who have already had all the children they want or who have decided that they don't want any children at all.

Advantages/Disadvantages of This Method

Sterilization's advantages and disadvantages are essentially the same: it should be considered a permanent method of birth control, one that cannot be easily, if ever, reversed. For a mature married couple who have either had all the children they want or who have made the decision not to have children at all, this can be an excellent method of birth control. For anyone else, especially teens, this really isn't a reasonable option in most instances. With other highly effective methods of birth control available, why close off permanently the possibility of having children in the future?

IN AN EMERGENCY . . .

In most cases, of course, sex is *not* an emergency. There is always time for a responsible couple to take adequate birth control precautions. However, condoms can break. Diaphragms can get dislodged. Couples can get carried away with the passion of the moment. And, unfortunately, rape and sexual assault can happen. In these instances, what can you do after the fact to prevent pregnancy?

The most common method is two elevated doses of oral contraceptives twelve hours apart, beginning within three days of unprotected intercourse. If you have been sexually assaulted, of course, you need to go immediately to your local hospital emergency room for follow-up treatment. In other instances, call your doctor for an emergency prescription or for his or her directions for the dosage you should take from your regular supply of birth control pills if your pill brand is one of the six approved in 1997 by the Food and Drug Administration for emergency contraception. If you live in the state of Washington, you may buy emergency contraception directly from a pharmacist without a doctor's prescription.

These pills must be started within three days (72 hours) of unprotected intercourse. You take one dose, wait twelve hours, and then take the second. Because these elevated doses can cause nausea and vomiting, many health-care providers suggest taking an anti-nausea medicine (like Dramamine II or Benadryl) one hour before each dose of emergency contraception. If you vomit within one hour of taking one of your two doses, you may need to take another dose (but check with your doctor first).

The following chart shows the brands of oral contraceptives and dosages used for emergency contraception.

19 APPROVED PILLS AND DOSAGES FOR EMERGENCY CONTRACEPTION

Brand of Oral Contraceptive	Dose 1 (Within 72 Hours of Unprotected Sex)	Dose 2 (12 Hours After First Dose)
Ovral	2 white pills	2 white pills
Lo/Ovral	4 white pills	4 white pills
Levlen	4 light-orange pills	4 light-orange pills
Nordette	4 light-orange pills	4 light-orange pills
Tri-Levlen	4 yellow pills	4 yellow pills
Triphasil	4 yellow pills	4 yellow pills

Do not take more than the recommended dosage or you will increase your chances of nausea and vomiting.

Your period may be a little early or late. If it hasn't started within three weeks, see your physician. You may be pregnant. If you do get your period, plan to talk with your health-care provider about a reliable, regular form of birth control if you're not already using one.

For more information on emergency contraception, you can call the toll-free number (888) NOT-2-LATE. If you have access to the Internet, you can get further information about emergency contraception via the Emergency Contraception Web site at *http://opr.princeton.edu/ec/*.

BIRTH CONTROL OF THE FUTURE

I don't like what I see with birth control as it is today, even though my boyfriend and I do use it (condoms and foam). Are there any new methods coming up that we can look forward to?

Gillian G.

A number of new contraceptives are currently undergoing research and, in some instances, clinical trials. The process is a long and painstaking one, but some fascinating new birth control methods may be available in the future.

Vaginal Ring

This small silicone ring contains a synthetic preparation of the hormone progesterone (or a combination of estrogen and progesterone) and would be placed around the cervix and worn three weeks each month. This method would deliver a constant dose of these hormones into the bloodstream through the vaginal tissue. In testing, it has a high effectiveness rate.

■　■　■

Transdermal Patches or Gel

Both gel and patch contain Nesterone, a synthetic form of the hormone progesterone, which suppresses ovulation. The gel is rubbed on the abdomen. The patch is put on for four days while the hormone enters the bloodstream through the skin.

Protectaid Sponge

This new barrier form of contraception is currently available without prescription in Canada. This polyurethane sponge contains several spermicides and is an effective barrier contraceptive and may also help to prevent the transmission of some STDs. If approved for use in the United States, as expected within the next three years, the Protectaid would replace the Today contraceptive sponge, which was taken off the market in 1995 largely due to manufacturing costs. The Protectaid has a different combination of spermicides and has two finger slots to aid in removal.

Improved Cervical Caps

Two are currently undergoing testing. One is the FemCap, easier to insert than the current available brand, and less likely to become dislodged. The Lea Contraceptive is a silicone cervical cap with a valve for venting (this improves the seal between the cap and the vagina wall) and a loop for easy removal.

Unipath Contraceptive System

This aid to natural family planning electronically monitors a woman's level of hormones via a series of urine tests (done on small strips). When a woman begins her menstrual period, she pushes the "M" button on the device and this information is entered into the memory so that her cycle as well as hormonal levels are tracked. When the device shows a red light, she needs to abstain from sex. A green light means it's safe to have sex, and a yellow light is a request for another urine test. This device, already available in Europe, is currently undergoing testing in the United States.

Combination Once-a-Year Shot and Implant for Men

This hormonal form of birth control for men works two ways: the shot deactivates GnRH, a hormone that is crucial to sperm production, while the implant, a small capsule placed under the skin of the upper arm, delivers a synthetic type of testosterone, a male hormone that suppresses sperm production while maintaining normal sexual desire.

Birth Control Pill for Men

This may be a way off. Currently undergoing development is a pill combining two steroids that suppress sperm production. Testing with this pill has shown that when men stop taking this pill, sperm production resumes at normal levels. (Previous pills tested, using a different formula, permanently impaired fertility in about 20 percent of men in test groups.)

Unisex Birth Control Pill

Now being researched at the Salk Institute, this pill, using the hormone *inhibin,* would block sperm production in males and ovulation in females. If successful in tests, it could be available within a few years.

Contraceptive Nasal Sprays

Used by a man or a woman, this promising new birth control method is now being studied at the National Institutes of Health and other research centers around the world. It uses hormonal proteins called *peptides* instead of steroids such as estrogens (currently used in the birth control pill). Peptides seem to have fewer adverse effects on the human body. The first peptide tested, LHRH, acts on the pituitary gland at the base of the brain. This gland regulates women's ovaries and men's testes. The contraceptive will be inhalable because peptide pills are absorbed and deactivated too quickly by the digestive system. No side effects are evident yet, but researchers are cautious; it may take some years of testing before this product will be available to the general public.

While many exciting birth control advances seem to be on the horizon (or years away) there is a great deal you can do *today* to prevent an unplanned, unwanted pregnancy. It's true that, right now, there is no perfect method of birth control. But there are effective—and reasonably convenient—methods. It's important to keep in mind that your own motivation to *use* whichever birth control method you choose is a vital part of its success. Personal responsibility is the most important ingredient in any method of birth control.

QUICK SCAN

BIRTH CONTROL: AN OUNCE OF PREVENTION

✔ If you want to prevent an unwanted pregnancy, you must use a reliable method of birth control **every time you have sex, including the first time.**

✔ While abstinence is the only 100 percent guaranteed way to prevent pregnancy, birth control methods such as oral contraceptives (the Pill) and the Depo-Provera three-month injection are very close to 100 percent effective, when used correctly.

✔ Unless you and your partner were both virgins going into your relationship or unless

continued

you were both tested for various sexually transmitted diseases before entering your five-years-or-longer exclusive relationship, you need to use a condom and spermicide to help prevent some sexually transmitted diseases as well as pregnancy.

✔ Emergency contraception is available if you have unprotected sex (a condom breaks, a diaphragm slips, you are sexually assaulted, or you just get carried away by the moment). The most common form of treatment would be two prescribed larger-than-usual doses of one of six brands of birth control pills. But you must call your doctor and begin the prescribed treatment within three days (72 hours) of unprotected intercourse. This is fine for an emergency but not for regular birth control, since these larger-than-usual doses of oral contraceptives can cause nausea. For more information on emergency contraception, you can call the toll-free number (888) NOT-2-LATE or check out the Emergency Contraception Web site at *http://opr.princeton.edu/ec/*.

CHAPTER FOURTEEN
Pregnancy and Parenthood

CONSIDERING PARENTHOOD

I'm 14 years old and I want to have a baby. I try to be very sensible and think of the unfairness it would bring to a child and to my family, but I still want to get pregnant. If I do have a baby, do you think it might be abnormal because I'm so young? Do you think I could take care of it? I'm pretty mature for my age and I've got a way with children. I love kids a lot and I'd be willing to get a job and support my child. I don't know what to do. I want a child very badly, but I want the best for it.

Anonymous

One of the most amazing developments of the turn of the century has been watching the sharply declining numbers of teenage pregnancies after decades of soaring rates. There are a lot of theories about why this may be so, including better, more comprehensive sex education, or (according to some) sex education with a greater emphasis on abstinence; greater teen knowledge about and access to reliable methods of birth control; and, perhaps, a gradually strengthening economy that gives more young people a glimmer of hope for their own futures.

Some ethnic groups, however, continue to have high rates of teen pregnancy, especially Latina teens with ancestral ties to Mexico. It has been the-

orized that a complex combination of cultural traditions and religious beliefs may be a factor in the reality that Latina teens are much more likely than African American or white teens to become young parents.

Whatever your dreams for your future, whatever your ethnicity, parenthood—or nonparenthood—is one of the most important choices you'll ever make. It can affect your life tremendously and, if you're a parent, the life of a child as well. This is a decision that must be made with care, NOT left to chance!

Whether you're single or married, in adolescence or young adulthood, there are some vitally important questions to ask yourself if you're thinking about having a baby.

1. *What are my plans for my own future?* Do you have specific educational, career, or lifestyle goals? What will it take to achieve them? If you don't have clear-cut goals beyond early parenthood, have you thought realistically about how you will support yourself and your child? If you have only vague ideas about this, think twice. Your parents may not be thrilled—or even able—to help you out. Public assistance does not go far. And the wages that a young person with less than a high school education can earn—even if he or she can get a job—are inad-

equate for supporting a family, however small. If marriage seems like the way to go, think twice, too. Teenage couples have a notoriously high divorce rate.

You need to have a viable plan for your future before you even think of bringing a baby into your life. Don't you want your future child to have as good a life as possible? To achieve that goal, you may need to wait until you have a good education, job skills, and at least a minimum amount of financial security. Think about getting a truly marketable skill and *at least* a high school diploma.

This will give you more choices in life and will help make parenthood, when it comes, an active, positive choice, not something that just happens because you have nothing else to do with your life.

2. *Why do I want a baby?* People have babies for all kinds of reasons, many of them very personal; we're not saying one reason or the other is right or wrong. But if you hear yourself saying things like "I want someone who will love me no matter what!" or "I want people to look up to me," or "I want to prove my love to my boyfriend and for us to be together forever," you may be setting yourself up for disappointment.

It's true that, in many schools, pregnant teens get a lot of attention, and friends may look at you in awe. But once the baby is here and you're tied down with so many responsibilities, your friends may move on to hang out with people who have more ordinary teen lives and fewer, if any, major responsibilities.

A baby isn't a proof of love, of manhood, or of womanhood. A baby is a person. You can show love to your boyfriend in a myriad of ways, but, statistically speaking, early parenthood may be more likely to divide you than bring you closer together.

And while babies are wonderful, loving little people, they also make enormous demands on you and on your time, energy, and patience. Parenthood is much, much more about what you can give your child than about what the child can give you.

3. *What do I expect of my baby?* If you envision an invariably angelic, cuddly, cooing, sweet-smelling baby, you may be in for a shock. A baby, especially in the first few months of life, is by necessity self-centered and demanding. A baby is a separate person who may or may not resemble you, who may or may not live up to your dreams for him or her. A baby cannot even help itself, let alone your relationship with its father or your unmet emotional needs.

Could you love a child of either sex? A child who is average or even physically or mentally challenged? What you will give this little person is much more important that what you'll get.

4. *What can I give my baby?* Most of us want the best for our children. Can you offer your baby the best right now? What do we mean by best? We're not talking private schools or trips to Europe or fancy suburban homes. We're talking unconditional love, a fair amount of economic security, freedom from hunger, and, ideally, the emotional support of two parents who are committed to the child and to each other.

The ideal, of course, is not always possible. Many single-parent homes are rich with love, commitment, and caring. But when a family is headed by an unmarried teenager, the children involved start out with some strikes against them. They're more likely to grow up in poverty, more likely to fail in school, and more likely to grow to become teen parents themselves.

Parenthood can be a difficult job for a man or woman of any age. Although a baby may bring you very special joy, you will also have many challenges. In many instances, the child's needs will have to come before yours. The hardships and sacrifices involved are not always easy for anyone, but may be especially hard to take if you're still in the process of growing up and are feeling really needy, too.

5. *Am I ready for the responsibilities of parenthood?* Parenthood is a 24-hour-a-day, 18-year commit-

ment at the very least. But most parents come to realize that their child is forever—and that the emotional commitment to parenting never really ends.

The active parenthood it takes to raise a baby and toddler takes a very special commitment, however. It may involve giving up a lot of personal freedom, curtailing your social life, and being constantly aware of and concerned for your child's needs.

Are you ready to plan most of your current life around a baby? Are you ready to give up the freedom to come and go as you please?

These are important points to consider before you become a parent.

Keep in mind, we're not down on parenthood at all. To the contrary, we see it as one of the most wonderful, challenging, scary, and rewarding life experiences one can have. Because being a parent is probably the most demanding and important job a human being can have, it's important to be truly ready for meeting its challenges and savoring its joys.

IF YOU THINK YOU MIGHT BE PREGNANT

Please help me. I had sex for the first time and did not get my period this month. What's going on? Am I pregnant? I am only 14 years old and very scared. I'm afraid to tell my mom that I had unprotected sex!

Kris

What if you think you may be pregnant? What are the symptoms?

- *A missed menstrual period.* This is usually, though not always, your first clue that you might be pregnant. However, you may skip a period if you're not eating properly or if you're under a great deal of stress.
- *Fatigue.* You feel tired all the time, even when you've had enough sleep.

- *Breast changes.* Your breasts feel tender and swollen, much like they may feel just before your period, only this feeling doesn't go away after a few days.
- *Urinary and vaginal discharge changes.* These would include more frequent than usual urination and a heavier vaginal discharge.
- *Morning sickness.* This queasiness and nausea can happen at any time of day (especially when you smell food cooking) but it is most likely to strike just as you're getting out of bed in the morning. This sickness is triggered by *HCG* (human chorionic gonadotropin), which the fetus produces at an especially high level during the first three months. This is why morning sickness is most likely to occur in early pregnancy.

If you have one or more of these symptoms, do check with your physician. Many people use home pregnancy tests first. That's fine. But then you need to see a physician *right away*. This is important whether your pregnancy is planned or unplanned, wanted or unwanted. You may choose to go to a private physician, an adolescent clinic, a school clinic, a free clinic, or Planned Parenthood. But it's important to get your pregnancy confirmed by a physician. The physician will note changes in the size and firmness of the uterus as well as a bluish hue to the cervix. All of these may be signs of pregnancy.

Once your pregnancy is confirmed, you and your physician or another medical professional at the practice or clinic can discuss your plans. If you plan to continue the pregnancy—whether you will marry the father, be a single parent, or place your baby for adoption—you need to take precautions such as avoiding drugs, alcohol, and other habits so that your baby will get a healthy start to life. If you plan to terminate the pregnancy, the earlier this is done the better. Many clinics will not perform abortions after the first trimester (twelve weeks or beyond). And late abortions are not legal in a number of states. So if you are thinking of having an abortion, you need to seek help sooner rather than later.

MAKING DECISIONS ABOUT YOUR PREGNANCY

You have four basic options:

- Having the baby and marrying the father
- Having the baby and raising it yourself as a single parent
- Having the baby and giving it up for adoption
- Terminating the pregnancy by abortion

No one of these options is right for everybody. Not all will be available or acceptable to everyone. Not one of these is an *easy* option. But one may be best for you, given your unique circumstances.

You may find that those around you have a lot of opinions about what you should do. Some teens have told us that their friends put a lot of pressure on them to keep their babies—and are highly critical of classmates who have abortions or relinquish their babies for adoption. Other teens tell us that their parents (and their boyfriends) often assume abortion is the only option.

While it's important to listen to those who love you—especially to your parents (whose lives may well be profoundly affected by this decision, too)—it's important to listen to your own feelings, too, and to get professional counseling if you're having difficulty making a decision that feels right for you. Consider the direction you want your life to go, what you could or could not offer as a parent, and talk about this with those close to you. Together, you may work toward making a decision you can live with.

We're not advocating one option above another. We will simply review the four choices that you may be facing, giving you brief information about each choice with comments from teens who have made those choices.

Having the Baby and Marrying the Father

Teen marriages, especially those prompted by pregnancy, have a rough time, with a divorce rate twice that of couples even a few years older. However, some teen couples are making it. It helps if you have finished high school and are in your late teens. It helps if your families are supportive. It also helps if you had plans to be married anyway, pregnancy or not. And it helps if both of you have above-average maturity and commitment. Teen couples who make it seem to have a lot of love, a mutual commitment to struggle and share, as well as supportive others: families, friends, counselors, and physicians.

In making the decision whether to try marriage and parenthood simultaneously at a young age, it's important to determine whether you are both willing to try and whether you have outside help available for the difficult times.

Voices of Experience

Greg and I have always loved each other, but had a hard time right after we were married and our daughter Jennifer was born. He felt left out and jealous when I spent time with the baby. Now that she's a little older and is really attached to him, it's better. We felt pretty trapped at first: Greg as the breadwinner and me as a stay-at-home mother. Finally, my mother agreed to watch the baby several hours a day so I could work part time. Now Greg and I both work, take college courses at night, and share caring for the baby. We're lucky to have parents who help us, our education and skills, a healthy baby, and a wonderful doctor. But it still isn't easy. My school friends have kind of drifted away. I'm very young to be a wife, let alone a mother. Sometimes, even though I'm rarely alone, I get lonely.

Vicki, 17

My marriage only lasted a year and a half. My husband was a nice person, but too restless and young to be married. I had such stars in my eyes when I was 16 and pregnant. I was happy to drop out of high school and say goodbye to my dreams for the future. I thought Joe and I would be happy forever. Now I'm trying to finish high school, get a job, and get off welfare. I really love my child, but I miss my youth and I feel like it is gone forever.

Janelle, 19

Having the Baby and Raising It As a Single Parent

This option has become increasingly common among teens in the last 20 years.

The advantage, of course, is that you can grow to be a parent to your child (quite possibly with help from your own parents and extended family).

Some pitfalls of single parenthood for a teen: the risk of being undereducated and impoverished as well as having difficulties with the daily demands of parenthood. It's very hard to finish school and to get the education you need to adequately support yourself and your child when you have parenting responsibilities at such a young age. (But some young people, particularly those whose parents are supportive of them and/or those who are fiercely determined, do manage to get educated and fully employed.) It can also be very hard to give up your freedoms (maybe freedoms you took for granted) when you assume the very adult role of parent at such a young age.

Voice of Experience

My mother takes care of my baby when I'm at school and she'll do the same when I go to community college to study to become a nurse next year. But as soon as I get home from school, the baby is MY responsibility. I fit homework and everything else in between caring for her. Between those two things—school and taking care of my baby—I don't do anything. I don't go out at all anymore. I love my daughter more than anything, but being a mother means a lot of responsibility and loss of freedom. People need to KNOW that beforehand.

Johanna, 17

Having the Baby and Giving It Up for Adoption

This used to be one of the most common choices of unmarried mothers, but is less frequently the *first* option chosen these days. Unfortunately, some teens choose this option second—after trying to be a single parent for a time and feeling totally overwhelmed. Then they put their babies up for adoption. Since later relinquishments can be a trauma for both mother and child, and since a child's chances of being adopted decrease as he or she grows out of the infancy stage, it is far preferable to make the choice for adoption either before the baby is born or as soon as possible after birth.

An advantage of choosing adoption, of course, is that your baby has a chance for a new life with a family that wants him or her very much. The primary disadvantage has been that you relinquish your child forever to another family—in many instances, never knowing what has become of him or her. This has been changing, however, with the growing popularity of open adoption.

Open adoptions, often arranged through an attorney, mean that birth parents can play an active role in choosing adoptive parents. In some open adoptions, birth parents continue to be informed about their child's progress and some even have continued contact with the child. Even in some of the more traditional agency adoptions, there seems to be a more open attitude in terms of the birth mother and adoptive families having more knowledge of each other.

Voice of Experience

I felt a mixture of terrible grief and great relief when I gave my newborn baby boy up for adoption. It was the hardest thing I've ever done. But I feel I gave BOTH of us a chance at life. I know that the two parents who wanted him enough to go through all that screening will give him more than I could right now. It hurts me to admit that, but I know it's true. And I can pick up my life and go to college. If I had kept the baby, that wouldn't have been possible and I might have come to resent the baby for that.

Sandi, 17

■ ■ ■

Having an Abortion

Despite the storm of controversy surrounding it, abortion *is* legal in the United States as a result of the U.S. Supreme Court's *Roe vs. Wade* decision in 1973. And it *is* an option chosen by many young women. It is estimated that about one-third of abortions in the United States are performed on teenagers.

It's important to know that many people have strong moral issues about abortion, while others feel that it is a reasonable option in a difficult situation. It's also important to know that abortion is NOT a substitute for a responsible use of reliable methods of birth control. It is a legal alternative for pregnant women who feel that their best choice—of several difficult ones—is to terminate the pregnancy.

Women in this position have historically sought abortions whether these were legal or not, and many women have died as the result of illegal abortions performed by incompetent practitioners or of attempts to self-induce an abortion. Making abortions legal has meant that they're safer for you and, in some cases, considerably less expensive.

Abortions may be surgical or medical. The so-called surgical abortions *don't* involve making an incision. The most common type is the vacuum aspiration method. After a local anesthetic is administered, the physician inserts a small tube (connected to a suction device) through the cervix, and the contents of the uterus are, in effect, vacuumed out. This needs to be done by the twelfth week of pregnancy. So-called medical abortions, also done in the first trimester of pregnancy, mean that an injection or pills end the pregnancy. This might be the high dose of birth control pills used within three days of unprotected intercourse (see Chapter 13) or an injection of methotrexate, which is being used as an abortion drug in cities across the United States.

One of the newest methods of abortion is the use of ultrasound to spot a fertilized egg (referred to at this point as a *gestational sac*) a week to ten days after conception. Here the sac, no larger than the head of a match, is removed via a syringe placed in the cervix. The procedure takes two minutes and is less likely to cause bleeding or cramping afterward than the other two methods. Although this technique is quite new, it is an increasingly popular option among women seeking help very soon after unprotected intercourse (sometimes before they have missed a menstrual period).

Women who have first-trimester abortions are usually home the same day and, typically, experience little physical discomfort except perhaps for some brief, menstrual-like cramps.

It is much more difficult—legally, medically, and emotionally—to have an abortion in the second trimester. The health risks are greater, the doctors willing to perform the procedure are fewer, and the expense and pain are considerably more. These abortions are often done using an injection of saline or prostaglandin solution into the uterus, replacing the amniotic fluid. This results in the death of the fetus, followed by labor and delivery of the dead fetus. In many areas, such an abortion is done only in case of dire need, and many states have laws setting time limits—often 20 to 24 weeks of gestation—after which time an abortion may not be performed.

Voices of Experience

I was just relieved afterward. I felt I was making the right decision. But it's a decision I never want to have to make again. Still, I don't feel guilty or like my life has been scarred by the abortion.

Ellen, 18

I cried afterward even though everyone was very nice and it wasn't physically painful. I wondered what the baby might have been like and if I had made the right decisions. One of my girlfriends calls me a "murderer" and won't speak to me. I feel terrible about that. But my parents have helped me a lot. So did the counselor at the clinic. I felt depressed for a time. It still hurts to think about it. Maybe it always will. Still, I feel like I probably made the right decision.

Beth, 17

If you are seriously considering abortion, seek help from your physician or call Planned Parenthood in your area immediately. Your local Planned Parenthood office can give you information about local laws and resources.

WHY FOLLOW-UP MEDICAL CARE IS VITAL—WHATEVER YOUR CHOICE

Whether you choose to continue or to terminate your pregnancy, good follow-up medical care is vital.

If You Are Continuing Your Pregnancy

- Regular visits to your physician or clinic are REALLY important. The doctor needs to monitor your health and your baby's health and growth during the months. As a teen mother, you're physically at high risk. So regular medical care and monitoring is especially important.
- Don't take any drugs—even aspirin—without checking with your doctor first. A number of drugs can be harmful to the baby, especially during the early months of pregnancy when the baby's internal organs, arms and legs, teeth, and eyes and ears are forming. Some physicians caution against drinking beverages containing caffeine—colas, coffee, tea—during pregnancy.
- Stop smoking. Smoking can have harmful, even lethal, effects on a fetus. Women who smoke during pregnancy are twice as likely to miscarry or have a stillborn child or a low-birth-weight infant. Low-birth-weight babies tend to have twice as many physical and mental handicaps as other newborns and are more likely to die in infancy.
- Don't drink alcohol. Abstaining from alcoholic beverages during pregnancy can help protect your baby against fetal alcohol syndrome (FAS) or fetal alcohol effects (FAE).

These devastating, alcohol-induced conditions can mean lifelong disabilities, including impaired vision or hearing, facial abnormalities, spinal curvature, lack of coordination, and emotional or behavioral problems. Researchers have found that a woman who has only a few drinks a week may be at risk of having a baby with at least some of these symptoms.
- Eat a balanced diet, take iron and other vitamins as your physician may direct, and exercise. A well-nourished, well-toned body can help make pregnancy and childbirth easier. But, before you try anything on your own, check with your doctor.
- Report troublesome symptoms such as bleeding, swelling or puffiness of your face or limbs, sudden weight gain, blurred vision, or a severe headache to your doctor immediately. He or she may be able to prevent these symptoms from growing into serious complications.

If You Are Terminating Your Pregnancy

- Make a follow-up visit to your doctor or Planned Parenthood to discuss your use of a reliable method of birth control. Abortion (along with the three other options) is a difficult choice to make. You don't want to have to face such a situation again.
- While most women indicate that they do not need post-abortion counseling, do consider seeing a therapist if you have persistent depression or other troubling feelings and find it difficult or impossible to discuss these with those close to you.

LIVING WITH YOUR CHOICE

None of the choices we have discussed is easy. But with the support of those you love—as well as medical and mental health professionals when you need them—you can make the best of whatever choice you have made.

If you have chosen to postpone parenthood by having an abortion or giving your baby up for adoption, you have the chance to go on with your life plans now and opt for parenthood later if you choose and feel, at last, ready to nurture a child. Yet in a sense, you may feel forever changed by your pregnancy and by your difficult choice. The experience may give you greater will and momentum to go on to accomplish your dreams—and to safeguard them by using a reliable method of birth control.

If you have chosen to embrace parenthood as a single or married parent, you may well have your hands full. Seek help and support from those around you. And, while nurturing your child to the best of your abilities, take some time to nurture yourself: stay in school, get crucial job skills, and equip yourself educationally and emotionally to take the best possible care of yourself and your child. And use a reliable method of birth control so that you don't have another child too soon—before you are physically, financially, or emotionally ready to take on the considerable challenge of two or more small children. (When it comes to small children, one plus one does not equal two—but about ten! Give yourself and your child a break!)

Parenthood can be exhilarating and exhausting. It can be one of the most challenging, taxing, painful, and joyous roles you'll ever fill. It's far too important to be left to chance.

PREGNANCY AND PARENTHOOD

✔ Symptoms of pregnancy include a skipped period, fatigue, persistent tenderness and swelling of breasts, heavier vaginal discharge, frequent urination, and morning sickness. If you have some or all of these symptoms, see your doctor. Don't just rely on home pregnancy tests. You need good medical care and advice immediately, whatever decisions you make about your pregnancy.

✔ None of the options you face with an unplanned pregnancy are easy ones. No one option is right for everyone. Seek help from those you love and trust and from medical professionals in making your decision.

✔ Good follow-up medical care, including getting reliable birth control, is important whether you give birth or have an abortion.

✔ Parenthood is one of the most life-changing decisions you'll make. It's too important to be left to chance.

CHAPTER FIFTEEN

Help! When You Need It

(And How to Ask for It)

I heard that a girl is supposed to go to a doctor if she has had sex, no matter what her age is. Is that true? WHY? And what can I tell my mom about why I need to go to the doctor? She doesn't know I'm having sex. I only did it twice. Do I still have to go to the doctor?

Courtney L.

Going to a doctor may be scary, especially if you have never been in the habit of seeking medical care on a regular basis. However, asking for help when you need it is an excellent health safeguard.

Please don't take this personally, but I don't like doctors! It's not that I hate them. I've never had a physical exam that I can recall. What can I do not to be afraid of doctors?

Petrified

When do you need help? In a variety of situations.

IN AN EMERGENCY

An emergency doesn't mean just a serious injury or unmistakable signs of an appendicitis attack. Severe depression and suicidal feelings constitute an emergency. So do symptoms of a serious or potentially serious medical condition—such as diabetes. If, for example, on reading Chapter 10, you noted similarities between your symptoms and those of the medical problems discussed, it is a very good idea to consult a physician.

Don't hope that such symptoms will just go away. Don't adopt an "I'll wait and see!" attitude. In the long run, you'll be far less scared if you seek medical help, testing, and advice. You may find that you do have a special medical need. In that case, you will benefit a great deal from early diagnosis and treatment.

On the other hand, you may find that your condition is not as serious as you had feared. The sooner you find this out, the less time you will spend agonizing over the possibilities.

Many teens, however, are afraid of what the doctor might think of them if they do turn out to be healthy after all. "The doctor will think I'm dumb . . . hysterical . . . a hypochondriac . . . a nuisance . . . " are often-voiced fears. While we can't speak for all doctors, we have found that most doctors won't feel this way at all. Your doctor will think that you're wise for being concerned about your body and for seeking help promptly when it seemed that something might be wrong. Your doctor will also be just about as relieved as you are that nothing serious is wrong.

IF YOU'RE SEXUALLY ACTIVE

Both males and females who are sexually active should be aware of the availability of confidential testing and treatment for sexually transmitted diseases and birth control services. Certainly, if you note any symptoms that might mean you have a sexually transmitted disease, do get tested and treated immediately. These diseases *don't* just go away! And even if you have no symptoms, it is important to be tested twice a year for chlamydia, a sexually transmitted disease that is an epidemic among teens and has become one of the major causes of infertility.

If you are extremely sexually active with multiple sex partners, besides rethinking your lifestyle in view of the fact that some sexually transmitted diseases today are not only health- and fertility-threatening, but also life-threatening, you also need to get routine tests every two to three months for a variety of sexually transmitted diseases.

Birth control, as we've seen in previous chapters, is another concern that must not be neglected. Also, sexually active females should have pelvic examinations and Pap smears once a year. If you're taking oral contraceptives, your physician may want to see you every six months.

Many teens fear seeking such medical help because they're afraid that a doctor will be judgmental about their sexual activity. Some doctors may be judgmental, but, especially if you seek help from a youth-oriented free clinic or youth clinic, a school-based clinic, a family planning service such as Planned Parenthood, or a physician who specializes in adolescent medicine, chances are excellent that you will receive competent and nonjudgmental help. These health-care professionals, who care primarily for adolescents, are likely to be sensitive to your needs and difficult, if not impossible, to shock.

Adolescent-medicine specialists (called *ephebiatricians*) are often physicians with basic training in pediatrics or internal medicine who have done special additional training in the subspecialty of adolescent medicine. They may be found in a number of clinics or in private practice where they may combine practice of adolescent medicine with pediatrics, internal medicine, or another specialty; in some cases, they may see adolescents exclusively. These physicians, who genuinely like and actively choose to work with young people, may be particularly in tune with your feelings and needs.

Of course, there are nonjudgmental doctors in all specialties and settings—from clinics to private practice. If you have bad luck with one doctor, don't give up on finding one who will understand you and help you.

AS PART OF YOUR REGULAR HEALTH MAINTENANCE

Preventive medicine is a growing concept in health care these days, but it isn't really such a new idea. Seeking competent medical advice for relatively minor complaints such as colds or flu may help keep these from becoming major problems and may enable you to care for yourself more effectively.

Routine physical examinations are vitally important, too. If you're under 18, you should have yearly physical examinations. After age 18 and through the twenties, you should have a physical once every two years. However, a woman 18 or older—or a younger woman who is sexually active—should have a gynecological exam and a Pap test once a year.

These routine checkups are important. They will enable you and your doctor to spot any possible problems before you experience a major health crisis. These examinations can also help make you more aware of your body and how it works. They offer you an opportunity to ask questions and share ideas with your physician about what you can do to enhance and maintain your health and fitness.

IF YOU HAVE QUESTIONS ABOUT YOUR BODY

A health professional—a doctor, nurse, or nurse practitioner—is an excellent person to consult if you have any questions at all about your growth, development, or body in general. "But I'd feel like a total dork!" you may be saying. "I'd hate to bother a person like that with questions they might think are seriously clueless. They might say 'I don't have time for you.'" It could happen that you encounter a health professional who has neither the time nor the inclination to answer your questions; if so, he or she is obviously not the person for you. But many of those who treat adolescents—primarily or exclusively—tend to be extremely sensitive to the special needs you may wish to discuss.

LEGAL ASPECTS OF YOUR MEDICAL CARE

One question that many teenagers have (and are almost afraid to ask) is, "Can I be treated without my parents' knowledge or consent?" or "Will everything I say here get back to my parents?"

There are instances where you can get medical treatment without parental consent. For example, if you have or feel you might have a sexually transmitted disease or any other reportable communicable disease, you can get medical testing and treatment on your own and on a confidential basis if you're 12 or over.

Many states allow minors who are legally *emancipated* (living away from home, supporting themselves, and so forth) or "partially emancipated" (their parents have lost control over them in a certain area) to receive birth control help without parental knowledge or consent. In many places, too, there is recognition of the "mature minor" concept. That means that you are capable of understanding medical treatment and are thus able to give your own consent to it.

In practice, some doctors and/or clinics will take your word for it—without asking for proof—that you're emancipated. Others will be more cautious and ask that you get parental consent or have a parent accompany you. If parental consent would be a problem for you, it's a good idea to find out immediately what the policies of a particular doctor or clinic are while you are considering your health-care alternatives.

In recent years, some states have passed laws requiring parental consent and involvement in certain instances—most notably abortion—that involve a teenager. In every state, this mandatory parental consent can be bypassed via a legal process that your physician or clinic counselor can help you initiate. If you live in a state where such laws exist and, especially if you're pregnant and want to have an abortion, you need to seek help early so that you can either make use of the judicial bypass or get help in telling your parents.

What are the laws in your area? The following chart, adapted from information from the American Medical Association, will give you an idea of the state-by-state situation as of this writing. Please note that, in states where there is no law addressing the consent of minor to a particular treatment, the minor may often give consent to treatment. The difficulties come in parental consent (PC) or parental notification (PN) states.

Under ideal circumstances, all of these laws and regulations should not be necessary. Ideally, teens in a crisis would feel they could tell their parents. But the fact, as we all know, is that teens who feel they can talk with their parents, especially in a crisis, will do so on their own without being required by law. And those who can't talk with their parents often have very good reasons for not pursuing communication and seeking support that doesn't exist. Ideally, parents will be involved. Realistically, not everyone has parents who can or will help them through a crisis. But help, often confidential help, *is* available to you.

■ ■ ■

This chart will give you information on what confidential medical and psychological services are available to you in your state with or without parental notification or consent. This is what the letters mean:

NL= No law found regarding this (so you probably can get confidential treatment)
MC= Minor consent accepted for confidential treatment
PC= Parental consent required
PN= Parental notification required
The "Adult" column lists the age at which you cease to be a minor and are considered an adult.

Laws do change from time to time, so check with your health-care provider for the latest update on the legal aspects of your medical care.

State	Adult	Birth Control	STD	Abortion	General Medical	Psycho-therapy
Alabama	19	NL	MC	PC	MC	MC
Alaska	18	MC	MC	NL	MC	NL
Arizona	18	NL	MC	NL	NL	NL
Arkansas	18	MC	MC	PN	MC	NL
California	18	MC	MC	NL	NL	MC
Colorado	18	MC	MC	NL	NL	MC
Connecticut	18	NL	MC	MC	NL	NL
Delaware	18	MC	MC	NL	NL	NL
District of Columbia	18	MC	MC	MC	NL	MC
Florida	18	MC	MC	NL	NL	MC
Georgia	18	MC	MC	PN	NL	NL
Hawaii	18	MC	MC	NL	NL	NL
Idaho	18	MC	MC	PN	NL	NL
Illinois	18	MC	MC	NL	MC	MC
Indiana	18	NL	MC	PC	NL	NL
Iowa	18	NL	MC	NL	NL	NL
Kansas	18	MC	MC	NL	MC	NL
Kentucky	18	MC	MC	NL	MC	MC
Louisiana	18	NL	MC	PC	MC	NL
Maine	18	MC	MC	MC	NL	MC
Maryland	18	MC	MC	NL	MC	MC
Massachusetts	18	NL	MC	PC	MC	MC
Michigan	18	NL	MC	PC	NL	MC
Minnesota	18	NL	MC	PN	MC	NL
Mississippi	21	MC	MC	NL	MC	NL
Missouri	18	NL	MC	PC	MC	NL
Montana	18	MC	MC	NL	MC	MC
Nebraska	19	NL	MC	PN	NL	NL
Nevada	18	NL	MC	NL	MC	NL
New Hampshire	18	NL	MC	NL	MC	NL
New Jersey	18	NL	MC	NL	NL	NL
New Mexico	18	MC	MC	NL	NL	MC
New York	18	MC	MC	NL	MC	MC
North Carolina	18	MC	MC	NL	NL	MC
North Dakota	18	NL	MC	PC	NL	NL
Ohio	18	NL	MC	PN	NL	MC
Oklahoma	18	MC	MC	NL	MC	NL
Oregon	18	MC	MC	NL	MC	MC
Pennsylvania	18	NL	MC	NL	MC	NL
Rhode Island	18	NL	MC	PC	NL	NL
South Carolina	18	NL	NL	PC	MC	NL
South Dakota	18	NL	MC	NL	NL	NL
Tennessee	18	MC	MC	NL	NL	MC
Texas	18	NL	MC	NL	NL	MC
Utah	18	NL	MC	PN	NL	NL
Vermont	18	NL	MC	NL	NL	NL
Virginia	18	MC	MC	NL	NL	MC
Washington	18	NL	MC	NL	NL	MC
West Virginia	18	NL	MC	PN	NL	NL
Wisconsin	18	NL	MC	MC	NL	NL
Wyoming	19	MC	MC	PC	NL	NL

COMMUNICATING WITH YOUR DOCTOR

I don't know if this is a normal problem or whether it's just me or maybe it's because my doctor is part of an HMO and is totally busy, but this is the problem: By the time I get the nerve to ask him a question or tell him a problem, he's half out the door and I feel really stupid. But at the same time, I'm mad because I'm not getting as much as I should out of seeing my doctor. What can I do?

Frustrated

Good communication with your doctor is vital. There are several ways you can help your doctor—and help yourself at the same time.

- *Be honest.* Don't lie to your doctor about symptoms, sexual activity, or anything else he or she may ask you. Don't be afraid. Your confidential relationship should be respected. And doctors are notoriously difficult to shock. A doctor is there to help you, not to pass judgment.

    If a doctor asks you a specific question, it may be important to his or her diagnosis. Your lie might make a correct diagnosis more difficult—and vital treatment could be delayed significantly or not given at all. So it's to *your* benefit to be honest.

How much are you supposed to tell a doctor? This doctor I went to when I had a problem with my period asked if I'd ever been pregnant. He also wanted to know if I was sexually active and sort of acted like it would be okay if I had sex with a man OR a woman! What's it to him? Besides, I'm grossed out because I'm not having sex with anybody and he should have known that!

Grossed Out

- *Don't expect your doctor to be a mind reader.* Some doctors are very perceptive and can sense sometimes that you really want to talk about something. Some others, who are still sensitive to your needs, may not know you well enough to discern this or may get confusing signals from you.

    The doctor may be in a tough spot. He or she may realize that you have unexpressed areas of need, but may also be aware that if he or she seems overly inquisitive, you may be offended. So you can both help each other a bit here. If you want to talk about something, but find it difficult, say so; your doctor may be able to help you to discuss your concern.

- *Don't be afraid to ask questions.* Asking questions can help you learn and better understand your body and whatever treatment you may be getting. Most doctors would *prefer* that you ask questions. They will probably think that you're intelligent and concerned to ask, not dumb or troublesome.

    Ask about specific treatments, medications, or tests you're getting. Why are these being given? Are there any side effects? How can you help increase the effectiveness of the treatment? How long should you take medications? Will the tests hurt? Will they be expensive?

    Ask about any bodily function or aspect of development that you don't understand. Most doctors will be happy to explain this to you. If you understand your body, it will help the two of you to communicate better and will also help you take better care of yourself.

    If you don't understand a direction or suggestion your doctor has given you, *ask* him or her to clarify the point. Don't pretend to understand if you really don't. That's not fair to you. All medical conditions can be explained in plain English, so if your doctor gets carried away with long Latin phrases and other medical jargon, call a halt and ask for an instant replay—in *English*!

    And again, if your doctor is not askable, maybe you need to see a new doctor.

- *Give a good medical history.* This is one of the most important ways you can help your doctor to help you. Some of the questions the doctor might ask will seem dumb, such as ones about your family's medical history, but these can be important, since certain medical conditions can run in families.

If your doctor asks about your sexuality, he or she isn't trying to be nosy or to embarrass you. Your sexual activity, birth control method, possible pregnancy, STD risk, and so forth may all impinge on your health.

Some questions asked may take a little research on your part. You may have to check which immunizations you have had, for example, or look at a calendar and do some counting to recall the first day of your last menstrual period.

What are some of the questions a doctor is likely to ask you?

- What brings you here today?
- How long have you had this (problem or symptom)?
- How old are you?
- Has anyone in your family had cancer? Diabetes? Heart disease? High blood pressure? Allergies? Tuberculosis? Kidney disease? Asthma? Any other serious health problems?
- Do you have (or have you had) German measles (rubella), red measles, mumps, chicken pox, allergies, pneumonia, bronchitis, tonsillitis, diabetes, or epilepsy? If so, when? Other health problems or diseases?
- Do you have any of the following (never, sometimes, or frequently): sore throats, colds, headaches, dizziness, ear infections, constipation, diarrhea, excessive weight loss or gain, excessive thirst, difficulty in concentrating, feelings that trouble you, or suicidal thoughts? Any other troublesome feelings or physical symptoms?
- Have you ever been hospitalized? If so, when? Why?
- How much sleep do you get each night?

- Do you eat a balanced diet? Do you eat breakfast?
- Do you smoke? Drink alcohol? Drink coffee, tea, or colas? In what amounts?
- Have you experimented with drugs or taken drugs on a regular basis? If so, which ones?
- Are you taking any medications now (either prescription or over-the-counter drugs)? If so, what are you taking and for what reason?
- Are you sensitive to any particular drug?
- Have you had immunizations for polio? Measles? Rubella? Mumps? Chicken pox (Varicella)? Hepatitis B? Tetanus-diphtheria? When did you have your last tetanus-diphtheria booster? (*Note:* This is recommended between ages 14 and 16 and every ten years thereafter.)
- When did you first begin to develop physically?
- At what age did you begin to menstruate?
- Are your periods regular?
- What date did your last period begin?
- How many days does your period last?
- Is the flow light, medium, or heavy? (How many pads or tampons do you use per day?)
- Do you have cramps? If so, how long have you had them? How severe are they? Do you have nausea with these cramps?
- Do you have premenstrual symptoms (tension and irritability, weight gain, tender breasts, a bloated feeling, headaches)? How long do these symptoms last?
- Do you ever spot or bleed between periods?
- Are you sexually active?
- If so, what method of birth control do you use? Have you ever had any problems or symptoms stemming from this method?
- Have you ever been pregnant? If so, how long did the pregnancy last and how did it end (abortion, miscarriage, stillbirth, live birth of a premature baby, live birth of a full-term baby)?
- Have you ever had any operations or surgical procedures? If so, why and when?
- Do you have any pain when you urinate?
- Have you had any discharge from your penis?

THE PHYSICAL EXAMINATION

I'd like to know what happens during a physical. Do you have to get a blood test? A urine test? What's the difference between a physical for a man and one for a woman? I don't mean to sound ignorant, but I don't think I've ever had a real physical before and now I have to have one before I go to camp and I want to know what to expect.

Robin

The physical examination is, with the medical history, one of the best ways for a physician to assess your health. It's important that the examination be thorough, covering the body quite literally from head to toe. Every physician has his or her own way of performing a complete physical, but there are many similarities. The following rundown will give you a general idea of what to expect.

The General Examination

After you finish talking to the doctor, you will go to an examining room (after stopping off at the bathroom to leave a sample for urinalysis). You will usually be able to undress and put on an examining gown before the doctor knocks on the door, asks if you're ready, and enters the room.

First, the doctor will usually measure your height, weight, blood pressure, and pulse, and perhaps even take your temperature. Then the top-to-toe examination will begin. The thoughtful physician will, as a courtesy to you, only uncover one area of your body at a time, keeping the rest covered. If your doctor doesn't do this and/or makes you feel like "Exhibit A: Nonperson," tell him or her that you're feeling uncomfortable and embarrassed. This is important for you and for the doctor, who may not mean to be thoughtless. Your gentle reminder may help him or her to be more considerate now and in the future.

First, the doctor will examine your skin for any abnormalities—such as any moles that may have increased in size, any rashes, or any signs of bleed-

ing under the skin. Next, he or she will examine your head, starting with your hair. (Some diseases may cause changes in the texture of the hair or significant hair loss.) The doctor will probably examine your ears with an ear speculum, which enables him or her to see into the ear canal. A hearing test may also be included.

The doctor will check your eyes by shining a light into them to check pupil reaction and then will ask you to follow his or her moving finger with your eyes. This enables the doctor to see whether you have any weakness in the eye muscles. He or she may also examine your retina with a special instrument. This test is extremely important, since disorders such as diabetes, high blood pressure, and brain tumors may be, in many cases, diagnosed by examining the retina in this way. The doctor may also check your vision, by asking you to read a special chart on the wall.

In examining your nose, the doctor will look to see whether there are any abnormalities of the nasal bones or the nasal cavity itself. When examining your mouth, the doctor will look carefully at your teeth, gums, tongue, and throat. Although the doctor usually does not have dental training, he or she can tell whether the teeth are in fairly good condition or whether you need immediate dental care. Also, some diseases have symptoms that can appear in the mouth. Moving to your neck, the doctor will feel for an enlargement of the lymph glands or an enlargement or abnormality of the thyroid gland.

Examination of the chest area—breasts, lungs, and heart—follows. The breast examination for the female is extremely important. The doctor will gently feel the breasts (in the circular motion we described in Chapter 2) to detect any lumps, dimples, or other abnormalities of the breast tissue. He or she will probably also gently squeeze the breasts to see if any fluid comes from the nipples. (If such fluid is present, it could be a sign of a breast disease.) The doctor will probably also check the underarms for any lymph gland enlargement, which can be a sign of a breast disease or tumor.

Then the doctor will listen to your lungs with a stethoscope, checking for any signs of lung disease, such as asthma, which may manifest itself with a wheezing sound, or pneumonia or chronic lung disease, which may have symptoms such as decreased air exchange. The physician will also use the stethoscope to listen to different areas of your heart.

As your doctor begins to examine your abdominal area, it's important to relax, since tense abdominal muscles can make an accurate examination difficult. In this part of the physical examination, the doctor will check the size of the liver and spleen as well as look for any signs of tenderness of these organs. He or she will also gently examine this area for any evidence of abdominal masses, tumors, or tenderness. The doctor will also probably examine the lower back for any sign of kidney tenderness, which can be a sign of kidney disease. If the doctor touches a ticklish spot, don't be ashamed to giggle; we all have such spots. You're normal. So giggle, then take a deep breath and try to relax.

Often, in doing the abdominal exam, the doctor may feel or press the area where your bladder is located. It's a good idea, then, to empty your bladder (perhaps after giving a sample for urinalysis) before the examination begins. This is especially true for women, since direct pressure may be placed on the bladder during the pelvic examination.

Examination of the genitals usually follows.

Male Genital Examination

In the male, this includes an examination of the penis to see if there are any abnormalities. If you are uncircumcised, the doctor will check to see if your foreskin retracts easily. He or she will also look for any signs of abnormal growths, such as small skin tumors or genital warts on the penis.

It is very common for the adolescent male to have an erection during the genital exam part of a physical examination. If this happens to you (or if you're just afraid it will and have been avoiding the doctor because of this fear), it may help to know

that the physician sees this as a very common, non-specific, automatic reaction—not as an indication of sexual interest in him or her! Think about all the erections you have each day that aren't related to any stimulation. This is just another one of those. And your doctor will understand this if it happens in the examination room. This may help to ease, if not totally eradicate, your embarrassment.

The testicles will also be examined for any signs of tumors, unusual pain, or signs of hernia. Here the doctor will ask you to cough or exert pressure (as if you were moving your bowels) to enable him or her to see if there is any evidence of a possible hernia.

Female Pelvic Examination

In the female, the doctor will do a pelvic examination after putting your feet in stirrups. Many women find this position an embarrassing one, but it seems to be the best way to do an adequate pelvic examination.

The doctor will first examine the labia for any signs of growths, cysts, rashes, or other irritations. Then he or she will put a gloved finger into your vagina to ascertain which size *speculum* may be needed. This instrument, which helps the doctor to see and examine your cervix, comes in a variety of sizes, from infant to adult size. Before inserting the speculum, the doctor may warm it with water and then gently insert it into the vagina, taking great care not to hurt or pinch you.

A pelvic examination with a speculum enables the physician to see the cervix. A wooden stick is used to collect cells for a Pap smear.

A Pelvic Examination

With the speculum in place, the doctor can see the cervix clearly and can note any abnormalities, such as redness, erosion, cysts, polyps, or irritation. A bluish hue to the cervix may indicate pregnancy.

A *Pap test* will be done with the speculum still in place. The doctor will insert a very small, specially designed wooden applicator to obtain a small sample of the superficial lining around the mouth of the cervix. (Or, to get a better sampling, he or she will put a small, soft brush into the cervical *os*, or opening.) This procedure does *not* involve cutting, but simply gentle scraping, and it is painless. After obtaining the sample, the doctor places the spatula/applicator on a slide and sends it to a pathologist for examination.

The Pap test is important, since it can detect changes in the superficial cells, which can reflect changes in the cervix itself. These changes may vary from inflammatory changes that happen with a vaginal infection such as trichomoniasis to abnormal cells that may be a sign of cervical cancer. This cancer is quite treatable if caught early, and regular Pap tests can detect such cancer early. Also, if a Pap smear microscopically shows signs of genital warts on the cervix, you will be called back for a laser treatment to remove these. This is important, since the virus that causes genital warts has been linked to cervical cancer.

This test is usually not done during menstruation, so if you are scheduled for a physical examination and get your period, let the physician know. He or she may want to reschedule your exam or your Pap test. However, if you're experiencing pelvic pain, it's important to get an exam whether or not you're on your period. At the time of the Pap smear, the doctor may also put a cotton swab in the cervix to test for chlamydia and gonorrhea. (A new urine test for chlamydia and gonorrhea, called the LCR, is simple and does not require a pelvic exam. It involves very new technology, so not all doctors do this test, but it's very convenient and often used with adolescents these days.)

After the Pap test, the doctor gently removes the speculum from the vagina and begins the bimanual examination of the uterus and ovaries. He or she will insert one or two fingers into the vagina until they touch the cervix while placing his or her other hand on the abdomen above the uterus. In this way, the doctor can examine the uterus for position, shape, size, and tenderness. He or she will examine the ovaries for enlargement, cysts, tumors, or tenderness in much the same way.

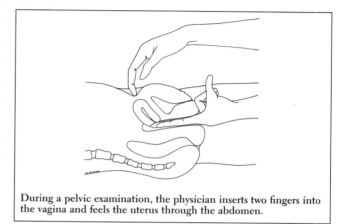

During a pelvic examination, the physician inserts two fingers into the vagina and feels the uterus through the abdomen.

Bi-Manual Pelvic Exam

If a woman has a uterus that is tipped toward the back, the doctor may need to insert a second finger into the rectum (with one remaining in the vagina) to adequately examine the uterus. If you're tense, this can be painful, so do try to relax.

Relaxation is important for the whole pelvic examination. If you're tense, it can be uncomfortable. If you breathe deeply, even closing your eyes, and try to relax, the procedure should not cause any real discomfort. Most doctors try to be as gentle and considerate of your feelings as possible during this examination.

Rectal Examination

Rectal examination is important for both males and females. Here, the doctor will check for hemorrhoids, rectal diseases, or fissures (splits in the skin of the rectum). He or she may also examine the male's prostate gland through the rectal wall for an enlargement or tenderness.

To detect whether you have any bleeding in the

intestinal tract, the physician may get a small stool sample on his or her glove for further examination. This may be a bit embarrassing, but can be of critical importance, since intestinal bleeding can be an early sign of possible major health problems.

Continuing the General Examination

After a thorough check of your genital organs and rectum, the doctor will look carefully at your extremities—your arms, legs, hands, and feet—for any signs of joint swelling or bone deformities, and will often examine your back (spine) for any signs of abnormal curvature, since scoliosis can be a problem for a number of teenagers.

A neurological examination, where the doctor checks your reflexes, coordination, sensory and motor functions as well as cranial nerves, may conclude the physical examination.

Lab Tests

Certain lab tests—blood and urine—may follow, if they didn't precede the examination. The urinalysis, of course, is painless and can help detect a number of problems such as kidney disease, urinary infections, and diabetes. The blood test may be a bit painful and scary for some, but it is very brief and is an important way of checking for anemia and other blood disorders.

These two tests are done routinely when you have a physical examination. There may be other lab tests—for example, for gonorrhea, chlamydia, or syphilis—that your doctor may suggest or that you may request. These diseases may not be detected during the regular examination and lab tests. The test for syphilis is a blood test—either the traditional VDLR or the newer RPR. The tests for both gonorrhea and chlamydia are cultures taken with a cotton-tipped applicator from possible sites of infection, such as the penis, cervix, rectum, mouth, or throat. These tests are a very good idea if you're sexually active with multiple partners and/or you have had any unusual symptoms that may indicate

you have been infected with one of these sexually transmitted diseases. Also, if you think you may be pregnant, you will need to request a special test.

GETTING HELP FROM MEDICAL WEB SITES

I've found some great health Web sites that tell me everything I need to know about medical and health stuff. My mom still insists I have to go have a physical and see my doctor once a year. What I want to know is, why? Everything I want to know, I can find on the Internet. It's not like my doctor likes to spend all that much time explaining things to me anyway. How can I convince my mom to agree with me?

Tyler

The wealth of information available on the Internet is one of the true wonders of the dawning new century! As you will see in the appendix, we're big fans of medical and health-oriented Web sites. These can be a really helpful source of information for people of all ages.

However, just as books (even this one) can't substitute for a thorough examination and personalized advice from your own doctor, so the health Web sites can't substitute for in-person medical help. Ideally, information you get from a Web site or support you get from a chat group will supplement information you get from your doctor or bring up questions you can ask your doctor at the next visit!

Also, keep in mind that information you get from the Internet or from books is, by necessity, quite general. For the most specific and personally useful advice and information, there's no substitute for your own physician!

GETTING HELP FOR YOUR MENTAL HEALTH

My parents are going to make me see a shrink because my school counselor told them that I should go see one because I'm having trouble in school (getting into fights) and my grades are dropping and they all think I'm down because of my parents' divorce last year. The only thing I know is I don't want to see a shrink! What can I do about this?

B. G.

Getting help from a mental health professional may be even harder for you to imagine and to do than seeing a physician for a physical problem. It's even more difficult when going to see a mental health professional—a psychiatrist, psychologist, licensed clinical social worker, or marriage/family therapist—is not *your* choice, but someone else's. You may worry about what your friends would think if they ever found out. You may find it unnerving—at least at first—to talk about feelings that aren't even that clear to you with an adult you don't know. And you may wonder how talking to someone like that would be helpful when, after all, you do have friends who will listen.

For many crises and problems in your life, those who love you—your friends and your family—will be all the help you need. But it can be useful, too, to spend some time with a professional who can help you work through feelings and difficult situations when no one close to you has been able to help.

Why Do People See Therapists Anyway?

Most people see professional therapists after they've reached a point in their lives when old ways of handling feelings and difficult times aren't working anymore, or when changes or conflicts have caused an emotional crisis, or when someone close to them insists that they see a therapist. You might want to think about seeing a mental health professional if:

- You're feeling depressed and/or irritable most of the day, every day for more than two weeks.
- You've lost interest and pleasure in things you used to enjoy.

- You've having trouble concentrating—and maybe your grades have suddenly started dropping.
- A change in eating habits has led to a significant weight loss or gain (a change of 5 percent of body weight or more in a one-month period).
- You've been withdrawing from your friends or driving them away with your angry outbursts or relentless irritability.
- You're experiencing a change in sleep habits—either being unable to sleep or wanting to sleep all the time.
- You're feeling restless or totally slowed down.
- You're feeling persistent fatigue and your physician has found no physical reason for this.
- You experience feelings of worthlessness or persistent guilt or overwhelming hopelessness on a daily basis.
- You have recurring thoughts of death and suicide, perhaps even imagining a specific plan for committing suicide or even attempting suicide.
- You feel that you need to talk with someone about a problem that you're too embarrassed or afraid to bring up with your parents or even your friends.

All of these are very good reasons to see a therapist. But who *are* these people and how do you find one who's right for you?

Who Are These Mental Health Professionals?

There are several varieties of mental health professionals. The type you choose may depend on your particular problem or the therapy you would like to have or what kind of care your insurance company covers.

Who are these therapists and how do they differ?

- *Psychiatrist.* This is a medical doctor with specialized post–medical school training in treating mental and emotional illnesses. He or she can treat people with mild to severe disorders who may require medication. Right now, psychiatrists are the only mental health professionals who can prescribe medications such as anti-depressants. But this doesn't mean that you can't get these medications if your therapist is not a psychiatrist. Most nonphysician mental health professionals have cooperative relationships with psychiatrists who will see their patients for a one-time medication evaluation and write prescriptions as needed, with occasional follow-up visits. If you're thinking of going to a psychiatrist, look for one who is certified by the American Board of Psychiatry and Neurology, which means that he or she has had special training in psychiatry and has passed a series of special exams to determine his or her competence in the field.

- *Psychologist.* This doctoral-level professional usually has a Ph.D. or Psy.D. in clinical or counseling psychology. To be licensed as a psychologist, this person must have completed four to six years of graduate study plus several more years of supervised clinical training (a total of 3,000 hours) and must have passed a special licensing exam in order to practice. Psychologists are qualified to treat emotional problems and disorders. They are also generally experienced in testing and assessment, which can be useful when extensive testing is required, needed, or suggested as part of your treatment.

- *Licensed Marriage and Family Therapist (MFT, MFCC).* This professional has at least a master's degree in clinical or counseling psychology, and a number have doctorates. This therapist has had two to six years of graduate level training (at least two years for a master's, four to six years for a Ph.D. or Psy.D.) followed by a required number of hours of supervised clinical work. These hours required vary greatly by state—from 1,000 postdegree hours in Arizona to 3,000 postdegree hours in Cali-

fornia to as many as 5,000 hours in other states. (We're talking at least several years of doing therapy under the close scrutiny of a clinical supervisor.) This type of therapist may do well with individual emotional problems, or may be able to help you communicate better with your parents or other family members.

- *Clinical Social Worker (MSW, LCSW).* This professional also has at least a master's degree—and some have doctoral-level degrees—in clinical social work or psychology. He or she is especially trained to evaluate and work with emotional problems in a social context. Licensed clinical social workers, like other mental health professionals, have had supervised clinical experience and have passed state licensing examinations.

How Do You Find a Therapist?

If you're feeling suicidal and need help quickly, call your local suicide prevention center or hotline for help and referral for therapy.

If your situation is distressing, but not a suicidal emergency, you might seek a referral from:

- Your physician.
- Local branches of national associations for mental health professionals: American Psychological Association (psychologists), American Psychiatric Association (psychiatrists), the American Association for Marriage and Family Therapists (MFTs), or the Academy of Certified Social Workers (MSWs, LCSWs).
- The graduate psychology department of a local university or the alumni affairs department of the nearest graduate professional school of psychology.
- A friend or relative who has had therapy and whose therapist may be able to refer you to a colleague.
- Your local family service agency (see your telephone white pages) or your family's HMO or employee assistance program (EAP).

Once you have the name of one or more possible therapists, make an appointment to see if you might work well together. Don't get discouraged if you find that the first therapist you talk with just isn't for you. Don't stop looking. Mental health professionals, despite having much in common professionally, have different personalities and styles of working. Finding the right therapist for you may be easy—the first one may feel right—or it may take a little more time. But it will happen.

While it's common to feel a little uneasy if you've never had therapy before, you will know, deep down, whether a particular therapist will work well with you. Some questions to ask yourself:

- Does this person listen well?
- Does he or she encourage you to work at seeking your own solutions (instead of claiming to have all the answers)?
- Do you feel that, once you get over your initial uneasiness about being in therapy, you could work with this person?

If you answer yes to these, then you may well have a good match.

What to Expect/ How to Make the Most of Therapy

- *You can expect confidentiality.* If you're getting individual therapy, your therapist is not going to tell your parents anything and everything. Psychotherapists of all kinds follow certain ethical and professional codes, and one of the most important of these is confidentiality. In most states, this applies even if you're a minor (see Chart 20 for the details about your state). There are only a few instances where a therapist is bound by law to break confidentiality: first, if you are in immediate danger of harming yourself—for example, if you are suicidal and have a plan, the therapist may notify your family so that they can also help protect your life at this time. The therapist is also obligated

by law to report to the proper authorities anything you may tell him or her about physical or sexual abuse. Also, in some states, the therapist also has a duty to warn a potential victim or victims if you appear to pose a serious threat to the life of another. In all other instances, however, what you say to a therapist will (and must) stay between the two of you.

- *You can expect therapy to be relatively brief in duration.* Except in very unusual cases, people aren't in therapy continuously for years and years. Many HMOs authorize about 20 visits—which may translate into five months of treatment, tops. You may be in therapy a little longer or considerably less, depending on your problem or issues. But therapists these days are trained to make the most of the relatively short time you will have together. (This fact may help make the idea of therapy more appealing to you, especially if you're feeling forced to get help.)

- *You can expect that there will be times when you feel worse on the way to getting better.* While you're in therapy, you may be exploring some very painful feelings. These are not caused by therapy. They come up in therapy because this is a safe place to let them happen. These are the feelings that may be interfering with your life in a number of ways. By facing and working through these painful feelings in therapy, you will begin to heal and to feel better.

How do you make the most of therapy?

- *Give your therapy (and your therapist) a fair chance.* It takes time and effort to make changes in your life—from minor ones to major ones. Therapy isn't going to give you all the answers or change your life all at once. It's hard work—and that hard work is mostly yours (or your family's, if you're getting family therapy). The therapist works hard to help and encourage you, but you're the one who makes the changes and develops the insights. If you bail out after one or two sessions and announce that therapy isn't for you, you're not giving therapy—or *yourself*—a fair chance.

■ *Make a commitment to work constructively, even if being in therapy isn't your choice.* It can feel awful to feel forced to go see a therapist. You may be, quite justifiably, angry that you're being seen as the one with the problems when, really, it's your family that's all screwed up. You may well be right—and it may not take your therapist long to see that you are right and suggest family therapy. However, even if you're stuck with individual therapy you don't especially want, you've got the listening ear of a trained professional and an opportunity to gain some insights and, perhaps, to make some changes that *you* want to make. As long as you have to go, you might as well get something out of it for yourself. It can be tempting to sulk and refuse to talk in sessions, but that may not be as useful as telling the therapist how angry you are to be there and how you feel about your family or life situation or anything else you would like to talk about. Don't worry about hurting the therapist's feelings or shocking him or her. Mental health professionals have been trained to do just fine with angry patients and most have heard just about everything, so, like physicians, they are pretty hard to shock. It's also a good idea to resist the temptation to just blow off appointments and not show up. Think about it this way: Most therapy these days is pretty brief, so you won't be doing this for a long time. Why not show up and see if it might help you in ways *you* want?

■ *Don't try to impress your therapist—either with how bad you are or how blameless you are.* This is one relationship where it's important to be real. You can say whatever you want and express feelings you might not share even with friends, in a safe and confidential place. If you spend most of your time trying to convince the therapist that you're totally bad or that all your troubles are someone else's fault, you're missing a chance to take the power to improve your own life.

■ *Be open to the possibility of change.* We're not talking about therapy changing your whole personality or essentially who you are. What it can help you to change are patterns of feelings, thoughts, and beliefs you have about yourself and the world that could be keeping you from being the best *you* possible. This can mean growing to feel better about yourself. It can mean learning new communication skills so that you can discuss issues with your parents (and others) without huge and pointless arguments. It can also mean learning the skill to say no to those you love or to risk being different from your friends when you need to be.

Good therapy is all about helping you build the insight, courage, strength, and resourcefulness to hope and to plan for and make changes that will make a wonderful difference in your life, in small and in major ways.

GROWING TOWARD A HEALTHY FUTURE

You, your physician, and/or your therapist are ideally a team working in unison to keep your body and/or mind as healthy as possible. You are the most important member of this health-care team. Many people make the mistake of casting the doctor or therapist into the role of guardian of their health and well-being, giving him or her all the responsibility. But a doctor can only diagnose, treat, and advise. A therapist can advise, gently guide you toward new insights, listen to you, and support you emotionally during painful times. But *you're* the one who does the daily work to take good care of your health and to make beneficial physical and emotional changes.

You live in your body and you're the person most responsible for its care. Your body *is* you. And do you really want anyone else trying to make the choices that are yours alone?

You can make many choices that will influence your health. We have looked at many of them in this book. Some of the choices enabling you to safeguard your health include the following:

- Understanding your body's growth and functions.
- Eating a balanced diet and exercising regularly.
- Abstaining from harmful habits such as smoking, drug use, and alcohol use.
- Learning to manage stress and deal with other troublesome feelings in constructive ways.
- Accepting and caring for your special medical needs—so you can be free to do what you like and need to do.

- Using care and common sense when you make sexual choices. The dangers of irresponsible sex have escalated significantly in recent years. Making the right choices and taking proper precautions can be health-enhancing, even lifesaving!
- Asking for help when you need it—whether this is help from a parent, a friend, a health-care provider, or a therapist. Sometimes, asking for help is a greater sign of strength and courage than trying to ignore a problem.

We hope that this book has given you some vital information and new ideas about some of your health needs and choices. We wish you a full, healthy, and happy life. But only *you* can make this wish reality!

HELP! WHEN YOU NEED IT (AND HOW TO ASK FOR IT)

✔ Both males and females who are sexually active need to be aware of the availability of confidential testing and treatment for sexually transmitted diseases and birth control services.

✔ If you're under 18, you should have yearly physical examinations. After 18 and through the twenties, you should have a physical once every two years. However, if you're female and 18 or older or a sexually active younger teen, you need to have a gynecological exam and Pap test once a year.

✔ You can get valuable medical information on the Internet. However, this is no substitute for the personal care and information you need from your own physician.

✔ Take good care of your body with regular exercise, a healthy diet, good stress management, regular medical checkups and using common sense when you make sexual and other lifestyle choices. Making wise choices can be health-enhancing, even life-saving!

APPENDIX:
Help! Where to Find It

CRISIS COUNSELING

Boys Town National Hotline
(800) 448-3000
(800) 448-1833 TDD (for hearing impaired)
http://www.ffbh.boystown.org/
This national crisis line for girls as well as boys offers free, totally confidential counseling and referral to help in your own area.

GENERAL ADOLESCENT HEALTH

Adolescent Health On-Line
http://www.ama-assn.org/adolhlth/adolhlth.htm
This is an excellent Web site put together by the American Medical Association.

Adolescence Directory On-Line
http://education.indiana.edu/cas/adol/adol.html
This Web site is an electronic resource for teens and parents. The part for teens features zines, a directory to fun Web sites, and honest, reliable help with a variety of questions and problems.

Society for Adolescent Medicine
1916 Copper Oaks Circle
Blue Springs, MO 64015
http://cortex.uchc.edu/sam/introduction-index.shtml
By writing to this address or accessing this site, you can get referrals to physicians in your area who specialize in adolescent medicine.

Virtual Children's Hospital
http://www.vh.org/VCH/Patients/ForKids.html
This fascinating site has information on a variety of medical conditions and issues such as scoliosis, diabetes, alcohol and drugs, information on how teens can stop smoking, Crohn's disease, asthma, and the physical aspects of puberty in general. The Puberty 101 site has lots of good information and advice—and you can also submit questions.

GENERAL HEALTH

National Institutes of Health
http://www.nih.gov/
American Medical Association
http://www.ama-assn.org/
National Health Information Center
(800) 336-4797
http://nhic-nt.health.org/
Healthfinder
http://www.healthfinder.gov/
HealthGate
http://www.healthgate.com/
This site emphasizes wellness and healthy living and covers topics from allergies to STDs. It offers free Medline (biomedical database) access.

InteliHealth

http://www.intelihealth.com/

   This site is affiliated with Johns Hopkins Medical School.

Mayo Clinic HealthOasis

http://www.mayo.ivi.com/

   This site offers information on a variety of topics such as asthma, pregnancy, diet and nutrition, women's health, and prescription medications. It offers a medical library and lots of interesting quizzes and health assessments. There is a teen smoking quiz and a thorough explanation of medical tests and procedures.

KidsHealth

http://www.kidshealth.org/index2.html

   Looks at teen health with special info on chronic conditions—such as epilepsy—and common health concerns such as scoliosis.

Medscape

http://www.medscape.com/

Medical Matrix

http://www.medmatrix.org/

Thrive

http://www.thriveonline.com/

Self-Help Sourcebook

http://www.cmhc.com/selfhelp/

SPECIAL-NEEDS RESOURCES

Abortion

Planned Parenthood
810 Seventh Ave.
New York, NY 10019
(800) 829-7732 (for general information about abortion)
(800) 230-7526 (for referral to a clinic or clinics in your area that offer abortion services)
http://www.plannedparenthood.org/

Adoption

National Adoption Center
(800) 862-3678

http://nac.adopt.org/
Bethany Christian Services
(800) 238-4269

AIDS

The CDC National HIV/AIDS Hotline
AIDS Packet
P.O. Box 6003
Rockville, MD 20845
(800) 342-AIDS (342-2437)—24 hours a day, 7 days a week
(800) 344-SIDA (344-7432)—Spanish - 8 A.M. to 2 P.M. EST, 7 days a week
National AIDS Clearinghouse
(800) 458-5231
HIV/AIDS Treatment Information Service
http://www.hivatis.org/

Alcohol/Alcoholism

National Clearinghouse for Alcohol and Drug Information
P.O. Box 2345
Rockville, MD 20847-2345
(800) 729-6686
http://www.health.org/
Alcoholics Anonymous
P.O. Box 459, Grand Central Station
New York, NY 10163
   Check your local White Pages for the number of your local AA chapter.
http://alcoholics-anonymous.org/
Al-Anon Family Group Headquarters
(800) 356-9996
http://al-anon-alateen.org/

Alternative Medicine

National Center for Complementary and Alternative Medicine
National Institutes of Health
Suite 450, 6120 Executive Blvd.

Rockville, MD 20892-9904

(301) 402-2466

Write or call for a general information packet.

*http://altmed.od.nih.gov/nccam/clearinghouse/
#pubs*

Alternative Medicine Homepage

http://www.pitt.edu/~cbw/altm.html

This Web site is maintained by the Falk Library of Health Sciences at the University of Pittsburgh.

American Academy of Medical Acupuncture

(800) 521-2262

http://www.medicalacupuncture.org/general.htm

Anemia (Sickle Cell)

Sickle Cell Anemia Hotline

(800) 421-8453

Provides genetic counseling and an information packet.

Anorexia Nervosa, Bulimia, and General Eating Disorders

American Anorexic/Bulimic Association (AA/BA)

Suite 1R

293 Central Park West

New York, NY 10024

(212) 501-8351

**National Association of Anorexia Nervosa and
    Associated Disorders**

P.O. Box 7

Highland Park, IL 60035

(847) 831-3428

Anorexia and Related Eating Disorders

http://www.anred.com/

American Anorexia/Bulimia Association

http://members.aol.com/amanbu/index.html

National Eating Disorders Organization (NEDO)

http://www.laureate.com/nedointro.html

**The Something Fishy Website on Eating
    Disorders**

http://www.something-fishy.org

This is a comprehensive site on the general subject of eating disorders: signs and symptoms,

physical dangers, definitions, resources, and personal stories.

Athletes and Eating Disorders

http://www.mirror-mirror.org/athlete.htm

This site gives special attention to athletes at highest risk for eating disorders: those in gymnastics, figure skating, dance, and synchronized swimming.

Males and Eating Disorders

http://www.primenet.com/~danslos/males.html

Asthma

American Lung Association

1740 Broadway

New York, NY 10019

(212) 315-8700

http://www.lungusa.org/

Allergy and Asthma Network

2751 Prosperity Ave., Suite 150

Fairfax, VA 22031

(800) 878-4403

http://www.aanma.org/

alt.support.asthma

A newsgroup providing an on-line meeting place for people with asthma to share information.

**National Institute of Allergy and Infectious
    Diseases**

http://www.niaid.nih.gov/

Birth Control

Planned Parenthood

(800) 230-PLAN (to find the Planned Parenthood clinic nearest you)

http://www.plannedparenthood.org/

Diet, Nutrition, and Fitness

American Dietetic Association Hotline

(800) 366-1655 (for nutritional information)

http://www.eatright.org

This site gives online nutritional advice.

Women's Sports Foundation
(800) 227-3988

Information on women's sports, physical fitness, and sports medicine.

http://www.lifetimetv.com/WoSport/

Personal Nutritionist

http://www.ama-assn.org/insight/gen-hlth/pernutri/pernutri.htm

This is part of the AMA Health Web site and gives online nutritional and weight assessments.

Shape Up America!

http://www.shapeup.org/general/index.html

This Web site provides information about safe weight management and physical fitness.

Drug Abuse

Center for Substance Abuse Treatment and National Hotline
(800) 662-4357

http://www.samhsa.gov/csat/csat.htm

Affiliated with the National Institute on Drug Abuse. Offers treatment referrals.

National Clearinghouse for Alcohol and Drug Information
(800) 729-6686

http://www.health.org/

Epilepsy

The Epilepsy Foundation of America
(800) 332-1000

A hotline for patients and families that provides information on epilepsy and referrals to local chapters.

http://www.efa.org/

http://www.alt.support.epilepsy

A newsgroup providing an online meeting place for people with epilepsy.

Gay and Lesbian Teens

National Gay/Lesbian/Bisexual Youth Hotline
(800) 347-TEEN

Lyric Gay Youth Hotline
(800) 246-PRIDE

http://thecity.sfsu.edu/~lyric/

Out Youth Austin
(800) 96-YOUTH

Boston Alliance of Gay and Lesbian Youth
(800)42-BAGLY

http://www.bagly.org/

National Coalition for Gay, Lesbian, and Bisexual Youth
P.O. Box 24589
San Jose, CA 95118
E-mail: info@outproud.org

http://www.outproud.org/

Pen Pal Program—Youth Outreach
Los Angeles Gay and Lesbian Community Services Center
1625 N. Hudson Ave.
Los Angeles, CA 90029
(800) 773-5540

http://www.gay-lesbian-center.org/homepage.html

International Gay/Lesbian Pen Pal Program
P.O. Box 20716
Indianapolis, IN 46220

Parents, Families, and Friends of Lesbians and Gays (PFLAG)
1101 14th St., N.W.
Suite 1030
Washington, D.C. 20005
E-mail: pflagnt@aol.com

http://www.pflag.org/

Dimension Health Services for Queer and Questioning Youth

http://www.hify.com/glbtq_clinic.html

Grief

Grief Recovery Institute
(800) 445-4808

http://www.grief-recovery.com/

Headaches

National Headache Foundation

(800) 843-2256

http://www.headaches.org/

Call for literature on a variety of headache causes and treatments.

alt.support.headaches.migraines

Melanoma

NCI CancerFax Service

(301) 402-5874

(800) 624-7890 (assistance using CancerFax)

The code for the Melanoma Fact Sheet is 201302.

Mental Health

National Mental Health Association

(800) 969-6642

(800) 433-5959

http://www.nmha.org/

Referrals to mental health groups and general information about mental health and illness.

Depression Awareness

(800) 421-4211

Call for free literature regarding depression and where to get effective treatment. This hotline is operated by the National Institute of Mental Health.

American Academy of Child and Adolescent Psychiatry

http://www.aacap.org/

National Institute of Mental Health

http://www.nimh.nih.gov

Girl Power!

http://www.health.org/gpower/index.htm

This site is a public health initiative launched by the U.S. Department of Health and Human Services. It is designed to prevent risky behaviors in girls.

APA's Psychology in Daily Life

http://www.apa.org/pubinfo/

Parenting (New)

Baby Center

http://www.babycenter.com/

Storksite

http://www.storksite.com/

National Parenting Center

http://www.tnpc.com/

Plastic Surgery

Plastic Surgery Information Service

(800) 635-0635

http://www.plasticsurgery.org/

Call this number for a referral to a board-certified plastic surgeon. Referrals are available throughout the United States and Canada. You can also get brochures and pamphlets describing the procedures and the results. This hotline is sponsored by the American Society of Plastic and Reconstructive Surgeons.

PMS

PMS Access

(800) 222-4767

http://womenshealth.com/hotline.html

Call for research information on PMS.

Sex Education

Sexuality Information and Education Council of the United States (SIECUS)

(212) 819-9770

http://www.siecus.org

Dr. Ruth Online

http://www.drruth.com

This site offers a special category of teen questions. You may ask a personal question, but it may take Dr. Ruth up to eight weeks to reply, so be patient!

Safer Sex Page
http://www.safersex.org/
Not Me Not Now (Abstinence-Only)
http://www.notmenotnow.org/talking2.html
This site offers quizzes and feedback on answers and links to other abstinence-only Web sites.

Sexually Transmitted Diseases

National STD Hotline
(800) 227-8922
Tell them your zip code and they'll tell you where you can find help close to home. They also offer up-to-date information on sexually transmitted diseases.
National Herpes Hotline
(919) 361-8488
(800) 227-8922
Centers for Disease Control (CDC)
http://www.cdc.gov/nchstp/od/nchstp.html

Smoking

American Cancer Society
(800) 227-2345
For information regarding the "Fresh Start" program to stop smoking.
http://www.cancer.org/
alt.support.stop-smoking
A newsgroup for people trying to kick the tobacco habit.
Smoking, Tobacco, and Health Information Line
(800) 232-1311
Tips 4 Teens—Stop Smoking Help
http://www.cdc.gov/nccdphp/osh/tipsteen.htm

Stress

Stress Reduction Clinic
University of Massachusetts Medical Center
55 Lake Ave.
North Worcester, MA 01655
(508) 856-2656—M–F 8 A.M to 4 P.M. EST
This hotline offers referrals to meditation workshops nationwide.

Index

Page numbers with boldface indicate tables. Italicized page numbers indicate illustrations.

Abortion, 210–11, 230
Abstinence, 158, 159, 161, 167, 180, 184
Abuse, 54–56, 72
Academy of Certified Social Workers, 224
Acanthamoeba keratitis, 93
Accidents from drugs, 108, 112, 115, 116
Accutane, 86
Acne, 83–86, **85**, 109
Acquired immune deficiency syndrome.
    See AIDS
Acupuncture, 135, 136
Acyclovir, 174
Adolescent nipple, 14
Adolescent nodule/gynecomastia, 32
Adoption, 209, 230
Advil, 19
Aerobic exercise, 75, 76, **78**, 81
AIDS (acquired immune deficiency
    syndrome), 230
    and birth control, 187, 188
    sexuality and, 160, 162
    sexually transmitted disease, 167, 168–71,
        181, 183, 184
Albuterol, 142
Alcohol, 230
    problems with, 108, 115–16, 124
    and sexuality, 163, 166
    statistics about, 111–12, 124
Alcohol, Drug Abuse, and Mental Health
    Administration, 112
Alcoholics Anonymous, 122
Allergies, 138–39
Alternative medicine, 133–35, 136,
    230–31
Amerge, 128
American Academy of Medical
    Acupuncture, 135
American Academy of Ophthalmologists,
    92–93
American Academy of Pediatrics, 112,
    188
American Association for Marriage and
    Family Therapists, 224
American Association of Naturopathic
    Physicians, 134

American Cancer Society, 33, 123, 174
American College of Obstetrics and
    Gynecology, 188
American Dental Association, 94
American Health Foundation, 107
American Medical Association, 188, 215
American Psychiatric Association, 224
American Psychological Association, 157,
    224
Amphetamine highs, 119
Anabolic steroids, 79, 112, 119–20, 124
Anatomy, female, 7–8, 7–9
Anatomy, male, 27–29, 27–30
Anemia, 139–41, 231
"Angel dust" (PCP), 117
Anger, 46–47
Animal allergies, 138
Anorexia nervosa, 68, 130–31, 231
Antibiotics, 172
Antihistamines, 139
Anti-inflammatory drugs, 142
Areola, 12, *12*
Asthma, 141–42, 231
Athlete's foot, **90**
A-200 (pyrinate), 177
Aura phenomenon, 127
Azithromycin, 172
Azmacort, 142

Bacterial vaginosis, **23**, 171
Bad breath, 93–94, 115
Balanced diet, building, *64–65*, 64–66,
    64–67
Beauty aids, questionable, 106–7, 109
Bed wetting (nocturnal enuresis), 142–43
Benign scrotal masses, 34
BHT, 174
Binge drinking, 112, 116
Biofeedback, 134, 136
Bipolar disorder, 57
Birth control, 185–204, 231
    for acne, 86
    cervical cap, 194–95, 202
    condoms (female), 181, 182, 187, 188,
        197, 197–98, 204

condoms (male), 181, 182, 187, 188, *195*,
    195–96, 203
Depo-Provera, 191, 203
diaphragm, *193*, 193–94
emergency contraception, **201**, 201–2,
    204
excuses (lame) for not using, 185–86
men's birth control pill, 203
method, choosing, 188, **188**
nasal sprays, contraceptive, 203
natural family planning, 199–200
nonprescription methods for, 187
Norplant system, 192–93
obtaining, 187–88
pill (oral contraceptives), *189*, 189–91,
    203
pregnant, getting, 186, 203
prescription methods for, 187
Protectaid sponge, 202
and "safe sex," 187–88
and sexuality, 154, 161, 162, 164
shot and implant for men, 203
spermicide, 187, 188, *198*, 198–99, 204
sterilization, *200*, 200–201
transdermal patches or gel, 202
tubal ligation, *200*, 200–201
unipath contraceptive system, 202–3
unisex birth control pill, 203
vaginal ring, 202
vasectomy, *200*, 200–201
Blackheads, 84–85, **85**
Bleaching teeth, 96–97
Blisters, feet, **90**
Blood pressure, 132–33, 136
"Blue balls," 35
Body
    normal, 3–4
    odor, avoiding, 22, 105–6, 115
    piercing, 104, 109
    questions about, 215
    See also Man's body; Woman's body
Body Mass Index (BMI), 70, 71, **71**
Bonding teeth, 97
Bong (marijuana pipe), 117
Boredom, 48–49

Boston City Hospital, 116
Boys Town National Hotline, 60, 62, 230
Braces, invisible, 97
Breast
    cancer, 13–14
    developers, 12, 107
    development, 10, *10, 12,* 12–15
    enlargement/reduction (mammoplasty), **100**
    self-examinations, *14,* 14–15, 25
    swelling in males, 32
Bronchodilators, 142
Bulbourethral glands, 28
Bulimia, 68, 131, 231
Bunions, **90**
Bust developers, 12, 107

Calculus, 95
Cancer
    breast, 13–14
    oral, 115
    testicular, 33–34
Candidiasis (yeast infection), **23**
Ceasing to have periods (secondary
    amenorrhea), 17
Ceftriaxone, 176
Centers for Disease Control, 69, 112, 168
Certified hypnotherapist (CHT), 135
Cervical cap, 194–95, 202
Cervical dysplasia, 175
Cervix, 8, *8*
Chamomile for stomach and cramps, 134
Chat groups on Internet, 49
Chiropractors, 133
Chlamydia, 24, 167, 168, 171–72
Cholesterol and health, 108
CHT (certified hypnotherapist), 135
Circumcision, 29, *29*
Clindamycin lotions (Cleocin T), 86
Clinical Social Worker (MSW, LCSW), 224
Clitoris, 7, 8, *8*
Cocaine, 118
Comedo extractor, 84, *85*
Compulsive overeating, 132
Conception, 8
Condoms, 181, 182, 187, 188, *195,* 195–98,
    197, 203, 204
Condylomata acuminata (genital warts),
    174–75
Confidential health services, state, **216**
Contact allergies, 138
Contact dermatitis, 102
Contacts, 92
Contraception. *See* Birth control
Corns, feet, **90**
Cosmetic allergies, 138
Cosmetics, 101–3
Crack, 118
Cromolyn sodium, 142
Crystal methamphetamine, 118
Current Science, 107
Cystic acne, 86

Danazol, 32
Date rape, 55–56, 162–63
DDAVP (desmopressin acetate), 143

Delayed puberty, 12
Dental care, 93–98, *95–96*
Depilatories, 105
Depo-Provera, 191, 203
Depression, 56–59, 61–62, 126, 127, 134
Desensitization shots for allergies, 139
Desmopressin acetate, 143
Diabetes, 143–46
Diaphragm, *193,* 193–94
Diastolic (blood pressure reading), 133
Dieting dangers, 68–69, 73, 108
Dip (smokeless tobacco), 115
Divorce, 43–44
Doctor, communicating with, 217–18
Douching, 22
Doxycycline, 172
Drug allergies, 138
Drugs, drinking, smoking, 111–24, 232, 234
    accidents from, 108, 112, 115, 116
    alcohol, 108, 111–12, 115–16, 124, 230
    anabolic steroids, 79, 112, 119–20, 124
    binge drinking, 112, 116
    for coping with adolescence, 114
    decision making about, 120–24
    funneling, 112, 116
    habits, stopping, 121–24
    heroin, 111, 119
    inhalants, 118
    LSD and hallucinogens, 111, 119
    marijuana, 117–18, 124
    problems with, determining, 113–14
    reasons to say no to, 108, 111–13
    secondary amenorrhea (ceasing to have
        periods) from, 17
    smoking and smokeless tobacco, 108,
        111–12, 114–15, 124, 234
    stimulants, 118–19
    and women, 116, 119–20, 124
Dysmenorrhea (menstrual cramps), 19–20,
    25, 134
Dysthymic disorder, 57

EAP (Employee Assistance Program), 224
Ear piercing, 103–4, 109
Eating disorders, 129–32, 136, 231
Eating for good health, 63–74, 231–32
    anorexia nervosa, 68, 130–31, 231
    balanced diet, building, 64–65, *64–66,*
        64–67
    Body Mass Index (BMI), 70, 71, **71**
    bulimia, 68, 131, 231
    dieting dangers, 68–69, 73, 108
    Food Guide Pyramid, 64, *64–65,* 65
    hazardous foods, 66, **66–67**, 74
    improving eating habits, 66–67, **66–67**
    minerals, 65, **65**
    obesity, 70
    overweight, 68–70
    reasons for, 107–8
    steps to, 63, 74
    underweight, 67–68
    vegetarians, 65, *65*
    vitamins, 64, **64**
    weight loss, sensible, 70–74, **71, 73,** 108
    See also Exercise for good health; Mind-
        body connection

Echinacea for cold or flu, 134
Ecstasy, 118
Ectomorphs, 69
Eczema, 86
Eggs (ova), 9, 27
Ejaculation, 28, 35–36, 160
Ejaculatory duct, 28
Electrocautery, 87
Electrolysis, 105
Electronic anesthesia, 97–98
Elimite (permethrin), 177
Emancipated minor statutes, 187–88
Emergencies, help for, 213
Emergency contraception, **201,** 201–2,
    204
Emollients in cosmetics, 101
Emotional abuse, 54–56, 72
Employee Assistance Program (EAP), 224
Emulsifiers in cosmetics, 101
Endometrial walls, 8
Endometriosis, 18
Endomorphs, 69
Endorphins, 20
Environmental allergies, 138
Ephebiatricians, 214
Epididymis, 27, 28, *28*
Epilepsy, 146–47, 232
Epilepsy Foundation of America, 147
Epstein-Barr virus, 148
Erection (hard-on), 29, *29*
Erythromycin, 86, 172
Estrogen, 16, 17, 19, 202
Excedrin Migraine, 128
Exercise for good health, 75–81, 231–32
    aerobic exercise, 75, 76, **78,** 81
    anabolic steroids, dangers of, 79, 112,
        119–20, 124
    for dysmenorrhea (menstrual cramps),
        19–20
    injuries, *78,* 80, **80,** 81
    physical examination before, 76–77, 81
    for premenstrual syndrome (PMS), 18
    reasons for, 108
    RICE (Rest, Ice, Compression,
        Elevation), 80, **80**
    secondary amenorrhea (ceasing to have
        periods) from heavy, 17
    starting, 76–81
    strengthening exercise, 75, 77–78
    stretching exercise, 75
    supplements, dangers of, 79
    target heart rate, 78, 80
    tips for, 81
    See also Eating for good health; Mind-
        body connection
Eyes
    cosmetics, 101–3
    healthy, 92–93
    surgery, 93

FAE (fetal alcohol effects), 211
Fallopian tubes, 8, *8*
Family changes, coping with, 43–44
Family planning, natural, 199–200
Fantasies, sexual, 154, 166
FAS (fetal alcohol syndrome), 116, 211

FDA (Food and Drug Administration), 101, 102
Fear-of-obesity syndrome, 130
Feelings, 39–62, 232–33
    abuse, 54–56, 72
    anger, 46–47
    bipolar disorder, 57
    boredom, 48–49
    date rape, 55–56, 162–63
    depression, 56–59, 61–62, 126, 127, 134
    dysthymic disorder, 57
    about family changes, 43–44
    grieving a loss, 46, 57–58, 232–33
    infatuation, 45
    and Internet, 49
    about "isms," 52–53
    love, 44–45
    normal, 4
    about parents, 42–43
    rape, 54–56, 162–63
    self-defeating behavior, 51–52
    shyness, 47–48
    stress, 49–51
    suicide, 59–60, 62
    and your health, 60–61
    about yourself, 40–42
    See also Eating for good health; Exercise for good health; Mind-body connection
Feet, healthy, **90**, 90–91
Female. *See* Woman's body
FemCap, 202
Fetal alcohol effects (FAE), 211
Fetal alcohol syndrome (FAS), 116, 211
Feverfew for migraine headaches, 128, 134
Fiber (roughage), 129
Fibrocystic disease, 14
"Fight or flight" response, 132
Fitness. *See* Exercise for good health
Flaccid penis, 28, 29
Flagyl, 179
Floating testicle, 33
Flossing teeth, 95, 96, 96
Follicle-stimulating hormone (FSH), 9
Follow-up medical care, 211, 212
Food allergies, 138
Food and Drug Administration (FDA), 101, 102
Food Guide Pyramid, 64, *64–65*, 65
Foreskin problems, 34–35
Forgiveness, 46
FSH (follicle-stimulating hormone), 9
Funneling, 112, 116

Gay people, 155, 156–57
General examination, 219–20, 222
Genetic heritage
    and excess hair, 104–5
    and normal growth, 3, 25, 31, 37
    and Type I diabetes, 144
Genital herpes, 167, 168, 173–74
Genital warts (condylomata acuminata), 174–75
Genitals, female, 7–8, *7–9*
Genitals, male, 27–29, *27–30*
Gestational sac, 210
Ginger for upset stomachs, 134

Gingivitis, 94–95, 95
Glucometer, 144
Gonorrhea, 24, 167, 168, 175–76
Good Housekeeping Institute, 107
Gordon, Sol, 48
Grand mal seizures, 146
Grieving a loss, 46, 57–58, 232–33
Groin pain, 35, 37
Growth, normal, 3
Guided imagery, 134, 136
Gums. *See* Teeth and gums, healthy
Gynecomastia, 32

Habits (drug), stopping, 121–24
Hair, excess, 104–5
Hair, healthy, 91–92
Hallucinogens, 111, 119
Hammertoes, **90**
Hard-on (erection), 29, *29*
Harrington rod, 150
Hazardous foods, 66, **66–67**, 74
HCG (human chorionic gonadotropin), 207
Headaches, 126–28, 134, 136, 233
Health, 107–9, 226–27. *See also* Birth control; Drugs; Eating for good health; Exercise for good health; Feelings; Help; Man's body; Mind-body connection; Pregnancy and parenthood; Sexuality; Sexually transmitted diseases; *specific medical needs*; Woman's body
Health Maintenance Organization (HMO), 224, 225
Help, getting, 213–27, 229–34
    in an emergency, 213
    for body, questions about, 215
    doctor, communicating with, 217–18
    for health maintenance, 214
    for healthy future, 226–27
    if sexually active, 214, 227
    from Internet Web sites, 222, 227
    on legal aspects of medical care, 215–16, **216**
    for mental health, 222–26, 233
    physical examination, 12, 76–77, 81, 109, 214, 219–22, 227
    resources for, 229–34
Hematospermia, 36
Hepatitis (A, B, C), 179–80
Herbal remedies, 134
Heredity
    and acne, 84
    and allergies, 138
    and breast size, 12
    and migraine headaches, 127–28
Hernia, 35
Heroin, 111, 119
Herpes encephalitis, 173–74
Herpes Resource Center, 174
Heterosexuals, 155, 156, 166
High blood pressure (hypertension), 132–33, 136
Hirsutism, 105
Hives, 138
HMO (Health Maintenance Organization), 224, 225

Holistic view of health, 136
Holmes, Thomas H. III, 126
Homosexuals, 155, 156–57, 166, 232
Hormones
    and acne, 84, 85
    and feelings, 4
    and migraine headaches, 128
Hot waxing for excess hair, 105
HPV (human papilloma virus), 174
HTLV-III virus, 168, 169
Huffing (inhalant abuse), 118
Human chorionic gonadotropin (HCG), 207
Human papilloma virus (HPV), 174
Hydrocele, 34
Hymen, 8, *8*
Hypertension (high blood pressure), 132–33, 136
Hypnosis, 134–35
Hypoallergenic, 102
Hypoglycemic seizure, 145
Hypothalamus, 16, 27

IBS (irritable bowel syndrome), 128–29, 136
Icterus, 93
ImmuVir, 174
Imperforate hymen, 8
Infatuation, 45
Infectious hepatitis (hepatitis A), 179, 180
Infectious mononucleosis, 147–48
Ingrown toenails, **90**
Inhalants, 118
Inhalers for asthma, 142
Inhibin, 203
Injuries from exercise, **78**, 80, **80**, 81
Insecurities
    about man's body, 37
    about woman's body, 24–25
Instead (menstrual cup), *20*, 21
Insulin, 143, 144–45
Internet
    cautions about, 49
    help from Web sites, 222, 227
Intimacy versus sex, 165–66
Inverted nipples, 13, 14
Iron-deficiency anemia ("tired blood"), 140
Irregular periods, 17
Irritable bowel syndrome (IBS), 128–29, 136
"Isms," 52–53

Jock itch (tinea cruris), 178–79
Joint (marijuana), 117

Kaiser Permanente Medical Center, 171
Kinsey Institute, 155
Kurz, Craven, 97
Kwell (lindane), 177

Lab tests, 222
Labia majora/minora, 7, *7*
Lasers for drilling teeth, 97
LASIK, 93
LCR (ligase chain reaction), 171–72, 221
LCSW (Clinical Social Worker), 224

Lea Contraceptive, 202
LEARN-TM, 135
Legal aspects of medical care, 215–16, **216**
Lesbians, 155, 156–57
Licensed Marriage and Family Therapists
 (MFT, MFCC), 224
Ligase chain reaction (LCR), 171–72, 221
Lindane (Kwell), 177
Liposuction, **100**
Los Angeles County Epilepsy Society, 147
Love, 44–45
LSD and hallucinogens, 111, 119

Male. *See* Man's body
Mammoplasty (breast
 enlargement/reduction), **100**
Man's body, 27–37
 adolescent nodule/gynecomastia, 32
 anatomy, 27–29, 27–30
 benign scrotal masses, 34
 ejaculation, 28, 160
 ejaculation problems, 35–36
 foreskin problems, 34–35
 genital examination, 220
 groin pain, 35, 37
 insecurities about, 37
 pink pearly papules, 33
 prostatitis, 32
 puberty, 27, 29–31, **30–31**, 37
 short stature, 31–32
 testicular cancer, 33–34
 testicular self-examination, 34, *34*, 37
 undescended testicle(s), 33
 See also Birth control; Drugs; Eating for
 good health; Exercise for good health;
 Feelings; Help; Mind-body connection;
 Pregnancy and parenthood; Sexuality;
 Sexually transmitted diseases; *specific
 medical needs*
Marijuana, 117–18, 124
Marriage, 208
Marriage and Family Therapists (MFT,
 MFCC), 224
Masturbation, 160–61, 166, 180, 181
Maxalt, 128
Medical abortions, 210
Meditation, 135, 136
Melanin, 88
Melanomas, 88, 89, 233
Men's birth control pill, 203
Menstrual cramps (dysmenorrhea), 19–20,
 25, 134
Menstrual cup (Instead), 20, 21
Menstruation, 15–22
 cycle of, 8–9, *15*, 15–16
 dysmenorrhea (menstrual cramps),
 19–20, 25, 134
 endometriosis, 18
 irregular periods, 17
 premenstrual syndrome (PMS), 18–19,
 25, 233
 sanitary products, 8, *20–21*, 20–22
 secondary amenorrhea (ceasing to have
 periods), 17
Mental health, 222–26, 233
Mesomorphs, 69

Methotrexate, 210
Migraine headaches, 126, 127–28, 134
Migranal, 128
Milwaukee brace, 150
Mind-body connection, 125–36, 230–31, 233
 acupuncture, 135, 136
 alternative medicine, 133–35, 136,
 230–31
 biofeedback, 134, 136
 chiropractors, 133
 guided imagery, 134, 136
 headaches, 126–28, 134, 136, 233
 herbal remedies, 134
 holistic view of health, 136
 hypertension (high blood pressure),
 132–33, 136
 hypnosis, 134–35
 meditation, 135, 136
 music therapy, 134
 See also Stress
Minerals, 65, **65**
Moles (nevi), 14, 88, 88
Molluscum contagiosum, 176
Mononucleosis, 147–48
Motrin, 19
Mount Sinai School of Medicine, 22
Mozart Effect, 134
MSW (Clinical Social Worker), 224
Music therapy, 134

Nails, healthy, 91
Naprosyn, 19
Narcotics Anonymous, 122
Nasal sprays, contraceptive, 203
National Adolescent Health Information
 Center, 59
National Asthma Education and Prevention
 Program, 141
National Commission for the Certification
 of Acupuncturists, 135
National Council of Alcoholism, 116
National Institute of Drug Abuse, 118
National Institute of Mental Health, 130
National Institutes of Health, 141, 203
National Psoriasis Foundation, 87
Natural family planning, 199–200
Nevi (moles), 14, 88, 88
Nipples, 13, 14
Nix, 177
Nocturnal enuresis (bed wetting), 142–43
Normal, 3–5
Norplant system, 192–93
Nose job (rhinoplasty), **100**
NOT-2-LATE, 202, 204
Nuprin, 19
Nutrition. *See* Eating for good health

Obesity, 70
Onycholysis, 91
Ophthalmologist, 92
Opioid inhibitors, 131
Optometrist, 92
Oral
 cancer, 115
 contraceptives, *189*, 189–91, 203
 sex, 181, 182

Oregon Health Sciences University, 174
Orgasm, 160
Orientation, sexual, 154–58
Os, 8
Osgood-Schlatter disease, 148–49
Ova (eggs), 9, 27
Overweight, 68–70
Ovulation, 8, 16

Pads, sanitary, 20, 20
Pap test, 174, 214, 221
Paraphimosis, 35
Parental consent (PC) states, 215
Parental notification (PN) states, 215
Parenthood. *See* Pregnancy and parenthood
Parents, feeling about, 42–43
Parkinson's disease, 119
Patella, 148
PC (parental consent) states, 215
PCP ("angel dust"), 117
Peak flow diary cards, 141
Pediatrics, 9
Pelvic examination, 174, 214, 220–21,
 220–21
Pelvic inflammatory disease (PID), 167, 172
Penile corona, 33
Penis, 27–29, 28, 29
Peptides, 203
Periodontal (gum) disease, 94–95, 95
Permethrin (Elimite), 177
Perspiration, 22, 105–6
Petersen, Anne, 9
Petit mal seizures, 146
Philmosis, 35
Photo Refractive Keratomony (PRK), 93
Physical abuse, 54–56, 72
Physical development. *See* Puberty
Physicals
 examination, 12, 109, 214, 219–22, 227
 before starting exercising, 76–77, 81
Physicians, communicating with, 217–18
PID (pelvic inflammatory disease), 167, 172
Pill (oral contraceptives), *189*, 189–91, 203
Pimples. *See* Acne
Pineal gland, 27
Pink pearly papules, 33
Pituitary gland, 9, 27
Planned Parenthood, 161, 211, 214, 231
Plantar warts, 87–88
Plaque, 94, 95
Plastic surgery, 98–100, **100**, 109, 233
PN (parental notification) states, 215
Podofilox, 175
Ponstel, 19
Pregnancy and parenthood, 205–12, 230,
 233
 abortion, 210–11, 230
 adoption, 209, 230
 alcohol and pregnancy, 116
 choices for, 208–11, 211–12
 considering, 205–7
 follow-up medical care, 211, 212
 living with choice about, 211–12
 marriage, 208
 single parent, 209
 symptoms of pregnancy, 207, 212

Premenstrual syndrome (PMS), 18–19, 25, 233
Prepuce (foreskin), 27, 29
Preservatives in cosmetics, 101
Princeton Center for Dental Information, 98
PRK (Photo Refractive Keratomony), 93
Prodrome, 173
Progesterone, 16, 17, 19, 202
Prostaglandins, 18, 19
Prostate gland, 28, 28
Prostatitis, 32, 36
Protease inhibitors, 169–70
Protectaid sponge, 202
Proventil, 142
Provera, 17
Prozac, 131
Psoriasis, 86–87
Psychiatrists, 223–24
Psychogenic headaches, 126, 127
Psychologists, 224
Psychomotor seizures, 146–47
Psychosomatic disorders, 126
Puberty (physical development)
    female, 9–12, **10–11**, *10–11*, 25
    male, 27, 29–31, **30–31**, 37
Pubic lice, 177
Pyrinate (A-200), 177

Quadriceps, 148

Rape, 54–56, 162–63
Rectal examination, 221–22
Relationships and sexuality, 161–66
Remafedi, Gary, 156
Retin-A, 86
Retrograde ejaculation, 36
Rhinoplasty (nose job), **100**
Riboflavin for migraine headaches, 134
RICE (Rest, Ice, Compression, Elevation), 80, **80**
Roe vs. Wade, 210
RPR test, 178, 222

"Safe sex," 180–84, 187–88
Salk Institute, 203
Sanitary products, 8, *20–21*, 20–22
Scabies, 177
Scoliosis, *149*, 149–50
Scrotum, 27–28, 28, 34
Sebum, 84
Second trimester abortions, 210
Secondary amenorrhea (ceasing to have periods), 17
Secondhand smoke, 115, 118, 124
Self-defeating behavior, 51–52
Self-Hate Traps, 41–42
Seminal fluid/vesicles, 28, 28
Serotonin, 127
Serum hepatitis (hepatitis B), 179–80
Sexual abuse, 54–56, 72
Sexuality, 153–66, 232, 233–34
    and alcohol, 163, 166
    choices, making, 159–60
    date rape, 55–56, 162–63
    defined, 153, 166

and fantasies, 154, 166
    heterosexuals, 155, 156, 166
    homosexuals, 155, 156–57, 166, 232
    intimacy versus sex, 165–66
    masturbation, 160–61, 166, 180, 181
    orientation, sexual, 154–58
    as part of your life, 153–54
    and relationships, 161–66
    sex, ready for, 163–65
    sex education, 158–59, 233–34
    sex versus, 153, 154, 161–62, 166
    transsexuals, 156
Sexually active, help for, 214, 227
Sexually transmitted diseases (STDs), 167–84, 234
    bacterial vaginosis, 171
    chlamydia, 24, 167, 168, 171–72
    genital herpes, 167, 168, 173–74
    genital warts (condylomata acuminata), 174–75
    gonorrhea, 24, 167, 168, 175–76
    hepatitis (A, B, C), 179–80
    molluscum contagiosum, 176
    pelvic inflammatory disease (PID), 167, 172
    pubic lice, 177
    "safe sex," 180–84
    scabies, 177
    syphilis, 177–78
    tinea cruris (jock itch), 178–79
    trichomoniasis, 179
    See also AIDS
Shapedown, 132
Short stature of men, 31–32
Shot and implant for men (birth control), 203
Shyness, 47–48
Sialastic implant, 33
Sickle cell anemia, 140–41, 231
SIDS (Sudden Infant Death Syndrome), 115
Sinai Hospital, 175
Single parent, 209
Skin, healthy, 83–90
    acne, 83–86, **85**, 109
    eczema, 86
    moles (nevi), 14, 88, 88
    psoriasis, 86–87
    sun protection, 88–90, 108
    warts, 87–88
Smegma, 29
Smoking and smokeless tobacco, 108, 111–12, 114–15, 124, 234
Snuff (smokeless tobacco), 115
Social changes and feelings, 4
Social Worker (MSW, LCSW), 224
Solvents in cosmetics, 101
Special medical needs, 137–38, 151. *See also specific medical need*
Speculum, 220, *220*, 221
Sperm cells, 28
Spermatocele, 34
Spermicide, 187, 188, *198*, 198–99, 204
St. John's wort for depression, 134
Stabilizers in cosmetics, 101
STDs. *See* Sexually transmitted diseases

Sterilization, 200, 200–201
Steroids, anabolic, 79, 112, 119–20, 124
Stimate (desmopressin acetate), 143
Stimulants, 118–19
Stomach and stress, 128–29, 134, 136
Strengthening exercise, 75, 77–78
Stress
    acne from, 85
    anorexia nervosa from, 68, 130–31, 231
    bulimia from, 68, 131, 231
    compulsive overeating from, 132
    eating disorders from, 129–32, 136, 231
    fear-of-obesity syndrome from, 130
    illness from, 126, 136
    irritable bowel syndrome (IBS) from, 128–29, 136
    managing, 109
    migraine headaches from, 128
    perspiration from, 106
    and premenstrual syndrome (PMS), 18
    secondary amenorrhea (ceasing to have periods) from, 17
    and stomach, 128–29, 134, 136
    See also Mind-body connection
Stretching exercise, 75
Stroke, 132
Sudden Infant Death Syndrome (SIDS), 115
Suicide, 59–60, 62
Sun lamps, 90
Sun protection, 88–90, 108
Supplements, dangers of, 79
Syphilis, 177–78
Systolic (blood pressure reading), 133

Tampons, 8, *20–21*, 20–22
Tanner, J. M., 9, 31
Tanning, 90
Target heart rate, 78, 80
Tattoos, **100**, 104
T-cells, 169
TEEN magazine, 4
Teeth and gums, healthy, 93–99
    bad breath, 93–94
    bleaching, 96–97
    bonding, 97
    braces, invisible, 97
    electronic anesthesia, 97–98
    flossing, 95, 96, 96
    gingivitis, 94–95, 95
    lasers for drilling, 97
    periodontal (gum) disease, 94–95, 95
    plaque, 94, 95
    steps for, 95, 109
Tension headaches, 126, 127
Testicles, 27, 27–28, 28, 33
Testicular
    cancer, 33–34
    self-examination, 34, *34*, 37
    torsion, 35
Tetracycline, 86
THC, 117–18
Therapy, 222–26
Tibia, 148
Tinactin, 178–79
Tinea cruris (jock itch), 178–79

"Tired blood" (iron-deficiency anemia), 140

Tobacco. *See* Smoking and smokeless tobacco

Toenail fungus, **90**

Toxic shock syndrome (TSS), 22

Transcendental Meditation, 135

Transdermal patches or gel, 202

Transsexuals, 156

Trichomoniasis, **23**, 179

Triphasic birth control pills, 189

TSS (toxic shock syndrome), 22

Tubal ligation, *200*, 200–201

Tumors and inverted nipples, 13

Type I (insulin-dependent) diabetes, 143, 144

Type II diabetes, 143–44

Tyramine, 128

Underweight, 67–68

Undescended testicle(s), 33

Unipath contraceptive system, 202–3

Unisex birth control pill, 203

University of California, 68, 175

University of Illinois, 117

University of Michigan, 116

University of Minnesota, 9, 156

University of North Carolina, 129

University of Washington, 116, 173

Urethra, 7, 8, *8*, 150

Urinary tract infections, 150

U.S. Bureau of the Census, 155

Uterus, 8, *8*

Vacuum aspiration abortions, 210

Vagina, 7, 8, *8*, 150

Vaginal
  health and infections, 22–24, **23**, 25
  opening, 8, *8*
  ring, 202

Varicocele, 34

vas deferens, 28, *28*

Vasectomy, *200*, 200–201

Vasopressin, 130

VDRL test, 178, 222

Vegetarians, 65, *65*

Venereal warts, 87

Ventolin, 142

Virgins, 8

Vitamins, 64, **64**

Vulva, 7

Wake Forest University, 117

Warts, 87–88

Washington University, 147

Waxing for excess hair, 105

Weight
  and breast size, 12
  loss, 70–74, **71, 73**, 106–7, 108
  secondary amenorrhea (ceasing to have periods) from change in, 17

Weight Watchers, 132

"Wet dreams" (nocturnal emissions), 36

Wide pulse pressure, 133

Woman's body, 7–25
  anatomy, 7–8, *7–9*
  breast cancer, 13–14
  breast development, 10, *10, 12*, 12–15
  breast self-examinations, *14*, 14–15, 25
  and drugs, 116, 119–20, 124
  insecurities about, 24–25
  pelvic examination, 174, 214, 220–21, *220–21*
  puberty, 9–12, **10–11**, *10–11*, 25
  scoliosis, *149*, 149–50
  urinary tract infections, 150
  vaginal health and infections, 22–24, **23**, 25
  See also Birth control; Drugs; Eating for good health; Exercise for good health; Feelings; Help; Mind-body connection; Pregnancy and parenthood; Sexuality; Sexually transmitted diseases; *specific medical needs*

Wrinkles, 90, 115

Yeast infection (candidiasis), **23**

Zits. *See* Acne

Zomig, 128

About the Authors

Kathy McCoy, Ph.D., is an award-winning author of eleven books. She is also a psychotherapist with Caring Connections, a group private practice in Pasadena, California, and assistant to the chancellor at the California School of Professional Psychology, Los Angeles. A former columnist for *Seventeen* magazine and a former editor of *'TEEN*, she has written hundreds of articles for national magazines, newspapers, and professional journals such as *Redbook, Reader's Digest, The New York Times, Family Circle, Woman's Day, New Woman, Ladies' Home Journal, Glamour, Mademoiselle, TV Guide,* and the *Journal of Clinical Child Psychology.*

A popular guest on national television shows, she has made numerous appearances on the *Today* show and has also appeared frequently on such programs as *The Oprah Winfrey Show, Geraldo, Hour Magazine, Sally Jessy Raphael,* and *Sonia Live.* She also appears frequently on the pages of *USA Today* as an expert on adolescent issues. Dr. McCoy is an on-line expert specializing in adolescent psychology for the National Parenting Center.

Charles Wibbelsman, M.D., the award-winning author of four books and former "Dear Doctor" columnist for *'TEEN* magazine, is a nationally prominent adolescent-medicine specialist. In addition to serving as chairman of the chiefs of adolescent medicine for the Permanente Medical Group of Northern California, he is chief of the Teenage Clinic at Kaiser Permanente, San Francisco, and is an associate professor of pediatrics at the University of California, San Francisco, Medical School. A past president of the Northern California chapter of the Society for Adolescent Medicine, Dr. Wibbelsman also serves on the Board of the Society for Adolescent Medicine and on the San Francisco Superintendent of Schools Advisory Committee.

Dr. Wibbelsman is also a popular guest on national television shows, including the *Today* show and *The Oprah Winfrey Show.* He appears regularly on *Parenting and Psychology* on BAY-TV in San Francisco and is an on-line expert specializing in adolescent health for the National Parenting Center.

M8234-TN